Essential
Clinical Medicine

Essential Clinical Medicine

Edited by

R. H. Salter BSc MB BS FRCP
Consultant Physician, Cumberland Infirmary, Carlisle
Associate Clinical Lecturer, University of Newcastle upon Tyne

Published by
P G Publishing Pte Ltd
Singapore ● Hong Kong

Originally published by
John Wright & Sons Ltd, 823–825 Bath Road, Bristol BS4 5NU, England.

British Library Cataloguing in Publication Data

Essential clinical medicine.
1. Pathology
I. Salter, R. H.
616   RB111

ISBN 9971 973 02 2

Published in 1984 by
P G Publishing Pte Ltd, 3. Mt Elizabeth #06-09, Mt Elizabeth Medical Centre, Singapore 0922.

Typeset by
Severntype Repro Services Ltd, Market Street, Wotton-under-Edge, Glos.

Printed in Great Britain by
John Wright & Sons (Printing) Ltd at The Stonebridge Press, Bristol BS4 5NU

Preface

The intention of this book is not to provide a comprehensive medical treatise competing with already well-established reference tomes. In contrast the approach is analogous to a laboratory bench-book—to be kept readily accessible and hopefully well-thumbed rather than gathering dust on a library shelf.

Each contributor has been asked to deal only with disorders which in his judgement are encountered with reasonable frequency in clinical practice and to concentrate particularly on the problems of diagnosis and management. The aim has been to provide a text dealing with common problems specifically for the doctor at the sharp end of medicine who needs to see the wood for the trees.

This approach has allowed a much fuller discussion of bread and butter medical problems, such as diabetes, than is possible in a more orthodox text. The importance of psychiatry in relation to clinical medicine has been recognized by its inclusion.

It is hoped that this book will be helpful to physicians in hospital practice or primary care, whether established or in training, and should also appeal to medical students.

R. H. S.

Contributors

D. Bates MA MB BChir FRCP
Senior Lecturer and Consultant Neurologist, Royal Victoria Infirmary, Newcastle upon Tyne

A. K. Clarke BSc MB BS MRCP
Consultant in Rheumatology and Rehabilitation, Royal National Hospital for Rheumatic Diseases, Bath

I. W. Delamore PhD MB ChB FRCP FRCPEd FRCPath
Consultant Physician, Manchester Royal Infirmary

J. R. Edge MB ChB MD FRCP
Consultant Physician, North Lonsdale Hospital, Barrow-in-Furness, Cumbria. Consultant Chest Physician, Barrow and Furness Group Hospitals

R. G. Henderson MD MRCP
Consultant Physician, Huntingdon County Hospital, Hinchingbrooke and Addenbrooke's Hospital, Cambridge. Associate Lecturer, Cambridge University Hospitals, Cambridge

R. D. Hill MB BS FRCP
Consultant Physician, Poole General Hospital

J. Crawford Little MD MB ChB FRCPEd FRCPsych
Lately Director of Clinical Research and Consultant Psychiatrist, Crichton Royal Hospital, Dumfries

R. H. Salter BSc MB BS FRCP
Consultant Physician, Cumberland Infirmary, Carlisle. Associate Clinical Lecturer, University of Newcastle upon Tyne

G. Terry MB BS FRCP
Consultant Physician, Dryburn Hospital, Durham

Contents

1 Common Cardiovascular Disorders

G. Terry

1.1 INTRODUCTION

In the diagnosis and assessment of patients with heart disease it is just as important to obtain a complete history and perform a full clinical examination as in any other branch of medicine.

Special attention should be paid to the following symptoms:

Chest pain

Exertional dyspnoea

Orthopnoea and paroxysmal nocturnal dyspnoea

Peripheral oedema

Palpitations

Syncope.

On physical examination the following features should be carefully examined:

Arterial pulse—including carotids and femorals

Arterial blood pressure

Jugular venous pressure and wave form

Inspection and palpation of the precordium to identify the cardiac apex, to detect the presence of ventricular hypertrophy and thrills

Auscultation for assessment of heart sounds and murmurs

Auscultation of the lung for presence of pulmonary congestion

Detection of oedema

Retinal examination.

These symptoms and physical signs will be discussed in the relevant sections of this chapter.

Cardiac investigations

Only those investigations which are available to most hospitals will be discussed here. They include:

Chest radiography

Electrocardiography including exercise testing and ambulatory ECG monitoring

Echocardiography

Nuclear cardiology.

Invasive investigation with cardiac catheterization and angiography is usually only available in specialist cardiac units and will therefore not be discussed in detail.

Chest radiology

Chest radiology gives useful information about cardiac size as well as specific chamber enlargement. The pulmonary vascularity can also be assessed and pulmonary congestion can be detected. The various components which make up the cardiac outline on the chest radiograph are shown in *Fig.* 1.1. It will be seen that the right ventricle does not contribute to the heart outline on the PA film but forms the anterior border on the lateral film.

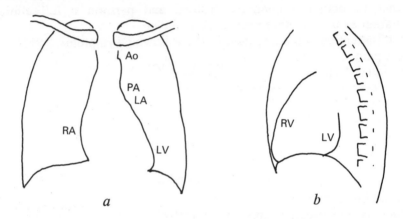

Fig. 1.1 Cardiac outline on (*a*) PA and (*b*) Left lateral radiograph. Ao, aortic knuckle; LA, left atrial appendage; LV, left ventricle; PA, pulmonary artery; RA, right atrium; RV, right ventricle.

Electrocardiography (ECG)

An ECG is essential in the diagnosis of arrhythmias but can also detect the presence of:

Ischaemia and infarction

Atrial and ventricular hypertrophy

Bundle-branch block and heart block.

The exercise ECG can show the presence of ischaemia when the resting ECG is normal and is an important investigation in the assessment of coronary artery disease. Ambulatory monitoring can detect the presence of intermittent rhythm disturbances.

Echocardiography

Echocardiography is a relatively new technique but is now available in most hospitals. The normal M-mode echocardiograms obtained from the heart are illustrated in *Fig.* 1.2.

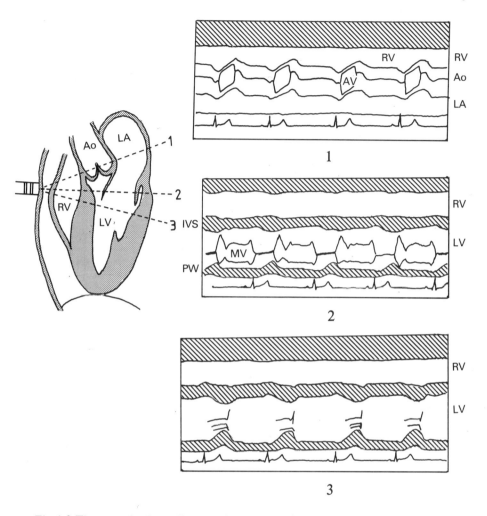

Fig. 1.2 The normal echocardiogram. Ao, aorta; AV, aortic valve; LV, left ventricle; LA, left atrium; MV, mitral valve; IVS, interventricular septum; PW, posterior left ventricular wall; RV, right ventricle.

Echocardiography is particularly important in showing:
Abnormalities of mitral, aortic and tricuspid valves
Left ventricular size and function
Right ventricular and left atrial size
Pericardial effusion
Cardiac tumours.
Two-dimensional echocardiography is now becoming available and gives additional information about congenital cardiac abnormalities and can even detect these abnormalities in utero.

Nuclear cardiology

Information can be obtained about heart size, function and myocardial perfusion using isotopic techniques. These include:

Gated blood-pool scan
Hot-spot scanning
Cold-spot scanning.

GATED BLOOD-POOL SCAN

This is performed by injecting an isotope which remains in the circulating blood (technetium bound to albumin). Once this has been distributed throughout the intravascular space a series of pictures can be produced of the intracardiac blood pool at various stages of the cardiac cycle, using a gamma camera.

The area of interest is the left ventricle and this can be shown from the views in *Fig.* 1.3.

Using computer analysis LV wall movement can be shown. This technique is useful in:

1. Determination of ejection fraction
2. Identification of regional wall abnormalities—after myocardial infarction
3. To outline a ventricular aneurysm.

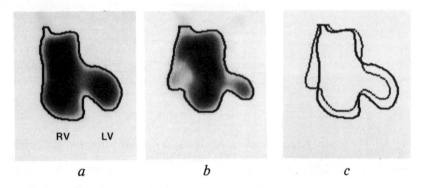

Fig. 1.3 Left anterior oblique projection. (*a*) End diastole; (*b*) End systole; (*c*) Wall motion, —————end diastole, ... end systole.

HOT-SPOT SCANNING

This is used to detect myocardial infarction. Pyrophosphate is taken up by infarcted myocardium and shows as a 'hot-spot'. The isotope is also taken up by bone, producing in addition a picture of the thoracic skeleton. This technique can identify myocardial infarction in the presence of left bundle-branch block.

COLD-SPOT SCANNING

This utilizes isotopes which have similar properties to potassium. Thallium is taken up by heart muscle relative to its blood supply. If an area of myocardium is under-perfused this will show as a 'cold-spot'. The LV makes up the major portion of the heart muscle mass and appears on a normal scan as a 'doughnut'. Patients with angina usually have a normal scan at rest but injection of the isotope during exercise can outline the ischaemic area and relate it to the coronary artery supply.

1.2 ISCHAEMIC HEART DISEASE (IHD)

This is the commonest form of heart disease in the adult population of developed countries and is a principal cause of premature death. Ischaemic heart disease is caused by atherosclerotic narrowing and occlusion of coronary arteries and may present in the following ways:

Sudden death
Angina pectoris
Myocardial infarction
Progressive heart (pump) failure.

Sudden death

Sudden death is defined as death occurring unheralded or within 24 h of the onset of cardiovascular symptoms.

The final event is due in the majority of cases to ventricular fibrillation and underlying coronary artery disease is a common finding.

Angina pectoris

Clinical aspects

Angina is a symptom which usually denotes the presence of underlying coronary artery disease. The patient with angina describes retrosternal pain or discomfort coming on with effort and settling within 2–10 min of rest. This is the classic description but the site and radiation of pain may vary considerably in different cases, but the site is remarkably constant in the same individual. The common sites of pain are shown in *Fig.* 1.4.

In stable angina pectoris the pain comes on after a given work load but may be precipitated by lessening degrees of effort as the disease progresses.

Unstable angina may come on at rest or may have an unpredictable pattern in relation to exertion.

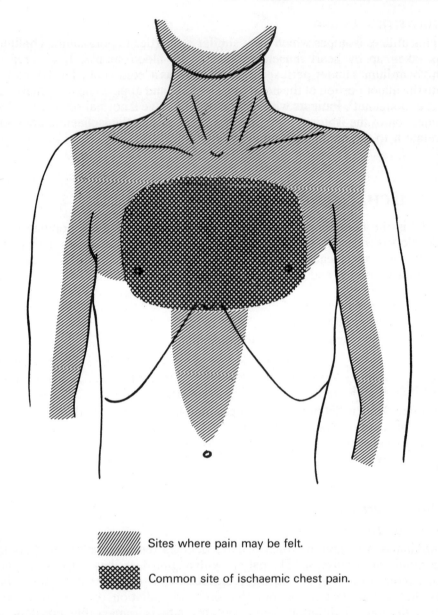

/////// Sites where pain may be felt.

▨▨▨▨ Common site of ischaemic chest pain.

Fig. 1.4 Distribution of ischaemic pain.

Physical examination in angina pectoris is often normal but it is important to exclude underlying causes such as anaemia, thyrotoxicosis or aortic valve disease which may cause anginal pain in the presence of normal coronary arteries.

Diagnosis

The diagnosis of angina can be confirmed by finding ischaemic changes on the ECG. The resting ECG is frequently normal and ischaemic changes may have to be induced by exercise.

Diagnostic ECG changes of ischaemia (*Fig.* 1.5) include:

Horizontal S–T segment depression greater than 1 mm

Downward sloping S–T segment

Symmetrical T wave inversion

S–T elevation (Prinzmetal variant angina).

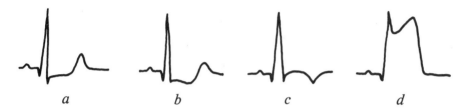

Fig. 1.5 Diagnostic ECG changes of ischaemia. (*a*) Horizontal S–T depression; (*b*) Downward sloping S–T segment; (*c*) Symmetrical T wave inversion; (*d*) S–T elevation (Prinzmetal variant angina).

The exercise stress test should only be carried out by trained personnel, with continuous ECG monitoring, in a location where full resuscitative facilities are available. A bicycle ergometer or treadmill are the two instruments in common use for this procedure.

The exercise is continued to a predetermined end-point i.e. target heart rate or symptoms of ischaemia. The test is terminated prematurely if the following features develop:

1. Dizziness
2. Fatigue
3. Sudden fall in blood·pressure
4. Atrial and ventricular arrhythmias
5. Gross S–T depression or S–T elevation on the ECG.

Interpretation of an exercise test can be difficult but in general a positive test will occur in about 75% of patients with significant coronary artery disease and 90% of those with negative tests will be found to have no significant disease.

In the variant type of angina described by Prinzmetal, attacks of pain often occur at rest and are associated with S–T elevation of the ECG (*Fig.* 1.5). Ventricular arrhythmias or heart block may accompany these events. Many of the patients with this type of angina are found to have relatively normal coronary arteries and coronary artery spasm has been demonstrated as the underlying cause. In other patients, severe critical coronary artery narrowing has been demonstrated and these patients are obviously at risk of developing myocardial infarction.

Management

This must include an explanation to the patient about the nature of his symptoms, so that precipitating causes can be avoided. The following methods of treatment are then employed:

1. Control of aggravating factors
     Reduce heavy physical work
     Correct obesity
     Control hypertension
2. Correction of risk factors
     Cessation of smoking
     Detection and treatment of hyperlipidaemia
3. Specific treatment
     Nitrates
     Beta-blocking drugs
     Calcium antagonists
     Coronary artery surgery.

Nitrates such as glyceryl trinitrate will give rapid relief from anginal pain and can be taken prophylactically before exertion to prevent angina. Nitrates may also be given orally or transcutaneously and can prevent angina, particularly in those patients with coronary artery spasm. Nitrates have a dilating effect on coronary and peripheral arteries. The peripheral effect reduces the cardiac work load and reduces oxygen demand.

Beta-blocking drugs are the standard medical treatment of angina. They slow the resting heart rate and limit exercise tachycardia. They also reduce the force of contraction of ventricular muscle and thereby reduce myocardial oxygen requirements.

Calcium antagonist drugs such as nifedipine or verapamil are an alternative form of treatment. They act by inhibiting the uptake of calcium into myocardial cells, thereby reducing the force of contraction. They also cause peripheral vasodilatation by reducing contractility of vascular smooth muscle and this reduces cardiac work. Calcium antagonists are particularly useful in patients with coronary artery spasm but are also used in stable angina.

If medical treatment fails to control angina, surgical treatment should be considered. Coronary arteriography must first be performed. A radio-opaque contrast medium is infused directly into each coronary artery via a special catheter. The number of vessels and branches which are diseased can be seen and their suitability for surgical repair assessed. The operation of coronary artery bypass grafting consists of inserting a length of saphenous vein between the aorta and the coronary artery, distal to the point of obstruction. Vein grafts are usually inserted into all diseased vessels. The operation is an effective method of relieving symptoms in patients with angina and in some cases it can also improve mortality by preventing myocardial infarction.

The indications for referral of patients for coronary arteriography include:

1. Angina failing to respond to medical treatment.

2. Determination of the extent of coronary artery disease in patients with angina or following myocardial infarction, as those with severe disease have a worse prognosis and are better treated surgically. This indication is particularly relevant in young patients.

3. To establish the diagnosis of ischaemic heart disease in individuals with non-specific symptoms or ECG changes, particularly when this diagnosis is important to their occupation e.g. airline pilots, heads of state, etc.

Myocardial infarction

Myocardial infarction is produced by occlusion of a coronary artery previously narrowed by atheroma. About half the patients will have had preceding angina. The usual mode of presentation is severe pain similar in site and distribution to angina but the pain is prolonged (more than 1 h) and fails to respond to nitrates. It may be accompanied by sweating, vomiting, lightheadedness and a sensation of impending death. In some cases myocardial infarction may be painless and is only diagnosed at a later stage if an ECG is recorded. Other patients may present with acute pulmonary oedema, the severe dyspnoea overshadowing the pain.

On examination in the early stages following myocardial infarction the patient is often pale, sweating and anxious. Signs of heart failure may be present with raised venous pressure and basal rales. Inspection of the precordium will sometimes reveal an area of systolic pulsation distinct from the apex beat. Auscultation will frequently reveal third or fourth heart sounds. If presentation is delayed physical examination may be entirely normal.

Diagnosis is confirmed by the ECG—the classic changes of infarction are shown in *Fig.* 1.6. The initial ECG may be normal and in these cases if the clinical history is suggestive the patient should be admitted to hospital.

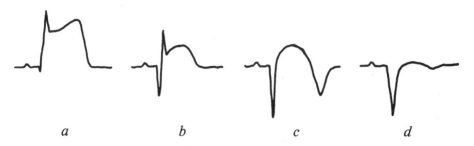

a   b   c   d

Fig. 1.6 Evolution of ECG changes with myocardial infarction. (*a*) Early changes, 0–12 hours; (*b*) 12–24 hours; (*c*) Beyond 24 hours; (*d*) Changes of old infarction.

Confirmatory evidence:

1. Rise in cardiac enzymes (*Fig.* 1.7)
2. Raised white cell count and ESR
3. Fever—temperature is normal for first 24 h then rises and may remain elevated for 1 week
4. Pericardial friction rub may be audible in the days following myocardial infarction and may be accompanied by further chest pain of pericardial type (*see* p. 46).

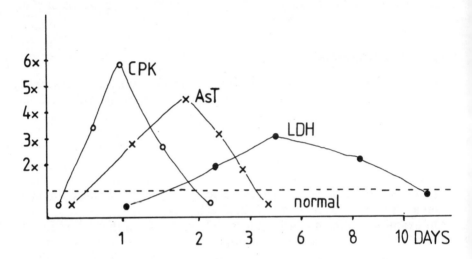

Fig. 1.7 Changes in cardiac enzymes with myocardial infarction. CPK, creatinine phosphokinase; AST, aspartate transaminase; LDH, lactic dehydrogenase.

Early management

Oncc the patient arrives in hospital he should be transferred to a Coronary Care Unit without delay where heart rhythm can be constantly monitored and serious disturbances of rhythm can be detected and treated. Relief of pain can usually be achieved by diamorphine, given i.v. 5–10 mg, together with cyclizine to prevent vomiting induced by the opiate. Diamorphine should be repeated until pain is relieved. The dangers of addiction should not be considered when only short-term use is envisaged. Oxygen should be administered if the patient is breathless or if signs of left ventricular failure are present.

Anticoagulants are not used routinely but in those patients with severe infarction complicated by heart failure where prolonged bed rest may be necessary, treatment with warfarin should be considered. Subcutaneous heparin 5000 u 12-hourly may also reduce the risk of deep vein thrombosis and pulmonary embolism.

COMPLICATIONS

Complications of myocardial infarction can be divided into:
1. Electrical— cardiac arrhythmias
heart block
2. Mechanical— heart failure
cardiogenic shock
disruption of anatomy (i.e. ventricular septal defect).

Cardiac arrhythmias of all types can occur after myocardial infarction; they fall into the following categories:
1. Cosmetic blemish on the ECG
Most isolated ectopic beats fall into this group and should not be treated. Most antiarrhythmic drugs have an adverse effect on ventricular function.
2. Arrhythmias which cause a haemodynamic disturbance
Extremes of tachycardia and bradycardia have an adverse effect on cardiac output; effective treatment is therefore required for sinus bradycardia, complete heart block, rapid atrial and ventricular arrhythmias and frequent ectopic beats.
3. Life-threatening arrhythmias
These rhythm disturbances may indicate a liability to develop ventricular fibrillation. They include:
   a. R on T ventricular ectopics
   b. Frequent multifocal ectopics
   c. Pairs of ventricular ectopics
   d. Paroxysmal ventricular tachycardia.

If these are seen, prophylactic antiarrhythmic drugs may prevent ventricular fibrillation. Management of arrhythmias will be discussed in the relevant section of this chapter.

The development and severity of heart failure is directly related to the extent of myocardial damage and carries an adverse prognosis.

Signs of heart failure in myocardial infarction include:
1. Sinus tachycardia
2. Gallop rhythm
3. Basal crepitations
4. Raised jugular venous pressure
5. Tachypnoea
6. Radiological evidence of pulmonary congestion.

Cardiogenic shock is present when the cardiac output is low, in the absence of pulmonary congestion. Clinical features include:
1. Systolic BP <90 mmHg
2. Cold and cyanosed periphery
3. Poor urine output
4. Impaired cerebral function.

This clinical state is seen in cases with severe myocardial damage and carries a very poor prognosis.

Rupture of the infarcted ventricular wall may occur causing death from cardiac tamponade. Rupture of the ventricular septum causes a ventricular septal defect and rupture of a papillary muscle causes severe mitral regurgitation. Distinguishing these two events can be difficult as both present with a pansystolic murmur and the sudden severe deterioration of the patient's condition with further pain and heart failure. Both of these complications can be repaired surgically but the patient needs intensive supportive measures. The prognosis is poor.

LV aneurysm may complicate myocardial infarction. A balloon-like expansion of the infarcted LV wall occurs and may produce the following features:
1. Intractable heart failure
2. Ventricular arrhythmias
3. Repeated embolic episodes.

The condition can be recognized by finding a bulge on the left heart border on radiography or persistent S–T elevation on the ECG.

Surgical excision should be considered if symptoms cannot be controlled by medical treatment.

Late management

Most patients with uncomplicated myocardial infarction can be mobilized within a few days and be discharged home after 1 week. Outpatient follow-up in 4–6 weeks is important to identify:
1. Presence of heart failure
2. Recurrence of angina
3. Late onset of arrhythmias
4. Ventricular aneurysm.

At this visit, future activities including return to work can be discussed and advice about correction of risk factors can be reinforced.

Secondary prevention

Although many studies have shown a benefit from giving β-blocking drugs following myocardial infarction, their widespread use has not been established.

1.3 HYPERTENSION

There is no clear-cut level of blood pressure above which hypertension can be diagnosed, although it is established that in adults below the age of 50, BP levels greater than 140/90 mmHg carry an increased morbidity and a reduced life expectancy. The causes of death in hypertension are:
1. Heart failure
2. Renal failure
3. Stroke
4. Myocardial infarction.

each of which occurs with much greater frequency than in normotensive individuals.

Severity of hypertension is usually determined by the level of diastolic pressure:

Mild 90–105 mmHg
Moderate 105–120 mmHg
Severe >120 mmHg
Malignant >120 mmHg + papilloedema.

Although elevations of systolic pressure alone carry an increased risk, systolic hypertension may be difficult to control.

Clinical features

Most hypertensives are asymptomatic—the raised BP being discovered by coincidence. In cases of severe or long-standing hypertension symptoms of heart failure, ischaemic heart disease or renal impairment may be present. Headaches and mental impairment are a feature of accelerated (malignant) hypertension. Examination may reveal signs of cardiac enlargement with left ventricular hypertrophy. The presence of a fourth heart sound is common in severe cases. Examination of the fundi gives a clue to the severity and duration of hypertension.

Fundal changes are classified:
Grade 1. Narrow arteries (silver wiring)
Grade 2. A–V nipping
Grade 3. Haemorrhages and exudates
Grade 4. Papilloedema.

Investigations

Investigations in hypertension are performed in order to determine:

1. Evidence of target organ damage
2. The presence of an underlying cause of the hypertension.

A summary of these investigations is given in *Table* 1.1.

In most cases investigations are limited to:
Blood count
Urea and electrolytes and serum creatinine
Urinalysis, microscopy and culture
Chest radiography
ECG.

More extensive investigation should be considered in the following:

1. Young patients with severe hypertension of sudden onset
2. Malignant hypertension
3. Paroxysmal hypertension
4. Features of Cushing's syndrome
5. Low serum K^+

Table 1.1 The investigation of hypertension

1. *To determine end-organ damage*

Organ	Investigation	Finding
Heart	ECG	LV hypertrophy; ischaemia; infarction
	Chest radiograph	Cardiac enlargment; pulmonary congestion
Kidney	Blood urea	Evidence of renal functional impairment
	Creatinine	
	Creatinine clearance	

2. *To determine an underlying cause for hypertension*

Cause	Screening test	Definitive investigation
Renovascular disease	IVP	Arteriography
Pyelonephritis	Urine culture	IVP
Glomerulonephritis	Urine microscopy	Renal biopsy
Polycystic kidneys	Plain radiograph	IVP
		Ultrasound scan
Cushing's syndrome	Plasma cortisol	ACTH
	Urinary corticosteroids	CAT scan
		Surgery
Primary hyper-aldosteronism	Serum potassium	Renin, aldosterone levels
		CAT scan
		Surgery
Phaeochromocytoma	Urinary catecholamines	CAT scan
		Surgery

6. Indication of renal abnormality—history of urinary tract infection or presence of an abdominal bruit
7. Failure to respond to standard treatment.

It is also important that coexisting risk and aggravating features be identified and treated. For example:

1. Obesity
2. Cigarette smoking
3. Hyperlipidaemia
4. High salt intake.

Management

Before starting a patient on long-term hypotensive treatment serial blood pressure recordings should be taken.

MILD HYPERTENSION

Drug treatment of a patient with a diastolic BP below 100 mmHg has not been shown to be effective in reducing complications or mortality. Non-pharmacological measures are therefore advisable in these cases and include correction of obesity, reduction of salt intake and encouragement of regular exercise. Follow-up BP recordings are important.

Table 1.2 Standard 'triple' therapy in hypertension

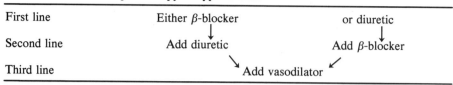

First line	Either β-blocker	or diuretic
Second line	Add diuretic	Add β-blocker
Third line	Add vasodilator	

MODERATE HYPERTENSION

Treatment in these cases is beneficial but the non-therapeutic measures should be employed initially. Standard 'triple' therapy is outlined in *Table* 1.2.

SEVERE HYPERTENSION

Severe hypertension is treated along the same lines as moderate hypertension but there is a greater degree of urgency to bring the BP under control—particularly if target organ damage is present, e.g. heart failure, renal failure, stroke, encephalopathy.

MALIGNANT HYPERTENSION

Malignant hypertension is a medical emergency and requires urgent control of BP. Preliminary investigation should not interfere with this aim. Urgent lowering of BP can be achieved by:
    Labetolol 50–200 mg i.v. slowly
    Hydralazine 15–40 mg i.v.
    Diazoxide 300 mg i.v.
    It is also advisable to administer frusemide 80–160 mg to promote a rapid diuresis.
    The aim is to bring the diastolic pressure down to a 'safe' level <110 mmHg. These drugs can be repeated as necessary but standard hypotensive drugs should be introduced and further investigations carried out.

Failure of hypertensive patients to respond to therapy

The possibility of poor compliance should be excluded. If β-blockers are being prescribed a normal pulse rate may suggest poor compliance.
    Admission to hospital and maintenance of the same regime will identify some of the compliance failures.
    If this is discovered—careful explanation is required about the aims of therapy and the drug regime should be simplified if possible.
    Most hypotensive agents can be administered either once or twice per day.
    True failure to respond requires more extensive investigation to try and identify an underlying, treatable cause for the hypertension. This often needs

referral to a specialist centre for renal arteriography and renal vein catheterization. Other investigations should include:

1. IVP rapid sequence
2. Isotope renogram
3. VMA or HMMA to detect a phaeochromocytoma.

If an underlying cause is still not discovered alternative hypotensive agents should be used. These include:

Captopril (an angiotensin-converting enzyme inhibitor)

Calcium antagonists—nifedipine

Minoxidil (powerful vasodilator which may cause severe fluid retention and hirsutism).

1.4   HEART FAILURE

Heart failure exists when the cardiac output falls below a level consistent with normal body function.

Cardiac output is influenced by:

1. Filling pressure (preload). Increased filling pressure causes greater stretching of myocardial muscle fibres and this enhances the force of contraction (Frank–Starling law)
2. Contractility describes the functional state of the myocardium
3. Peripheral resistance (afterload), the resistance against which the heart has to work.

The relationship between cardiac output and filling pressure is shown in *Fig.* 1.8.

In the normal heart, exercise increases venous return by the pumping action of muscles on veins. The raised filling pressure so produced increases cardiac output. In heart failure the cardiac output for a given level of filling pressure is lower. Modest amounts of exercise may increase the filling pressure to the point where congestive symptoms occur (usually >25 mmHg). In severe heart failure cardiac output is very low (cardiogenic shock) and attempts to increase cardiac output even at rest, by raising filling pressure, will cause congestive symptoms.

The clinical features of heart failure are related to both reduced cardiac output and congestive symptoms.

Signs of low output are similar in both left and right heart failure and include:

1. Tiredness on exertion
2. Lethargy
3. Cold periphery
4. Peripheral cyanosis.

High output failure can occur in anaemia or thyrotoxicosis. In these cases a high cardiac output is necessary to meet the increased demand but in attempting to achieve this the filling pressure may rise to a level where

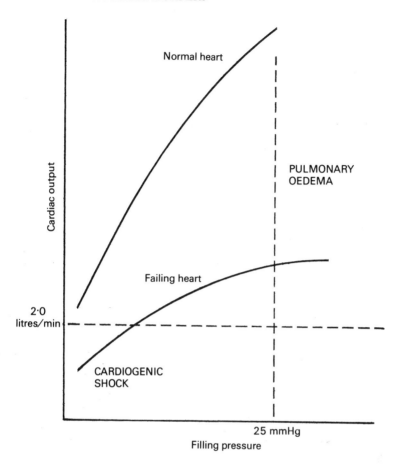

Fig. 1.8 Relationship between filling pressure and cardiac output.

congestive signs are produced. These patients therefore have a warm periphery with a bounding pulse.

Congestive signs differ in right or left heart failure:

Right	*Left*
Raised JVP	Exertional dyspnoea
Oedema	Orthopnoea
Hepatomegaly	Nocturnal dyspnoea
Ascites	Pulmonary oedema

The common causes of heart failure include:

Right	*Left*
Secondary to LHF	Ischaemic heart disease
Cor pulmonale	Hypertension
Pulmonary hypertension	Aortic and mitral valve disease
Constrictive pericarditis	Cardiomyopathy

Management of heart failure

This can be achieved along the following lines:

1. Treatment of the precipitating cause:
   Treatment of infection
   Control of arrhythmias
   Correction of anaemia
2. Treatment of the underlying cause
   Valvular surgery in aortic and mitral valve disease
   Control of hypertension
3. Symptomatic treatment
   Reduction of physical activities
   Treatment of sodium and water retention (diuretic)
   Reduction of afterload (vasodilators)
   Increase of contractility (digitalis)
   Reduction afterload (arterial vasodilators)

Treatment of chronic congestive heart failure usually commences with diuretics. Thiazides are used in mild cases, but loop-diuretics such as frusemide are needed in more severe cases. Potassium supplements are important with these drugs. In cases resistant to this treatment the addition of a potassium-sparing diuretic (e.g. spironolactone) enhances the diuretic effect and prevents potassium loss.

Digitalis is used initially in cases with atrial fibrillation, its most important effect being the reduction of ventricular rate. Digoxin does increase the contractility of the failing heart in cases of sinus rhythm and helps to relieve congestion.

The addition of vasodilators, either nitrates (venodilator) or prazocin (mixed arterial and venous dilator), can be beneficial.

Treatment of acute pulmonary oedema is a medical emergency. Immediate treatment with a loop-diuretic is needed (frusemide 40–80 mg i.v.). Doses up to 250–500 mg can be given if a diuresis is not induced within 30 min. Patients are often extremely anxious with pulmonary oedema and i.v. opiates, e.g. diamorphine 2·5–5·0 mg, can help to relieve this.

Oxygen therapy should also be administered.

If these measures are not immediately effective the use of venous vasodilators should be considered. An i.v. infusion of isosorbide dinitrate will lower filling pressure but the dose must be carefully monitored. Invasive measurements of pulmonary wedge pressure and cardiac output are desirable in this situation but are not essential in the emergency situation.

USE OF VASODILATORS IN HEART FAILURE

Vasodilators are divided into:

1. Venous dilators
2. Arterial dilators.

Venous dilators act on the venous capacitance vessels and cause pooling of large quantities of blood, reducing venous return and lowering filling pressure. When given in pulmonary oedema they lower venous pressure with little or no change in cardiac output. Once the pressure has fallen further vasodilatation will lower the cardiac output.

Arterial dilators act on the peripheral arteriolar vessels, reducing resistance to flow. When used in patients with a low cardiac output, the cardiac output increases with little or no change in filling pressure.

The use of drugs with both venous and arterial dilating properties will have a combined effect.

1.5 ARRHYTHMIAS

Abnormalities of sinus rhythm

Sinus bradycardia (<60 per min) or sinus tachycardia (>100 per min) are either physiological variants or may reflect underlying heart disease. Treatment is aimed at the underlying cause. Symptomatic sinus bradycardia after myocardial infarction can be temporarily treated with atropine intravenously. Inappropriate sinus tachycardia can be reduced by β-blocking drugs but should be used with extreme caution in patients showing signs of heart failure or after recent myocardial infarction.

Sino-atrial node disease (sick sinus syndrome) is characterized by:
1. Sinus bradycardia
2. Sinus arrest, producing syncope
3. Various escape rhythms
4. Atrial tachyarrhythmias.

This is a difficult condition to treat as the drugs which suppress the tachyarrhythmia aggravate the bradycardia. In many cases permanent pacing is required together with the use of antiarrhythmic drugs.

Atrial arrhythmias

Paroxysmal atrial tachycardia (PAT) is a common rhythm disturbance occurring in individuals who often have no underlying structural heart disease. The rate is 160–200 per min and the QRS is usually narrow, unless bundle-branch block is present. The patient is aware of rapid regular palpitations, the onset is sudden and attacks can often be terminated by a Valsalva manoeuvre or by self-induced vomiting.

PAT may be treated in the following ways:
1. Carotid sinus massage (*Fig.* 1.9)
2. Intravenous verapamil (not to be used with β-blockers or if recent myocardial infarction is suspected)
3. D.C. cardioversion

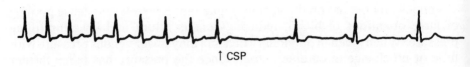

↑ CSP

Fig. 1.9 Paroxysmal atrial tachycardia—corrected by carotid sinus pressure (CSP).

Table 1.3 Doses of antiarrhythmic drugs

Drug	Intravenous dose	Oral maintenance dose
Amiodarone	5 mg/kg body weight over 20 min	600 mg/day for 1 week, reducing to 200–400 mg/day
Atropine	0·3–1·0 mg can be repeated (max. dose in 24 h = 3·0 mg)	
Beta-blockers	Practolol 5–10 mg slowly Atenolol 2·5 mg slowly	Propranolol 40–160 mg/day in divided doses Atenolol 50–100 mg/day Metoprolol 50 mg twice daily
Digoxin	0·5 mg (only if oral route impracticable)	Loading 0·5 mg for three doses Maintenance 0·0625–0·5 mg/day depending on renal function
Disopyramide	2 mg/kg slowly	300–800 mg/day in divided doses
Flecainide	2 mg/kg over at least 10 min	100–200 mg twice daily
Lignocaine	50–100 mg 2–4 mg/min infusion	
Mexiletine	100–250 mg over at least 10 min	200 mg 8-hourly
Procainamide	25 mg/min (max. dose = 1·0 g)	1 g 8-hourly (durules)
Verapamil	Up to 10 mg	40–120 mg 8-hourly

4. Prophylaxis against future attacks can be achieved with:
   Disopyramide ⎫
   Procainamide ⎬ Doses of all antiarrhythmic drugs are shown in *Table* 1.3
   Amiodarone ⎭

Atrial fibrillation is usually associated with underlying heart disease and often presents with a rapid (120–160 per min) and irregular ventricular rate (*Fig.* 1.10). The sudden onset of atrial fibrillation often causes a significant haemodynamic deterioration in those with heart disease, especially in cases of mitral stenosis.

The common underlying causes include:
1. Rheumatic mitral valve disease
2. Following myocardial infarction
3. Hypertensive heart disease
4. Cardiomyopathies
5. Thyrotoxicosis.

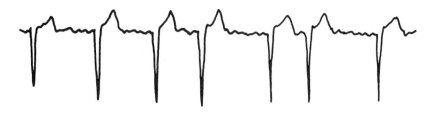

Fig. 1.10 Atrial fibrillation.

Initial management consists of controlling the rapid ventricular rate by slowing conduction through the AV node. Digoxin is effective but β-blocking drugs may have to be added if the ventricular rate remains high. Cardioversion may be considered in established atrial fibrillation once the underlying cause has been treated (i.e. after thyroidectomy or mitral valve surgery). Atrial fibrillation following myocardial infarction is often transient and may recur so drug therapy is preferable to d.c. cardioversion.

Paroxysmal atrial fibrillation is an extremely difficult arrhythmia to treat, as the ventricular rate is always rapid at the onset of attacks despite digoxin therapy. Disopyramide may reduce the frequency of attacks. Amiodarone is often very effective in these cases. Anticoagulant therapy should be considered when established atrial fibrillation complicates underlying cardiac disease especially in:

Mitral valve disease
Cardiomyopathies
After myocardial infarction.

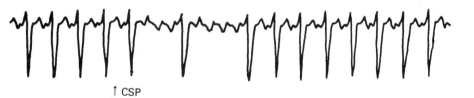

↑ CSP

Fig. 1.11 Atrial flutter with 2 : 1 block—showing the effect of carotid sinus pressure (CSP).

Atrial flutter occurs in the same situations as atrial fibrillation. The atrial rate is 300 per min and this is usually conducted to the ventricle in a 2 : 1 response. The ventricular rate is usually close to 150 per min. The typical saw-tooth pattern can be seen on the ECG (*Fig.* 1.11). Carotid sinus massage may temporarily increase the degree of AV block making the diagnosis clear. Digitalization is the treatment of choice but near-toxic doses are often required to slow the ventricular to 100 or 75 per min.

If the patient is showing signs of severe haemodynamic disturbance electric cardioversion should be considered first, together with diso-pyramide or procainamide to prevent recurrence. If digitalis fails to control the ventricular rate β-blockers can be added and elective cardioversion can still be considered provided digitalis toxicity can be excluded (urgent serum digoxin levels may be helpful in these cases).

Arrhythmias associated with Wolff–Parkinson–White syndrome

The Wolff–Parkinson–White syndrome is a congenital abnormality of the conducting pathway between the atria and ventricles. It allows rapid excitation to occur between these chambers in addition to the slower conduction through the AV node (pre-excitation). This rapid excitation is usually through an additional anatomical pathway. The presence of pre-excitation can be shown on the ECG by a short PR interval and the presence of a delta-wave in some leads (*Fig.* 1.12).

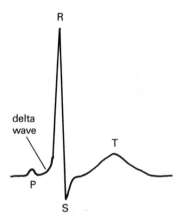

Fig. 1.12 ECG complex in Wolff–Parkinson–White syndrome.

Two varieties of rhythm disturbance can occur:
1. Paroxysmal supraventricular tachycardia
2. Atrial fibrillation.

Paroxysmal supraventricular tachycardia is produced by excitation proceeding along the AV node and returning to the atria via the additional pathway. The circus rhythm that is thereby set up causes rapid regular depolarization of the ventricules at a rate of 160–250 per min. Initial management is the same as for paroxysmal atrial tachycardia.

When atrial fibrillation occurs in Wolff–Parkinson–White syndrome the rapid atrial rate can be conducted down the aberrant pathway producing a rapid irregular ventricular response with rates between 150 and 450 per min. Those patients who can produce a very rapid ventricular response are in danger of developing ventricular fibrillation. In this situation digoxin is contraindicated as it may further speed conduction in the aberrant pathway. Disopyramide is the drug of choice, though cardioversion is often needed in urgent cases. Disopyramide also has a prophylactic effect and can be used long-term. Amiodarone is also very effective in the prevention of this life-threatening arrhythmia.

Ventricular arrhythmias

Isolated ventricular ectopic beats are extremely common in the normal population and may produce symptoms in some individuals. The awareness of 'missed beats' or palpitations often causes great anxiety and this tends to increase the frequency of ectopic activity. If underlying heart disease can be excluded then explanation of the symptoms and reassurance are all that is needed.

Ventricular tachycardia

Ventricular tachycardia is a condition where three or more consecutive ventricular ectopics occur. The ventricular rate is between 150 and 250 per min. The ECG shows broadened, abnormal QRS (*Fig.* 1.13) complexes in most leads. Independent sinus node activation of the atria may be observed and this will establish the diagnosis.

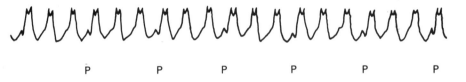

Fig. 1.13 Ventricular tachycardia—showing independent sinus node activation of the atria (P).

In established ventricular tachycardia, treatment should be along the following lines:
1. Bolus lignocaine, followed by i.v. infusion if sinus rhythm is achieved.
2. Intravenous disopyramide
3. D.C. cardioversion. Relatively small amounts of energy are required to convert this arrhythmia (25–100 joules). Cardioversion should be considered immediately if the patient is showing signs of severe haemodynamic decompensation.

Prophylaxis against further attacks should be mexiletine, disopyramide, procainamide, flecainide or amiodarone. In paroxysmal ventricular tachycardia drug therapy has to be relied upon but ventricular pacing may be used to terminate prolonged paroxysms, if they recur frequently.

Ventricular fibrillation

Ventricular fibrillation is the commonest arrhythmia associated with cardiac arrest (*Fig.* 1.14).

Ventricular fibrillation can occur in the following situations:
1. Following acute myocardial infarction
2. Critically ill patients with heart disease
3. Severe electrolyte disturbances, especially hyperkalaemia
4. Poisoning with drugs: digoxin, tricyclic antidepressants
5. Hypothermia.

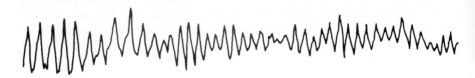

Fig. 1.14 Ventricular fibrillation.

The immediate treatment is d.c. shock but external cardiac massage and assisted respiration may have to be performed if defibrillation is not immediately available.

Following return to sinus rhythm the metabolic consequences of cardiac arrest should be corrected by i.v. $NaHCO_3$ 100 mEq. Further correction should depend upon analysis of arterial blood for pH, Po_2, Pco_2, HCO_3. When ventricular fibrillation complicates myocardial infarction anti-arrhythmic therapy with lignocaine should be given after restoration of sinus rhythm. If ventricular fibrillation has occurred in the early hours after myocardial infarction then prophylaxis is only required for 24–48 h. Late onset ventricular arrhythmias after myocardial infarction carry an adverse prognosis and often require long term prophylactic treatment.

Heart block

Heart block is caused by impaired conduction between the atria and the ventricles.

Various degrees of AV block are recognized:
First degree—prolonged PR interval >0·20 sec.
Second degree—
Wenckebach—increasing PR interval in successive beats terminating in failure to conduct (dropped beat) (*Fig.* 1.15).
Mobitz—dropped beats occur without a progressive increase in PR interval.
2 : 1 or 3 : 1 AV block—here only every second or third atrial beat is conducted to the ventricles.

Third degree (complete AV block) (*Fig.* 1.16)—There is no conduction between the atria and ventricles, both chambers beating independently. The ventricular rate in complete AV Block is between 20 and 50 per min.

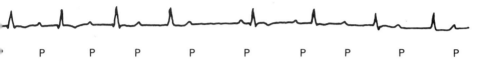

P   P   P   P   P   P   P   P   P

Fig. 1.15 Second-degree heart block (Wenckebach).

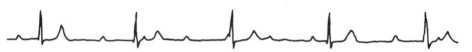

Fig. 1.16 Third-degree (complete AV) block.

Stokes–Adams attack

These attacks are a frequent feature of patients with heart block. They are due to a temporary cessation of ventricular contraction. In the majority of cases ventricular asystole (*Fig.* 1.17) is the cause, but in some cases, self-terminating ventricular fibrillation is found.

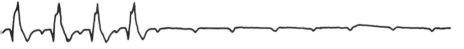

Fig. 1.17 Ventricular asystole (Stokes–Adams attacks).

Clinical features

The patient loses consciousness which may be preceded by dizziness. The attack usually lasts between 10 and 30 sec and convulsions may occur. The patient is often observed to be pale and pulseless but when the heart beat is restored, flushing is both observed and felt by the patient.

The ECG between attacks frequently shows abnormalities of AV conduction or bundle-branch block. Confirmation of the nature of the attack can often be obtained by 24-h ambulatory ECG monitoring. Even if the patient is symptom-free during the period of the tape, the ECG may show abnormalities of AV conduction or ventricular arrhythmias.

The implantation of a permanent pacemaker is indicated if syncope has occurred or if the ventricular rate is so low that symptoms and signs of cardiac failure are present.

Bundle-branch block

Isolated bundle-branch block can occur in a wide variety of cardiac conditions and may occasionally be found in *normal* subjects. Bundle-branch block may indicate the presence of AV conduction abnormalities even in patients in sinus rhythm. Usually more than one division of the bundle-branch system is affected (bi- or tri-fascicular block).

The commonest example of this is right bundle-branch block with left axis deviation (left anterior hemiblock).

Examples of right and left bundle-branch block are shown in *Fig. 1.18*.

Heart block following myocardial infarction

After inferior myocardial infarction, heart block may develop, due to ischaemia of the AV node. It frequently progresses through first and second degree block to complete heart block with ventricular rates between 20 and 50 per min. The QRS complex is usually narrow. This conduction disturbance recovers completely in the majority of cases but temporary pacing is necessary if the heart rate is below 50 per min or hypotension is present.

In anterior infarction the heart block is caused by damage to the ventricular Purkinje fibres involved in the infarcted area. Bundle-branch block is usually present when the patient is in sinus rhythm and the change to complete heart block is often sudden with periods of ventricular standstill. The association of heart block and anterior infarction has a high mortality but this is related to the extent of myocardial damage. Pacing is often required and may have to be permanent in those who survive the acute episode.

1.6   RHEUMATIC VALVULAR DISEASE

Mitral stenosis

Mitral stenosis may be congenital but usually occurs after rheumatic fever has damaged the endocardium of the mitral valve. A history of a previous attack of acute rheumatism or chorea is obtained in approximately 50% of patients with rheumatic valvular disease. Symptoms may take 5–15 years to develop after the attack of rheumatic fever.

Clinical features

The symptoms and signs of mitral stenosis are due to:

1. Reduced cardiac output—tiredness, cold and cyanosed periphery, mitral facies.

2. Raised left atrial pressure—exertional dyspnoea, orthopnoea, paroxysmal nocturnal dyspnoea, pulmonary oedema.

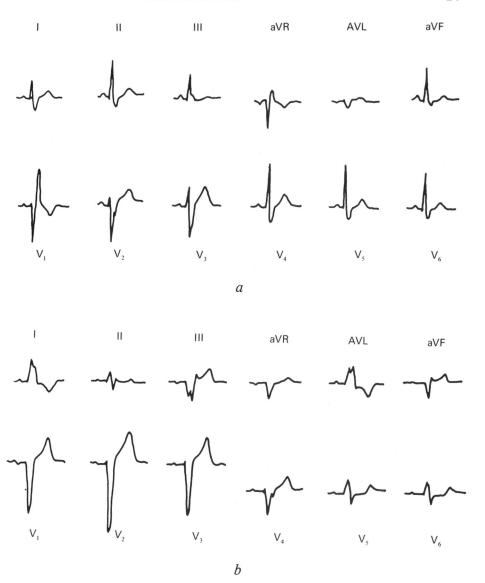

Fig. 1.18 ECG in (*a*) Right bundle-branch block; (*b*) Left bundle-branch block.

Patients with mitral stenosis have a higher incidence of chronic bronchitis and hypertension than the normal population. The onset of the above symptoms is usually very gradual but two events commonly precipitate the sudden onset of severe symptoms:

1. The onset of atrial fibrillation causing the loss of atrial contraction and shortening of the period of diastolic filling of the left ventricle.

2. Pregnancy and infection, by increasing the demands on a previously compensated circulation.

Physical examination may reveal a typical malar cyanosis (mitral facies). The pulse volume is small or normal and the jugular venous pressure may be raised. The apex beat is not displaced in pure mitral stenosis but the first heart sound may be palpable. A parasternal heave will be detected in most patients with significant stenosis, indicating the presence of right ventricular hypertrophy. The auscultatory features are shown in *Fig.* 1.19. The severity of stenosis can be determined by the closeness of the opening snap to the second heart sound and by the length of the diastolic murmur. The loudness of the first heart sound and opening snap indicate the pliance of the valve and its suitability for closed mitral valvotomy.

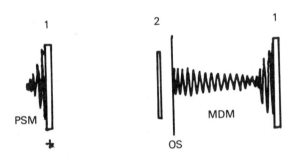

Fig. 1.19. Auscultatory features in mitral stenosis. PSM, presystolic murmur; MDM, mid-diastolic murmur; OS, opening snap.

The ECG will show evidence of left atrial hypertrophy (P mitrale). Right axis deviation and right ventricular hypertrophy will indicate the presence of reactive pulmonary hypertension. The chest radiograph will show slight prominence of the pulmonary conus and enlargement of the left atrial appendage. The left atrium may also be shown as a double contour, just inside the right heart border (*Fig.* 1.20). Dilated upper lobe veins may be seen together with pulmonary congestion (Kerley B lines) and pulmonary oedema in severe cases. Echocardiography will show the typical pattern of movement of the mitral leaflets seen in mitral stenosis (*Fig.* 1.21). It will also demonstrate valvular calcification and left atrial enlargement. Echocardiography should also help to exclude the possibility of a left atrial myxoma, which can present with many of the features of mitral stenosis.

Management

When symptoms and signs indicate the presence of severe mitral stenosis the patient should be referred for cardiac surgery. If pure stenosis is present and the valve is pliant and not calcified, closed mitral valvotomy can be considered. The presence of mitral regurgitation or calcification, previous

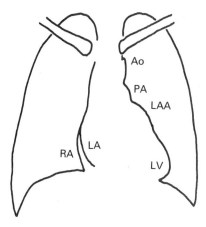

Fig. 1.20 Radiological features in mitral stenosis. Ao, aorta; LA, left atrium; LAA, left atrial appendage; LV, left ventricle; PA, pulmonary artery; RA, right atrium.

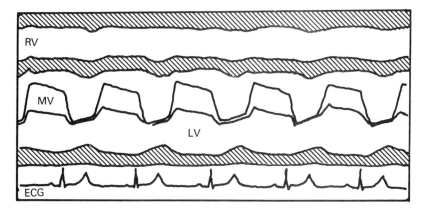

Fig. 1.21 Echocardiogram in mitral stenosis. LV, left ventricle; MV, mitral valve; RV, right ventricle.

valvular surgery or a history of embolic phenomena usually necessitates operation using cardiopulmonary bypass and often demands mitral valve replacement. Mild symptoms can be controlled by diuretic therapy. The onset of atrial fibrillation usually requires urgent treatment. The rapid ventricular rate is controlled by digoxin but the addition of β-blocking drugs may be necessary if the ventricular rate is still rapid despite full digitalization. The risk of peripheral emboli is high when atrial fibrillation complicates mitral valve disease and anticoagulant drugs are usually started at this time. Anticoagulation should also be considered in patients with significant mitral stenosis and a large left atrium even in the presence of sinus rhythm.

Mitral regurgitation

The causes of mitral regurgitation are:
1. Rheumatic mitral valve disease
2. Ruptured mitral valve chordae
3. Mitral valve prolapse
4. Papillary muscle dysfunction (ischaemia)
5. Papillary muscle rupture (infarction)
6. Dilatation of the mitral annulus secondary to left ventricular dilatation.

In rheumatic mitral valve disease, mitral regurgitation usually dates from the attack of rheumatic fever, although many years may pass before symptoms occur. Ruptured chordae or papillary muscle rupture occur as a sudden event often with the rapid onset of severe symptoms.

Clinical features

Significant mitral regurgitation causes volume overload of the left ventricle which compensates by dilatation and hypertrophy. The condition is often well tolerated and symptoms are a late feature unless ruptured chordae or papillary muscle is the cause. Increasing exertional dyspnoea and pulmonary oedema are the principal features but a significant degree of regurgitation will produce a fall in cardiac output, and fatigue will be a prominent symptom.

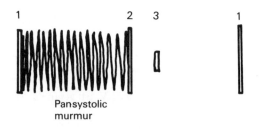

Pansystolic
murmur

Fig. 1.22 Auscultatory features of mitral regurgitation.

The pulse volume is normal or increased. The cardiac apex is forceful and displaced, indicating left ventricular hypertrophy and dilatation. The auscultation signs are shown in *Fig.* 1.22. The pansystolic murmur is best heard at the apex, is transmitted to the axilla and is often well heard over the back.

The ECG will show evidence of left ventricular hypertrophy. The chest radiograph will show dilatation of the left ventricle and atrium together with evidence of pulmonary congestion in severe cases. Echocardiography will also show evidence of left ventricular dilatation with normal left ventricular function (left ventricular volume overload). The underlying cause for the mitral regurgitation can frequently be identified by this technique (*Fig.* 1.23).

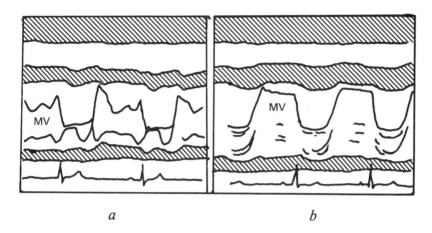

a   *b*

Fig. 1.23 Echocardiographic appearances in mitral regurgitation. (*a*) Mitral valve prolapse; (*b*) Ruptured chordae.

Management

The finding of significant mitral regurgitation usually necessitates the referral of the patient for invasive investigation as a preliminary to cardiac surgery. Mild symptoms will respond to diuretic therapy and the presence of atrial fibrillation will require digitalization and anticoagulant drugs.

Mitral valve prolapse

This is a common form of valvular disease, its frequent occurrence being demonstrated by echocardiography (*Fig.* 1.23*a*). Most patients are symptom-free and the degree of mitral regurgitation is often trivial but these patients are at risk of developing infective endocarditis. There is a common association of this condition with a history of atypical chest pain. T-wave abnormalities may be present on the ECG. Some cases may develop serious ventricular arrhythmias, with a risk of sudden death.

Aortic stenosis

Aortic stenosis may be congenital in origin, may result from rheumatic heart disease or may be the result of progressive sclerosis and calcification of a congenital bicuspid valve.

Clinical features

Significant aortic stenosis causes pressure overload of the left ventricle which compensates by marked hypertrophy. Dilatation of the left ventricle is a late, often terminal, feature.

The symptoms of aortic stenosis include:

Exertional dyspnoea—due to left ventricular failure on exertion.

Angina pectoris—due to relative lack of oxygen supply to the hypertrophied left ventricle, even in the presence of normal coronary arteries.

Faintness and syncope on exertion—due to failure to increase the cardiac output on exertion because of the fixed stenosis.

The pulse often has a characteristic slow upstroke (anacrotic) provided a major artery (i.e. carotid or femoral) is palpated. The blood pressure is normal or low but the finding of mild to moderate hypertension does not exclude the possibility of aortic stenosis. The cardiac apex is forceful but not displaced. The auscultatory signs are shown in *Fig.* 1.24. The murmur is

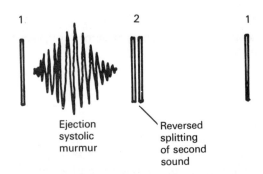

Fig. 1.24 Auscultatory features of aortic stenosis.

loudest over the base of the heart being transmitted to the carotid vessels but in some patients the murmur is well heard at the apex. Splitting of the second sound in expiration (reversed splitting) is an indication of significant stenosis provided left bundle-branch block is excluded. The ECG shows left ventricular hypertrophy (*Fig.* 1.25) but the presence of left bundle-branch block may mask this feature. The chest radiograph will show a 'bulky' left heart border due to left ventricular hypertrophy and there may be prominence of the ascending aorta (post-stenotic dilatation) (*Fig.* 1.26). Calcification of the valve may be seen on the lateral radiograph (*Fig.* 1.27) or by screening. Echocardiography will demonstrate a calcified or thickened aortic valve together with a thick-walled left ventricle.

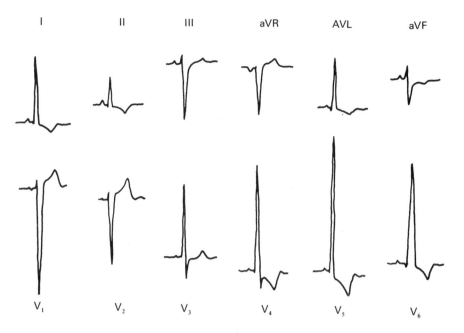

Fig. 1.25 ECG in left ventricular hypertrophy.

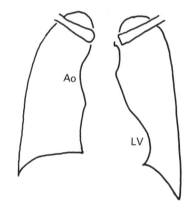

Fig. 1.26 PA chest radiograph in aortic stenosis. Ao, post-stenotic dilatation; LV, left ventricle.

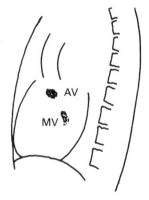

Fig. 1.27 Calcified mitral and aortic valves on lateral chest radiograph. AV, aortic valve; MV, mitral valve.

Management

The presence of many of the above symptoms and signs indicate significant stenosis and referral for surgery is necessary. Cardiac catheterization may not be necessary preoperatively but it is usual to perform a coronary arteriogram in all patients with aortic stenosis who complain of angina, to exclude coexisting coronary artery disease.

Aortic regurgitation

Aortic regurgitation can result from:
 1. Rheumatic heart disease
 2. Calcific aortic valve
 3. Ruptured aortic cusp (Marfan's syndrome; infective endocarditis)
 4. Syphilis
 5. Rheumatoid disease, ankylosing spondylitis
 6. Secondary to aortic dissection
 7. Severe hypertension.

Clinical features

Significant aortic regurgitation causes volume overload of the left ventricle which compensates by dilatation and hypertrophy. Aortic regurgitation is well tolerated unless it occurs suddenly (i.e. ruptured aortic cusp). Symptoms are, therefore, a fairly late feature and are usually due to progressive left ventricular failure. The pulse in aortic regurgitation has a collapsing character. The blood pressure demonstrates a wide pulse pressure and low diastolic pressure. Visible carotid pulsation is present and capillary pulsation can be demonstrated at the finger tips and by gentle compression of the finger nail. The cardiac apex is forceful and displaced indicating left ventricular hypertrophy and dilatation. The auscultatory signs are shown in *Fig.* 1.28. The murmur is best heard at the left sternal edge, with the patient

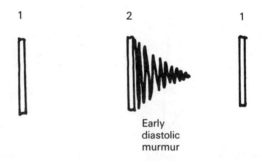

Early
diastolic
murmur

Fig. 1.28 Auscultatory features in aortic regurgitation.

sitting forward and with held expiration. In addition, a mid-diastolic murmur may be heard at the apex (Austin–Flint murmur). This is due to the regurgitant jet forcing the mitral valve leaflet to partially close, producing functional mitral stenosis. The ECG shows left ventricular hypertrophy. The chest radiograph will show dilatation of the left ventricle. Dilatation of the aorta will be seen if there is coexisting stenosis or if Marfan's syndrome, syphilis or dissecting aneurysm is present. Echocardiography will show vibration of the anterior mitral valve leaflet caused by the regurgitant jet, together with dilatation of the left ventricular cavity (*Fig.* 1.29).

The presence of significant aortic regurgitation is indicated by:
1. Low diastolic blood pressure
2. Marked left ventricular dilatation
3. Signs of left ventricular failure.

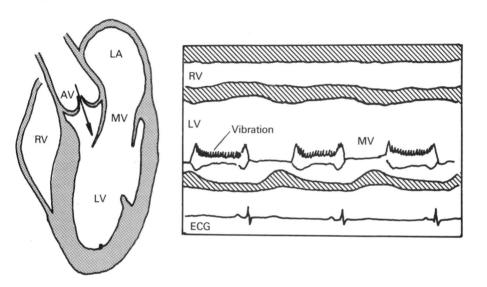

Fig. 1.29 Echocardiogram in aortic regurgitation. AV, aortic valve; LA, left atrium; LV, left ventricle; MV, mitral valve; RV, right ventricle.

Management

Although early symptoms can be controlled by medical treatment, the presence of significant regurgitation usually requires aortic valve replacement. Preoperative assessment of the severity of aortic regurgitation can be obtained by aortic root angiography.

1.7 CARDIOMYOPATHIES

A primary cardiomyopathy is a disorder of cardiac muscle of uncertain cause or association. Where a cause or association is present, e.g. alcohol or amyloidosis, it is preferable to refer to this as a specific condition, e.g. amyloid heart disease. The clinical presentation may be similar with a wide variety of aetiological factors.

A clinical classification into the following groups is the most practical method.
1. Hypertrophic cardiomyopathy
2. Congestive cardiomyopathy
3. Restrictive cardiomyopathy.

Hypertrophic cardiomyopathy

This is an inherited disorder, both dominant and recessive forms have been demonstrated. Affected members of a family may show varying degrees of severity. The pathological findings include massive hypertrophy of the left ventricular wall, particularly the interventricular septum. The bulging septum usually encroaches on the outflow tract of the left ventricle causing obstruction. The hypertrophied ventricular wall is stiff thereby interfering with left ventricular filling. Serious ventricular arrhythmias are an important complication and are responsible for sudden death, which is a feature of this condition. Symptoms include:
Syncope or lightheadedness on exertion
Typical anginal pain
Examination reveals a jerky pulse, a hyperdynamic apex beat, often with a double impulse: a mid-late systolic murmur at the lower left sternal edge with third or fourth heart sounds. The clinical findings may mimic aortic stenosis or mitral regurgitation.

The diagnosis can be confirmed by echocardiography which demonstrates a thick, relatively akinetic septum together with small left ventricular cavity. Abnormal anterior movement of the mitral valve leaflet can be seen in systole (*Fig.* 1.30).

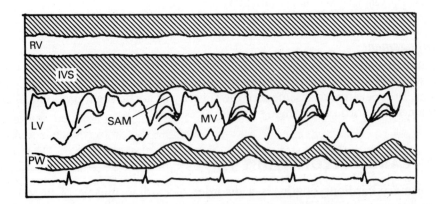

Fig. 1.30 Echocardiogram in hypertrophic cardiomyopathy. IVS, interventricular septum; LV, left ventricle; MV, mitral valve; PW, posterior left ventricular wall; RV, right ventricle; SAM, systolic anterior movement of mitral valve.

Management

Patients should be warned to avoid sudden severe exertion or lifting heavy objects. Beta-blocking drugs reduce the contractility of the hypertrophied left ventricle and are helpful in symptomatic cases. Calcium antagonists (verapamil) can also be helpful. A 24-h ECG recording should be performed to identify potentially serious arrhythmias and, if present, anti-arrhythmic drugs should be prescribed (amiodarone has been shown to be effective in this respect).

Congestive cardiomyopathy

This type of cardiomyopathy is the form most commonly seen, a similar clinical presentation being produced by many aetiological factors, e.g.
Alcoholic heart disease
Hypertensive heart disease
Ischaemic heart disease
Thyrotoxic heart disease.

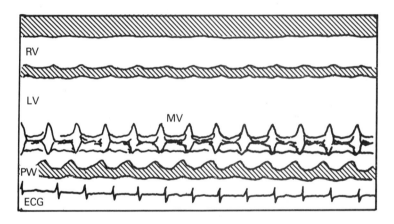

Fig. 1.31 Echocardiogram in congestive cardiomyopathy. LV, left ventricle; MV, mitral valve; PW, posterior left ventricular wall; RV, right ventricle.

The left ventricle is only moderately hypertrophied but grossly dilated. Contractility of the ventricle is greatly reduced. The main clinical features are those of congestive cardiac failure. Examination often reveals a gallop rhythm with an apical systolic murmur due to mitral regurgitation. The chest radiograph shows gross cardiomegaly with pulmonary congestion. The echocardiogram shows dilatation of LV with poor LV function (*Fig.* 1.31).

Management consists of treatment of congestive symptoms with diuretics, vasodilators and digoxin. Severe cases often require prolonged bed rest in hospital to relieve symptoms and in these cases anticoagulant therapy should be considered because of the risk of both systemic and pulmonary emboli. The prognosis of this condition is very poor and several cases have been referred for cardiac transplantation.

Restrictive cardiomyopathy

This condition is rare and closely resembles constrictive pericarditis in its presentation. Differentiation of the two conditions may require thoracotomy.

1.8   PULMONARY HEART DISEASE

The following forms of pulmonary heart disease will be considered:
Pulmonary embolic disease—acute mild pulmonary embolism, acute and subacute massive pulmonary embolism
Cor pulmonale
Pulmonary hypertension.

Pulmonary embolic disease

This is caused by thrombus originating in a peripheral vein, passing through the right side of the heart and blocking one or more branches of the pulmonary arterial tree. The severity of the condition is dependent on the degree of obstruction to pulmonary blood flow and the rapidity of onset. The thrombus usually arises in the iliofemoral or pelvic veins and its presence there may be clinically silent but may be accompanied by signs of venous thrombosis. It is convenient to consider the clinical features and management of venous thrombosis at this stage.

Venous thrombosis

The factors predisposing to venous thrombosis are:
1. Venous stasis—bed rest; immobilization of limbs in plaster; heart failure
2. Damage to veins—direct trauma or surgery
3. Increased coagulability of blood—pregnancy; oral contraceptives; trauma and surgery; polycythaemia; blood disorders and underlying malignancy.

Clinical features
The principal clinical features are pain and swelling of the affected leg. The calf region is commonly involved but swelling of the whole limb is seen in some cases of iliofemoral venous thrombosis. The affected limb is warm, the patient may be pyrexial and superficial venous dilatation may be seen.

Dorsiflexion of the affected foot may cause pain in the calf (Homans' sign) although this is not specific for venous thrombosis.

Management

Once the diagnosis of venous thrombosis is suspected bed rest is recommended until the pain subsides. Elevation of the foot of the bed is helpful if oedema is extensive. Heparin is given either by intravenous infusion or regular subcutaneous injection in doses which maintain the thrombin time or partial thromboplastin time (PPT) within the therapeutic range (2–2·5 × control). When symptoms and signs are subsiding, usually within 4–7 days, oral anticoagulants are substituted and are continued for at least 2–3 months. A history of recurrent venous thrombosis may require long-term treatment with anticoagulants.

Acute mild pulmonary embolism

In the majority of cases of this type, the acute event passes unnoticed and the first symptoms are due to the development of pulmonary infarction. This causes pleuritic chest pain. The degree of dyspnoea is often only mild and the patient may have haemoptysis. Examination may fail to show evidence of cardiac involvement, apart from sinus tachycardia, and initial examination of the chest is often negative. A radiograph taken soon after the onset of symptoms may also be normal but later films may show a segmental consolidation or an area of linear collapse. The development of a pleural effusion and elevation of the diaphragm on the affected side, are other features that may be seen. An isotope perfusion scan will frequently show a segmental area of underperfusion. If this is seen in the presence of a normal radiograph or ventilation scan, the diagnosis is usually certain.

Management

Powerful analgesia may be necessary to relieve pain. Subsequent treatment is aimed at preventing further emboli and this is achieved by anticoagulant drugs. Heparin is given by infusion for approximately 7 days followed by warfarin which is then continued for 3 months. Recurrent pulmonary emboli are usually an indication for long-term anticoagulant therapy.

Acute massive pulmonary embolism

In this type of pulmonary embolism more than 50% of the pulmonary artery tree is obstructed and the majority of symptoms and signs are due to the effects on the heart. It usually presents as an acute event, often with syncope. The patient is often anxious, with the feeling of impending death. Central constricting chest pain may be present, but dyspnoea is a common feature. Examination may reveal cyanosis with a rapid thready pulse. The pulse may diminish in intensity or disappear during inspiration (paradoxical pulse) and the blood pressure is often low. The jugular venous pressure may be raised and on auscultation a gallop rhythm may be heard over the right ventricle.

The ECG in these cases is frequently abnormal. The 'classical' $S_1 Q_3 T_3$ pattern with T-wave inversion in leads V_1–V_4 is due to acute right ventricular strain (*Fig.* 1.32). Right bundle-branch block may develop. In older patients changes consistent with left ventricular ischaemia may develop and may mislead the physician into diagnosing myocardial infarction. Atrial fibrillation may develop and frequent ventricular ectopics may be seen. The chest radiograph may be negative but areas of underperfusion may be seen by careful examination of the pulmonary vascular pattern.

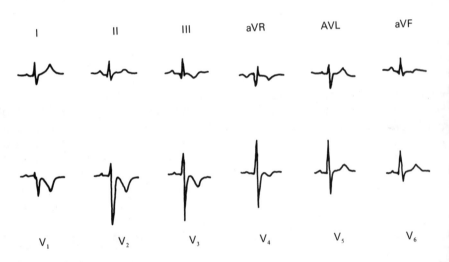

Fig. 1.32 ECG in acute pulmonary embolism.

The diagnosis is often easy when the above features are seen, but in doubtful cases pulmonary angiography should be performed and this will establish the diagnosis.

Management

From the onset of the acute episode there is a tendency for gradual improvement, with natural lysis of the embolus taking place.

The haemodynamic state of the patient at the time of presentation is important in deciding which course of action to take.

General measures such as alleviation of pain and anxiety with dia-morphine and the administration of oxygen are helpful. If the patient is haemodynamically stable and not shocked, treatment is aimed at lysis of the clot using streptokinase or urokinase. Streptokinase can cause allergic reactions and its lysing effect may be unpredictable. Urokinase, although more expensive is less likely to suffer from these drawbacks. A large loading dose of streptokinase, 600/000 u, is given over half an hour, followed by infusion of 100/000 u per hour. Treatment should continue for 24–48 h according to the response, and should be followed by heparin initially in low dosage and then full dosage.

If urokinase is used the loading dose is 4400/u per kg body weight given over 10 min followed by an infusion of 4400/u per kg body weight, per hour for 12 h.

If severe spontaneous bleeding occurs during treatment, this can be corrected by discontinuation of therapy and reversing its effects with epsilon-aminocaproic acid (EACA).

In patients who are shocked and unlikely to survive more than an hour, and those in whom thrombolytic therapy is contraindicated—e.g. following recent major surgery, in the puerperium, patients with known bleeding disorders or recent cerebrovascular disease—the only hope of survival can be achieved by pulmonary embolectomy under cardiopulmonary bypass if facilities for this procedure are available near at hand.

Subacute massive pulmonary embolism

This type is also associated with a greater than 50% occlusion of the pulmonary artery tree but this occlusion occurs gradually with repeated small emboli over a period of weeks.

The onset is insidious with increasing dyspnoea. Pleuritic chest pain may be present and cough, haemoptysis and fever may occur. On examination the patient is often cyanosed, the pulse may be rapid but the blood pressure is usually normal. Jugular venous pressure is often raised and a parasternal heave may be present. Auscultation may reveal a loud pulmonary component of the second sound which may be delayed. A gallop rhythm may be heard over the right ventricle. Other features of right heart failure will be present. The ECG will often show features of right ventricular strain and the radiograph may show dilatation of the main pulmonary artery with some cardiac enlargement. Right ventricular enlargement will be seen on a lateral film. The lung fields may show evidence of multiple emboli and these may also be detected on an isotope lung scan.

The diagnosis of this type of pulmonary embolic disease can be difficult. Right heart catheterization and pulmonary angiography will show the right ventricular and pulmonary artery pressure and angiography will show peripheral obstruction of the pulmonary artery branches.

Management

In this condition, heparin is the treatment of choice to prevent further embolism while the natural lysis of previous emboli takes place.

Cor pulmonale

Cor pulmonale is heart disease secondary to disease of the lungs. A variety of pulmonary conditions can have secondary effects on the right side of the heart causing pulmonary hypertension and right heart failure. They include:
1. Chronic bronchitis—particularly in cases with hypoventilation and carbon dioxide retention ('blue bloaters')
2. Pulmonary fibrosis including TB and pneumoconiosis
3. Chest wall deformities—kyphoscoliosis
4. Extensive lung resection
5. Gross obesity with hypoventilation (Pickwickian syndrome).

Longstanding vasoconstriction of pulmonary vessels will cause pulmonary hypertension and right ventricular hypertrophy. The first symptoms are usually due to right heart failure. Hypertrophy of the right ventricle is usually evident clinically and the venous pressure is usually raised. Auscultation may reveal accentuation of the pulmonary component of the second heart sound.

Right heart failure can be improved by diuretic therapy but digoxin is not very effective in cases in sinus rhythm.

Attempts at improving oxygenation in these patients may help to lower pulmonary artery pressure and improve the degree of failure. Oxygen should be used with caution in those patients with hypoventilation and the arterial P_{CO_2} should be monitored.

Idiopathic pulmonary hypertension

This is a rare condition which may occur in patients during the 2nd to 4th decades. It is more frequent in women. The aetiology is unknown but repeated micro-embolism has been suggested as a possible cause. The condition has a rapidly progressive course. By the time the diagnosis is made, the pulmonary artery pressure has often risen to systemic levels and right ventricular hypertrophy is evident clinically as well as on the ECG (*Fig.* 1.33). The main features are due to a low-output state with lassitude, peripheral cyanosis and occasionally syncope on exertion may occur. Eventually progressive right heart failure occurs with a fatal outcome within 2 years. There is no effective treatment at present but anticoagulants are often given. Hypotensive drugs which lower pulmonary artery pressure have been used but they do not seem to alter the prognosis.

1.9   INFECTIVE ENDOCARDITIS

Infective endocarditis can be caused by bacterial, fungal or rickettsial organisms becoming established on the endocardial surface of the heart. The valves of the left side of the heart are most frequently involved. The infective

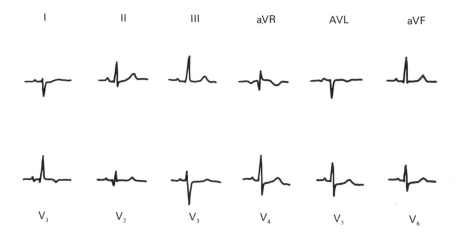

Fig. 1.33 ECG in right ventricular hypertrophy.

organism reaches the heart during bacteraemia from an infected focus elsewhere. There is usually previous endocardial damage on the surface of the valves though previously normal valves have become the site of infective endocarditis.

This condition is fatal if untreated, so it is vitally important to make the diagnosis, identify the infecting organism and give adequate treatment.

Clinical features

Infective endocarditis should be suspected in any patient with a fever and heart murmur. By the time the classic features of anaemia, weight loss, finger clubbing, splenomegaly, splinter haemorrhages, retinal lesions and petechiae appear, the disease has usually been established for many weeks. The serious complications of this condition include:

1. Destruction of heart valves causing severe heart failure
2. Embolic phenomena
3. Renal failure due to focal glomerulonephritis.

The common underlying cardiac lesions include:
1. Biscuspid aortic valve
2. Aortic regurgitation
3 Rheumatic mitral valve, especially mitral regurgitation
4. Mitral valve prolapse
5. Prosthetic valves.

The infecting organisms commonly encountered are:
1. Streptococcus—commonest in medical patients
2. *Staphylococcus albus*—seen in surgical patients with prosthetic valves, and 'main-line' drug addicts
3. *Coxiella burnetii* (Q fever)
4. Fungi—in immunocompromised patients

Table 1.4 Antibiotic therapy in infective endocarditis

Organism	Treatment	Duration	Comments
Streptococcus viridans (penicillin sensitive) MIC <0·1 μg/ml			
S. sanguis	Penicillin 12 megaunits/day i.v.		
S. salivarius			
S. mitior	Amoxycillin 1–3 g/day may be given after two weeks	4 weeks	Some organisms may be tolerant
S. mutans			
Streptococcus faecalis (relative penicillin resistance) MIC >0·1 μg/ml			
S. faecalis	Penicillin 20 megaunits/day i.v. +	6 weeks	Dose of gentamicin is dependent on renal function
S. bovis	Gentamicin 80 mg twice daily i.v.		S. bovis can occur in patients with bowel disease
S. durans	Amoxycillin can also be substituted after 2 weeks		
Staphylococcus pyogenes	Cloxacillin or flucloxacillin 1 g 4-hourly i.v.	6 weeks	Drug addicts
S. epidermidis			Prosthetic valves
			Surgery often necessary
Coxiella burnetii (Q fever)	Tetracycline Co-trimoxazole	'Indefinite'	
Fungi	Amphotericin B	Prolonged	Immunocompromised patients. High mortality
Culture negative	Treat as S. faecalis		

5. Virulent organisms such as *Streptococcus pneumoniae, Staphylococcus aureus* can cause rapid destruction of previously normal valves.

Management

The underlying cardiac lesion may be obvious on clinical examination but can often be detected by echocardiography which may also show the presence of vegetations.

The infecting organism can be identified by blood culture. It is important to take several cultures before antibiotics are given. The organism is easily isolated unless antibiotics have been given in recent weeks, and treatment can be started while the organism is being identified and its sensitivity determined. In culture-negative cases special culture media may be needed; it is therefore important to have a close liaison with the bacteriologist when cases of endocarditis are suspected. In culture-negative cases—serological tests for *Coxiella burnetii* (Q fever) should be performed.

Treatment requires bacteriocidal antibiotics in large doses for prolonged periods (*Table* 1.4). Back titration of the patient's serum against the original organism, will give a good guide to the efficacy of chemotherapy.

Surgical treatment—valve replacement—should be considered if heart failure develops, indicating destruction of valve tissue causing gross valvular incompetence.

Another indication for surgical intervention is the occurrence of repeated emboli despite apparently effective treatment.

Prevention of infective endocarditis

Many cases of infective endocarditis could be prevented if appropriate prophylactic antibiotics were given before any procedure which is liable to produce transient bacteraemia, in patients with known structural heart disease.

The cardiac lesions for which prophylactic antibiotics are given include:

1. Congenital heart disease, including bicuspid aortic valve
2. Mitral and aortic valvular disease including mitral valve prolapse
3. Patients with prosthetic valves, patch repairs of congenital lesions.
4. Hypertrophic cardiomyopathy.

The procedures liable to produce transient bacteraemia, the likely organism and the prophylactic antibiotic regime are shown in *Table* 1.5.

The antibiotic is given 1 h before the procedure and continued for 24 h.

1.10 DISEASE OF THE PERICARDIUM

Pericardial disease can be caused by a wide variety of factors. The common causes include:

Table 1.5 Antibiotic prophylaxis against infective endocarditis

Procedure	Antibiotic
Dental extraction	Penicillin 500 mg 1 h before, repeated at 8 and 16 h
Upper gastrointestinal endoscopy	Amoxycillin 3 g 1 h before (single dose) Erythromycin given in cases of penicillin allergy
Genitourinary investigations and surgery	Ampicillin 1 g + 1 h before, repeated at 8 and 16 h Gentamicin 100 mg
Abdominal surgery	Ampicillin 1 g + 1 h before, repeated at 8 and 16 h
Obstetric procedures	Gentamicin 100 mg

Infective—viruses and bacteria including TB
Uraemic pericarditis
Connective tissue disorders—SLE, rheumatoid disease
Pericarditis following myocardial infarction
Neoplastic pericarditis
Pericardial disease may present as:
1. Acute pericarditis
2. Pericardial effusion
3. Constrictive pericarditis.

Acute pericarditis

The commonest primary form of acute pericarditis is that related to virus infection.

The principal symptom of viral pericarditis is anterior chest pain. This pain is often sharp and stabbing in character, felt over the precordium or epigastrium with referred pain to the shoulder if the diaphragmatic pericardium is involved. The pain is exacerbated by deep inspiration and is worse when the patient is lying flat or on the left side. Auscultation usually reveals a pericardial friction rub. The patient is often febrile at the time of presentation and may give a history of upper respiratory tract infection in the preceding weeks. Investigations to confirm the presence of pericarditis include:

Chest radiograph
Echocardiography

The ECG classically shows S–T elevation (*Fig.* 1.34) involving most limb and precordial leads. In most chronic cases and also during recovery, T-wave inversion may occur making the differentiation from ischaemia difficult.

The chest radiograph will be normal in uncomplicated cases but an increased CT ratio raises the possibility of pericardial effusion. This can be confirmed by echocardiography.

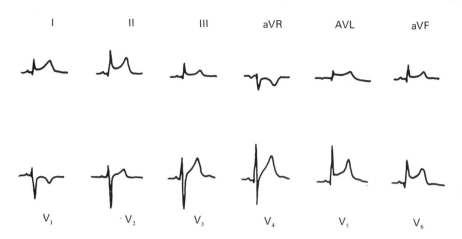

Fig. 1.34 ECG in acute pericarditis.

Other investigations are aimed at determining the underlying cause and include:
Virus antibodies
Autoantibodies
Rheumatoid factor
Blood urea.

Management

The pain of acute pericarditis can be relieved by aspirin, codeine or a non-steroidal anti-inflammatory drug (e.g. indomethacin). Severe pain may need opiates for relief. Steroids can be used in resistant cases (especially Dressler's syndrome and SLE) if the above measures are ineffective.

Most cases of acute viral pericarditis settle within 2–3 days although recurrent chest pains may occur in the following weeks.

Pericardial effusion

Pericardial effusion can complicate acute pericarditis from most causes but can also occur *de novo*. The rapid accumulation of 150–200 ml of fluid in the pericardial sac can produce severe symptoms whereas the gradual accumulation of over 1 litre of fluid may have little or no effect.

The principal causes of pericardial effusion are:
Infective—postvirus pericarditis; tuberculosis
Postmyocardial infarction (Dressler's syndrome)
Uraemia, especially during chronic dialysis
Neoplastic involvement of the pericardium
Connective-tissue diseases
Post-irradiation.

Clinical features

Pericardial pain may be a feature of pericardial effusion and large effusions also cause respiratory distress. The patient often dislikes lying flat and may obtain relief sitting forward or in the knee–chest position. If cardiac tamponade is present the patient is usually pale, shocked and peripherally cyanosed. Respiration is rapid and shallow. The pulse is rapid and a fall in pulse volume in inspiration may be detected (pulsus paradoxus). This sign is more easily demonstrated using a sphygmomanometer.

The venous pressure is often raised in significant effusions and a further elevation is seen on inspiration (Kussmaul's sign). On auscultation the heart sounds may be quiet though this is not universal. A friction rub may also be detected, despite the presence of large amounts of fluid.

The chief investigations are chest radiography which shows an enlarged heart shadow (*Fig.* 1.35) and echocardiography. With the patient supine and the echo beam directed vertically downwards even small amounts of fluid can be detected between the myocardium and pericardium (*Fig.* 1.36).

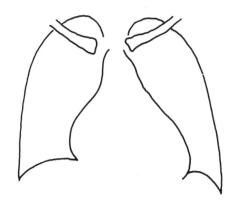

Fig. 1.35 Cardiac outline in pericardial effusion.

Management

Patients who demonstrate signs of cardiac tamponade should have fluid withdrawn by pericardial aspiration. This procedure is not without serious hazards and should only be undertaken by a skilled operator, unless it is a dire emergency and a large quantity of fluid has been demonstrated by echocardiography.

Removal of fluid for diagnostic purposes should only be performed by those with experience. More effective long-term treatment which also yields better diagnostic results can be achieved by creating a pericardial window through a limited thoracotomy.

Patients with few or no symptoms should be investigated to find the underlying cause and then treated appropriately.

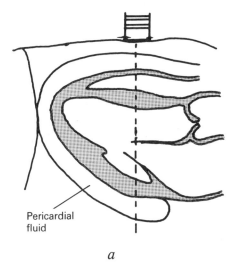

Pericardial
fluid

a

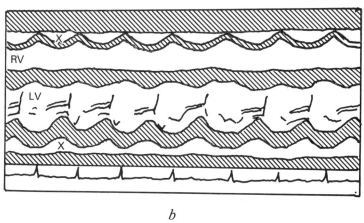

b

Fig. 1.36 Echocardiogram in pericardial effusion. LV, left ventricle; RV, right
ventricle; X, pericardial effusion.

Constrictive pericarditis

In this condition the heart is encased by a thick, rigid and often calcified
pericardium, the potential pericardial space often being obliterated. The
commonest cause is still related to previous tuberculous infection, but it can
also be seen after viral pericarditis and with connective-tissue disorders.

Clinical features

Patients insidiously develop symptoms and signs of gross right heart failure
with extensive peripheral oedema, hepatomegaly, ascites and dilated jugular
veins.

The precordium is quiet with soft heart sounds although a loud early third heart sound may be present. The jugular venous pulse shows inspiratory filling with a prominent 'Y' descent. Pulsus paradoxus can usually be demonstrated.

The ECG often shows low-voltage complexes.

The chest radiograph may reveal little or no cardiac enlargement and relatively clear lung fluids despite the gross degree of right heart failure. A lateral film may show calcification in the pericardium in about 50% of cases (*Fig.* 1.37).

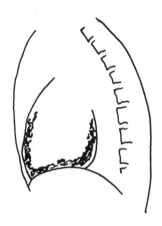

Fig. 1.37 Lateral chest radiograph showing pericardial calcification.

Definite diagnosis often requires invasive investigation with measurement of pressures in all heart chambers. Treatment consists of pericardectomy which is usually difficult. If TB is the cause standard anti-TB drugs are also given.

Differentiation of this condition from a restrictive cardiomyopathy can be extremely difficult and exploratory thoracotomy is often needed.

1.11   CONGENITAL HEART DISEASE IN ADULTS

The majority of cases of significant congenital heart disease are detected in childhood, either due to a murmur being discovered or due to symptoms such as heart failure or failure to thrive. The cardiac abnormality is then either corrected surgically if the condition is operable, or the child often fails to survive to adult life. This leaves only a relatively small number of conditions which can remain undetected during childhood and be discovered for the first time in an adult. Three categories of congenital cardiac abnormality will be briefly described.

1. Structural abnormalities without a shunt
    Aortic stenosis
    Pulmonary stenosis
    Coarctation of the aorta
2. Structural abnormalities with a left-to-right shunt (acyanotic)
    Atrial septal defect
    Ventricular septal defect
    Persistent ductus arteriosus
3. Structural abnormalities with a right-to-left shunt (cyanotic)
    Eisenmenger's syndrome
    Fallot's tetralogy
    Persistent truncus arteriosus

Abnormalities without a shunt

Aortic stenosis

Congenital aortic stenosis may be valvular, subvalvular or supravalvular. It may be discovered as a result of hearing a basal systolic murmur or in severe cases the symptoms will be similar to adults with acquired aortic valve disease. If the stenosis is at valvular level, a systolic ejection sound is often heard preceding the onset of the murmur.

Pulmonary stenosis

Pulmonary stenosis may occur at valvular level or may involve the outflow tract of the right ventricle (infundibular stenosis). Mild cases may present when a systolic murmur is discovered. Severe cases will have symptoms related to the inability to raise the cardiac output with exertion. Tiredness and fatigue are common symptoms together with light-headedness or syncope on exertion. Progressive right heart failure may develop. The pulse volume is small and the jugular venous pressure may be raised, often with a prominent 'a' wave. Right ventricular hypertrophy is evident clinically. The ejection systolic murmur which is best heard at the upper left sternal edge, increases in intensity with inspiration and may be preceded by an ejection sound. The ECG will show right atrial and ventricular hypertrophy in severe cases. The chest radiograph will sometimes show dilatation (post-stenotic) of the main pulmonary artery. Treatment is surgical after suitable invasive investigations have been performed.

Coarctation of the aorta

This condition should be suspected in any young person who is found to be hypertensive. Other presenting symptoms may be similar to cases with aortic stenosis. Examination will reveal hypertension in the upper limbs with a normal or low blood pressure in the legs. Marked arterial pulsation is visible in the neck but palpation of the femoral artery reveals a low volume, delayed pulse. Auscultation will reveal an ejection systolic murmur, best heard over the base of the heart or below the left clavicle. A continuous murmur may occasionally be heard by auscultation over the back, arising from the increased flow through intercostal arteries.

The ECG may show left ventricular hypertrophy.

A chest radiograph will show a hypertrophied left ventricle and notching of the lower rib margins may be seen, due to dilated intercostal arteries.

Angiography will demonstrate the size of the coarctation before surgical resection is performed. When the diagnosis and surgical treatment of coarctation are delayed until adult life, the associated hypertension may persist postoperatively and require medical treatment.

Abnormalities with a left-to-right shunt

Atrial septal defect (ASD)

Milder forms of this congenital defect often remain undetected until adult life and may in some cases only be discovered—after the fifth decade.

The left-to-right shunt in ASD causes volume overload of the right ventricle. Symptoms may include a restriction of exercise tolerance either by lassitude or dyspnoea. There may also be a history of repeated chest infections. The sudden worsening of symptoms in later life may be due to the onset of atrial arrhythmias. Examination may reveal a right ventricular impulse over the precordium and on auscultation the characteristic finding is wide, fixed splitting of the second heart sound. There is often an ejection systolic murmur in the pulmonary area due to increased flow in the pulmonary artery. More extensive left-to-right shunts may also produce a diastolic flow murmur arising from the tricuspid valve. The ECG usually shows partial or complete right bundle-branch block. Chest radiography will reveal a dilated main pulmonary artery with prominent lung vascular markings (*Fig.* 1.38).

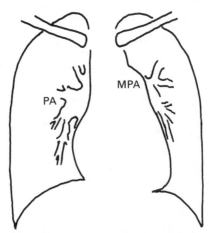

Fig. 1.38 Radiological features in atrial septal defect. MPA, main pulmonary artery; PA, dilated pulmonary arteries.

The echocardiogram will show the characteristic features of right ventricular volume overload, i.e. a dilated right ventricle with paradoxical septal movement (*Fig.* 1.39). Two-dimensional echocardiography will demonstrate the site of the defect in the interatrial septum. The diagnosis can be established by these investigations but cardiac catheterization is required to estimate the size of the left-to-right shunt and to determine the pulmonary artery pressure and vascular resistance. In the case of a moderate-to-severe shunt, operative closure is usually recommended provided the pulmonary vascular resistance is not significantly raised.

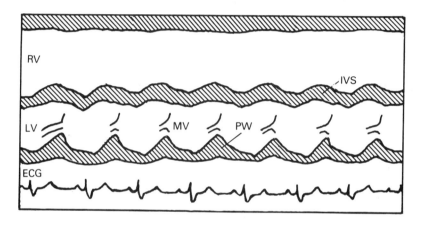

Fig. 1.39 Echocardiogram in atrial septal defect. IVS, interventricular septum; LV, left ventricle; MV, mitral valve; PW, posterior left ventricular wall; RV, right ventricle.

Ventricular septal defect (VSD)

Large ventricular septal defects cause significant problems in childhood and are usually repaired surgically. Smaller defects even though detected in childhood may be left alone in the hope that they may close spontaneously. Defects of this type are often discovered when a murmur is heard on routine examination. A large shunt from left to right will cause volume overload of the left ventricle, which will dilate and hypertrophy. The majority of adult patients with a VSD are asymptomatic but with larger shunts progressive exertional dyspnoea may occur. The main clinical finding is that of a pansystolic murmur which may be accompanied by a thrill—heard best over the lower sternum. Only in cases with a large shunt are the features of left ventricular hypertrophy seen on the ECG, radiograph and echo-cardiogram. Surgical closure of a VSD is usually indicated in patients with symptoms. It is reasonable to observe asymptomatic individuals provided precautions are taken to prevent infective endocarditis.

Persistent ductus arteriosus

The ductus arteriosus usually closes soon after birth but if it remains patent, it causes a left-to-right shunt between the aorta and pulmonary artery. The haemodynamic consequence of this is the development of left ventricular volume overload. Asymptomatic cases may remain undiagnosed until late childhood. The clinical features are usually diagnostic. The pulse is collapsing in character, associated with a large pulse pressure and low diastolic pressure. Visible pulsation of the carotid vessels is present. The left ventricle may be dilated and hyperactive. The murmur of a persistent ductus begins in early systole and continues through the second heart sound into diastole. The detection of a persistent ductus is an indication for its surgical correction.

Cyanotic congenital heart disease

The right-to-left shunt may be present at birth in conditions such as Fallot's tetralogy or truncus arteriosus; or may develop in some cases where the shunt was originally from left to right (Eisenmenger's syndrome). In cases with a large left-to-right shunt, the increased pulmonary blood flow causes vasoconstriction of the peripheral pulmonary vessels. This eventually causes structural changes in the pulmonary vessels which lead to irreversible pulmonary hypertension. There will be a consequent rise in pressure in the right-sided chambers with eventual reversal of the shunt from right to left. Once this stage is reached, the congenital defect is inoperable. Only symptomatic treatment can be offered to patients with cyanotic congenital heart disease at this stage. One important complication of cyanotic heart disease is worth mentioning, that is the development of a cerebral abscess. This occurs because infective material may travel in the venous blood, bypassing the lungs and enter the systemic circulation. The diagnosis should be considered in any patient with cyanotic congenital heart disease who develops a headache accompanied by fever. If these symptoms are neglected, localizing neurological signs will develop.

FURTHER READING

Julian D. G. (1977) *Angina Pectoris.* London, Churchill.
Opie L. H. (1980) *Drugs and the Heart.* London, Lancet.
Stock J. P. and Williams D. O. (ed.) *Diagnosis and Treatment of Cardiac Arrhythmias.* 3rd ed. London, Butterworths.
Wilkinson J. T. and Sanders C. A. (1977) *Clinical Cardiology.* New York, Grune & Stratton.

2 Common Problems in Respiratory Medicine

J. R. Edge

2.1 INTRODUCTION

Over the past three decades the overall pattern of chest disease has changed dramatically following the control of pulmonary tuberculosis, at least in advanced communities, by effective antibacterial therapy. (In many underdeveloped societies, however, modern methods of treatment have for a variety of reasons not been applied effectively; bearing in mind the rapid increase in global population over this period, there are very probably more patients with uncontrolled active tuberculosis in the world today than there were 30 years ago). During the same period there has been a remarkable increase in lung cancer, following several decades after the widespread adoption of cigarette smoking; it is interesting to observe the virtual absence of lung cancer from communities where cigarette smoking is not practised, or has only recently been introduced. Chronic bronchitis is likewise strongly related to cigarette smoking and carries a high annual mortality, comparable to that of cancer of the bronchus; its distribution also relates to atmospheric pollution.

It is clear that the control of lung cancer and bronchitis will depend on preventive and social measures, namely elimination of cigarette smoking and air pollution; and that improved education and increased financial resources in the developing countries will be the key to the eventual control of tuberculosis.

Table 2.1 shows the number of deaths due to these three diseases recorded in England and Wales in 1971 and in 1981 (by courtesy of OPCS, monitor DH2 82/3); whilst deaths due to pulmonary tuberculosis continue to fall steadily, and those from obstructive airway disease are decreasing modestly, the lung cancer rate continues to increase.

Bronchitis and emphysema accounted for a remarkable 27 million lost working days in 1975, the highest figure of any group of diseases including hypertension and ischaemic heart disease.

These three diseases of major importance are dealt with in Chapters 2.2, 2.3 and 2.6. Chapter 2.4 concerns immune disturbances, the study of which represents a major advance in the understanding of lung disorders in recent years. The importance of vascular disorders, discussed in Chapter 2.5, relates to the substantial advances in their recognition and management.

Table 2.1 Number of deaths in England and Wales

	1971	1981
Respiratory tuberculosis	925	433
Bronchitis, emphysema and asthma	28369	19129
Lung cancer	30754	34726

Occupational lung disease (Chapter 2.7) is a subject of increasing moment in an industrial society.

Pneumonias and their sequelae (Chapter 2.2) do not usually present problems unless they accompany some associated disorder, for example immune failure due to a debilitating illness. The control of asthma (Chapter 2.4), despite improvements in drug therapy, continues to present a major challenge, as does the recognition and control of disorders due to specific environmental hazards (Chapter 2.7).

Up to one-third of acute medical hospital admissions in the UK are due to chest illness; except in special centres their care is now largely in the hands of general physicians with a declared interest and training in the subject, rather than of whole-time specialists as was formerly the case. This change involves the possibility of an insufficiently aggressive approach to the particular problems of pulmonary tuberculosis.

Clinical assessment

History

Time spent on obtaining an accurate history in patients with lung disease is usually of greater value than that spent on clinical examination, as in many other branches of medicine. This is particularly the case in chronic bronchitis and in asthma, because in phases of remission, physical signs are likely to be absent, and investigations may be inconclusive.

Particular care is required to exclude environmental hazards, industrial or otherwise, and to assess the likely contribution of smoking. The possibility of reactions to drugs must also be kept in mind. Enquiry should always be made as to any prior radiological examinations; comparisons with an earlier film may rapidly settle the significance of a radiological abnormality and may obviate the need for further investigation.

Attention should also be directed to fear of cancer, particularly in smokers, many of whom suffer from chronic anxiety about the possible effects of their habit; this may be relieved by frank explanation and advice, and reassurance when appropriate.

Physical examination

Physical examination of the lungs provides useful but often limited information. In the lungs themselves, added sounds may help the recognition of obstructive airway disease where other investigations are inconclusive, and reduced breath sounds may indicate a lesion as yet invisible on radiography. In general, abnormal physical signs are more likely to help in relatively advanced disease, and the use of radiography to exclude the earlier stages of many diseases is mandatory.

A thorough general physical examination is essential, for example to detect metastatic disease or endocrine disturbance associated with bronchial carcinoma, to exclude heart failure in breathless patients, or to reveal evidence of system diseases which may present with chest symptoms.

Radiology

Routine postero-anterior and lateral radiography is essential not only to identify lesions not obvious on physical examination, but to provide a convenient permanent record. In this connection, a simple line diagram of the radiographic appearance entered in the case notes is not only a useful exercise in establishing in one's mind what is important on the film, but may be of greater historical value than a written report in the event of loss of the original radiographs.

Tomography is of value in assessing the diagnosis and activity of pulmonary tuberculosis, and the extent of nodal and pleural involvement as a guide to management of bronchial carcinoma.

Bronchography was widely used in the past to prove the diagnosis and extent of bronchiectasis prior to surgery, a method of treatment now rarely called for. It may be useful in demonstrating bronchial obstruction in carcinoma, but in this context has been largely replaced by fibreoptic bronchoscopy. It is an unpleasant investigation for the patient, and is now very rarely indicated.

Scanning

A scintiscan of the lung may reveal single or multiple filling defects when the radiograph is quite normal; the technique is of particular value in the diagnosis of pulmonary embolism, but tends to be unreliable in the presence of obstructive airway disease.

Pulmonary angiography, when facilities are available, is the only certain method of confirming the presence and extent of pulmonary embolism.

Lung function tests

Physiological testing is of value in establishing the degree as well as the nature of disturbance of function; it is directed at measuring both the mechanical functioning of the lung and the physiology of respiration at alveolar level.

Simple measurements of ventilation are readily available both in general and hospital practice; they enable assessment of overall ventilation, and provide a ready means of assessing the degree of airway obstruction and of its response to exercise and to therapy. This is most readily done by measuring the peak flow rate (PFR) using the Wright peak flowmeter.

A simple timed spirometer (respirometer or Gaensler Spirometer) will give a graphic representation of ventilation, namely the vital capacity, together with the amount of air expired in the first second of forced expiration (FEV_1); the latter is reduced in obstruction, the result being expressed as the FEV_1/VC ratio. Where ventilation is reduced in the absence of obstruction, a restrictive defect is present, due either to diffuse lung disease or pleural thickening, or impaired chest wall movement.

Using more sophisticated equipment, now available in most district general hospitals, the lung volumes can be measured. An increase in the residual volume after forced expiration is of particular help in the diagnosis of emphysema. The transfer of gas across the alveolar–capillary membrane is measured by observing the rate of absorption of carbon monoxide after inspiration of a weak mixture from a bag; the gas transfer (DCO) is impaired in peripheral lung disease, and carried out serially is a useful method of monitoring the effect of therapy.

Bronchoscopy

This examination is of major importance in the diagnosis of bronchial carcinoma, and in the assessment of its operability. It is also essential in the diagnosis and treatment of inhaled foreign bodies, for which a rigid bronchoscope is necessary; this instrument may also be useful for the removal of excessive secretions, for example after major surgery, but its use in diagnosis is limited by its restricted visualization of the bronchial tree, in particular of the upper lobes. Fibreoptic bronchoscopy has the advantage of deeper penetration into the bronchial tree, and of easy visualization of the upper lobe divisions. It is entirely practicable with local anaesthesia.

Laboratory investigations

Blood examination

Basic routine tests include a haemoglobin level, together with a white blood count as a pointer to infection, or to hypersensitivity states associated with eosinophilia. In advanced disease, measurement of the blood gases is essential in the diagnosis of pulmonary failure, and as a method of observing the response to treatment.

Sputum examination

Sputum culture is of value only if the sputum is purulent. Estimation of the antibiotic sensitivity of any pathogens isolated is of value in the treatment of infections. A routine search for acid-fast bacilli is wise in the presence of any radiological opacity, particularly as tuberculosis frequently presents atypically; culture on enriched media is required, but has the disadvantage of requiring several weeks.

Cytological examination of sputum for carcinoma cells is of value only in the hands of a highly experienced technician, i.e. in a major centre with a big turnover of cases. A false positive diagnosis is, of course, a major disaster.

Urine examination

Routine urine examination is also required particularly if there is any suspicion of tuberculosis.

Biopsy

In cases of diagnostic difficulty, particularly in diffuse interstitial lung disease, lung biopsy may be undertaken when other methods have failed. Histological evidence is of particular importance in establishing a firm diagnosis in sarcoidosis because of its very protean manifestations; in this and other system diseases, biopsy of liver, lymph nodes, or skin, are safe and would normally be done before a lung biopsy is considered. If the latter proves to be necessary, a formal approach through a reduced thoracotomy incision is required, as the risks of bleeding or air embolism following needle biopsy are usually unacceptable. Needle biopsy also invariably leads to pneumothorax, which in a patient with already limited lung function may be a serious complication.

Identification of cell type in bronchial carcinoma by either bronchial or scalene or axillary node biopsy is of increasing importance in particular as a guide to cytotoxic therapy.

Summary

A careful history will go a long way to establishing a diagnosis, but must always be backed up by routine radiography in addition to physical examination if early disease is to be detected. Apart from a routine blood count and measurement of FEV_1, no further routine investigation is usually called for in the majority of patients with chest symptoms unless a clinical clue is apparent. These simple measures are sufficient to reassure patients with anxiety symptoms, and can be carried out at a single consultation.

2.2 INFECTIONS OF THE UPPER RESPIRATORY TRACT AND BRONCHI

Coryza

The common cold is due to a wide variety of rhinoviruses, and is important in causing exacerbations of bronchitis in susceptible subjects. Treatment is limited to an antibiotic for secondary bacterial infection, commonly due to *Haemophilus influenzae*; the use of vasoconstrictors for the nasal obstruction is to be avoided, because they increase the risk of bacterial infection of the paranasal sinuses.

Acute pharyngitis

Epidemic sore throat may be due to a virus, or less commonly to β-haemolytic streptococcus which can be identified by throat swab and which may require antibiotic treatment if persistent.

Acute tracheitis

This usually follows an upper respiratory virus infection which lead to often severe substernal discomfort and initially unproductive cough: relief is experienced as the cough becomes productive of mucopurulent sputum. The disorder is self-limiting in the course of a few days, but may be associated with acute bronchitis.

Acute bronchitis

This also follows upper respiratory virus infections which leads to a dry cough with a variable degree of wheeze which is worse on waking. Production of purulent sputum follows, with relief of the wheeze, after secondary bacterial infection usually due to *H. influenzae* or *Streptococcus pneumoniae*. Initial attacks are usually brief, but if repeated become more prolonged with each attack, and may lead in due course to established chronic bronchitis (p. 83); because of this possibility the acute attack is best treated with a 5-day course of antibiotic. Ampicillin, 250 mg 6-hourly, or co-trimoxazole, tablets (960 mg) b.d. are suitable. Expectorant mixtures are ineffective: bronchodilator therapy may help (e.g. salbutamol 2–4 mg 3–4 times daily, or by aerosol, 2 puffs q.i.d.).

Pneumonia

Introduction

Pneumonia is an inflammatory process involving the parenchyma of the lung. Traditionally it is described either as lobar pneumonia or broncho-pneumonia, a classification which is now inadequate. Lobar pneumonia is a septicaemic illness due to infection with *S. pneumoniae,* which settles in the lungs and which leads to consolidation of one or sometimes two lobes: curiously, it has now become extremely uncommon, and when it does occur it may be due to a different organism. The term bronchopneumonia was in the past seemingly used to embrace all types of pneumonia other than lobar, but is probably best reserved for terminal patchy pneumonia associated with the ineffective cough and retained secretions found in debilitating disease or advanced age.

A more rational classification is based on identifying the causal agent, though it should be borne in mind that even the most careful laboratory investigation will be unproductive in about half the cases.

In all instances the possibility of pre-existing lung disease or other contributory factors must be kept in mind.

Clinical features

Symptoms directly attributable to pneumonia include fever, malaise, tachypnoea, cough sometimes going on to sputum production, with stabbing lateral chest pain on inspiration if the pleura is involved; in severe cases there may be delirium, peripheral circulatory failure, and central cyanosis due to pulmonary arterial blood passing through lung tissue which is no longer aerated.

Signs may include dullness to percussion, tubular breathing and localized râles, but radiography gives more reliable information.

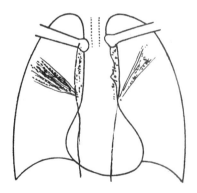

Fig. 2.1 Aspiration pneumonias with achalasia of the cardia; often upper zones; dilated oesophagus may be visible.

Aspiration pneumonia

The possibility of aspiration of infected material or vomit when the cough reflex is suppressed must be kept in mind (*Fig.* 2.1). This may occur in normal sleep, or during an epileptic fit, general anaesthesia, or acute alcoholic poisoning. Sources of infected material include dental sepsis and infected nasal sinuses, which should be identified and, when appropriate, treated; this is an important precaution before a general anaesthetic is given. Hiatus hernia with reflux, or oesophageal obstruction due to achalasia or carcinoma, also commonly lead to aspiration pneumonia, so that a barium meal is indicated particularly if one or more attacks of aspiration pneumonia do not have an obvious cause (*see also* Lipid pneumonia, p. 152).

Pre-existing disorders which may lead to pneumonia due to retention of secretions include bronchiectasis, bronchial obstruction due to carcinoma or foreign body, chronic bronchitis (p. 83), and mucoviscidosis (p. 149). The injudicious use of cough suppressants may be a contributory factor (*Fig.* 2.2).

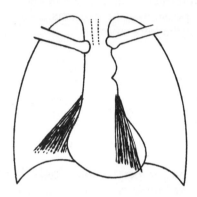

Fig. 2.2 Collapse of both lower lobes due to excessive linctus codeine for cough.

Acute complications include serous or purulent pleural effusion, pneumothorax or hydropneumothorax (particularly in infections due to *Staphylococcus pyogenes* or klebsiella) and lung abscess.

Investigations

These include chest radiography, with a lateral view as soon as the patient is well enough: this defines the anatomical site of the lesion, which is likely to be in a posterior segment for example in the case of aspiration pneumonia. The establishment of a bronchial (lobar or segmental) location may be a valuable help in differentiation from pulmonary embolism or infarction, where the lesions conform to the distribution of blood vessels, rather than segmental anatomy. This is not easily determined using the standard postero-anterior view alone.

Blood cultures taken before starting antibiotic treatment may be helpful, particularly if there is a history of rigor. A differential white blood count helps to distinguish bacterial from virus infections.

Smear and culture of any purulent sputum may also help to identify the causal organism and its sensitivity to bacterial agents. A search for *Mycobacterium tuberculosis* should not be omitted.

Serum cold agglutinins may be measured at intervals if *Mycoplasma pneumoniae* is suspected: this presents with an extensive soft X-ray shadow and constitutional rather than chest symptoms.

Serum precipitins confirm the diagnosis of legionnaire's disease, a toxic pneumonia carrying a high mortality; it occurs in epidemics through contamination of water supplies. The microbacterium *Legionella pneumophila* is not identifiable by the usual laboratory techniques.

Management

FLUIDS

A high fluid intake is required for any toxic or dehydrated patient: this may be given intravenously especially if hypovolaemic shock is present, as may occur particular in anaerobic infections.

PAIN RELIEF

Drugs for relief of generalized aches and pains should be limited to aspirin (300–600 mg 6-hourly) or paracetamol (0·5–1 g 6 hourly). For pleurisy a stronger analgesic such as pentazocine (25–100 mg 4 hourly) may be given, but opiates should be prescribed only with great caution because of the risk of suppression of the respiratory centre, with abolition of respiratory drive leading to respiratory failure. This is of especial importance in the presence of established obstructive airway disease.

Preparations containing codeine or diamorphine will suppress the cough reflex and may lead to sputum retention, and even to lobar collapse (*Fig. 2.2*) and should not be used.

OXYGEN

For the severely ill and cyanosed patient oxygen is given by nasal catheter at 2 litres per minute, or by Ventimask increasing from 24% to 28% as tolerated if chronic airway obstruction is present, when oxygen therapy must be monitored by regular blood Po_2 and Pco_2 levels.

STEROIDS

It is customary to give hydrocortisone empirically (200 mg 6-hourly i.m. or i.v.) in the presence of circulatory collapse, as may occur with anaerobic infections; and in particular in staphylococcal pneumonia following influenza, when steroids are life-saving in the presence of acute adrenal failure due to toxicity or infarction. This is not an easy matter to prove in the acute situation but steroids must be given in full dosage on suspicion, especially during an epidemic of influenza B, when adrenal involvement is a cause of sudden death in previously healthy young adults.

ANTIBACTERIAL AGENTS

The introduction of effective antibiotics and chemotherapy in the last few decades has reduced the mortality from uncomplicated pneumonia in the previously healthy to negligible proportions: a substantial problem remains, however, whenever there is a failure of host resistance. This may be due to a wide variety of associated factors, including malnutrition, chronic alcoholism, diabetes, or longstanding heart or lung disease. Immune incompetence may be due to congenital reduction or absence of gamma-globulins (*see* p. 110) to reticulosis or system disease or blood disorders, or the drugs used in their management, or to the immunosuppressive drugs required after transplant surgery.

The rational basis of antibacterial treatment depends on identification of the causal organism, as well as on clinical probabilities; results of blood or sputum cultures may inevitably be delayed, or uninformative, so that in the severely ill empirical therapy using multiple agents is mandatory.

A general guide to the choice of antimicrobial agent in relation to the clinical assessment and likely aetiology is given in *Table* 2.2 in relation to the previously healthy, and in *Table* 2.3 where there is pre-existing disease or immunity failure.

Lung abscess

Introduction

Lung abscess occurs when sepsis is followed by necrosis of lung parenchyma, most commonly following aspiration of septic material from the mouth, or of vomitus when consciousness is impaired. It is therefore more common in indigent populations with a high incidence of dental caries and of alcoholism than in the prosperous communities of the West.

It is more frequent in the elderly, and may be associated with oesophageal obstruction, or with ineffective cough in neurological conditions, such as bulbar palsy. It may also relate to bronchial obstruction, commonly from carcinoma, and much less commonly to an inhaled foreign body, such as a peanut.

Apart from aspiration or obstructive lesions, it may directly follow pneumonia due to *Staph. pyogenes* or to *Klebsiella pneumoniae* in which event perforation into the pleura is not uncommon, leading to a pneumo-thorax, usually further complicated by empyema. This is due to progressive enlargement of the cavity due to trapping of air within it on each aspiration, as may happen in tuberculosis (p. 73).

Infection of a pulmonary infarct may also lead to abscess formation so that pulmonary embolism must be considered if no obvious cause is apparent.

Clinical features

SYMPTOMS

A lung abscess is characterized by toxicity, fever and purulent sputum, with dyspnoea if a complicating pneumothorax or pleural effusion is present. The history of a choking attack whilst eating should always be sought, if there is

Table 2.2 Choice of antibiotic or chemotherapy for pneumonia in the previously healthy

Organism	Frequent clinical features	Antibiotic
A. Bacterial		
Strep. pneumoniae	Sometimes rigors. One of the commonest organisms causing pneumonia. Low mortality	Benzylpenicillin i.m. 2 megaunits 6-hourly
Klebsiella	Toxic prolonged course: high mortality up to 50%. Complications similar to *Staph. pyogenes* pneumonia	Streptomycin 1 g b.d. Co-trimoxazole 2 tab. (960 mg) b.d. Chloramphenicol 500 mg 6-hourly
Streptococcus Staph. pyogenes	Often follow virus infection, especially epidemic influenza. May lead to abscess, or pneumatocele, with or without pneumothorax or empyema	Flucloxacillin (effective against penicillinase +ve organisms) 250 mg q.i.d. with benzylpenicillin. Chloramphenicol 500 mg 6-hourly
Legionella pneumophila	Toxic: local epidemics, stemming from water supply	Erythromycin 250–500 mg 6-hourly
M. tuberculosis	May resemble septic pneumonia (without typical cavitation)	Isoniazid 200 or 300 mg daily. Rifampicin 10 mg/kg body weight. Streptomycin 1 g daily (0·75 g in elderly) Ethambutol 20 mg/kg body weight
B. *Viruses*	General rather than chest symptoms, due to viraemia (fever, diffuse aches and pains). Dry cough at first, later may develop secondary bacterial infection. Radiological shadowing may be extensive	None
C. *Rickettsial R. burnetii* (Q fever)	Travel to endemic areas	Tetracycline 0·5–1 g 6-hourly
Chlamydia psittaci (psittacosis or ornithosis)	Contact with birds. Prostration. Sometimes simultaneous hepatitis	Tetracycline 0·5–1 g 6-hourly
D. *Mycoplasma M. pneumoniae* 'primary atypical pneumonia'	Mild illness often with extensive radiological shadowing	Tetracycline 500 mg or erythromycin 250 mg 6-hourly

Table 2.3 Choice of antibiotic chemotherapy in pneumonia with pre-existing disease

Pre-existing disease	Likely organism	Antimicrobial
Bronchiectasis, muco-viscidosis, chronic alcoholism, debilitation, hypogammaglobulinaemia	Suspect gram-negative in addition to usual septic organisms Klebsiella	Streptomycin 1 g b.d. Co-trimoxazole 2 tabs. b.d.
	Pseudomonas	Gentamicin 2–5 mg/kg 8-hourly Carbenicillin 5 g 6-hourly i.v.
	E. coli	Co-trimoxazole 2 tabs b.d.
Immunosuppression due to reticuloses: antimitotic drugs: maintenance therapy after organ transplants	'Opportunist' organisms: i. Pneumocystis carinii	Co-trimoxazole 2 tabs. b.d.
	ii. Fungus (aspergillus)	Amphotericin 1 g 250 mg/kg i.v. Ketoconazole 200–400 mg daily orally
	iii. Cytomegalovirus	None
Severe overwhelming pneumonia, e.g. complicating major surgery, agranulocytosis	Multiple therapy giving wide spectrum required immediately, i.e. before cultures available: intravenously if shocked	Benzylpenicillin 2 M 6-hourly Flucloxacillin 250 mg 6-hourly Streptomycin 1 g b.d. Gentamicin 80 mg 8-hourly i.m.
		Also consider: Carbenicillin Metronidazole (Flagyl) 500 mg 8-hourly i.v.

any suspicion of inhaled foreign body. Enquiry must also be made as to any incident of disturbed consciousness, such as an epileptic fit.

SIGNS

Physical signs in the chest are usually unhelpful, the diagnosis depending on radiography: but associated lesions, such as dental sepsis or deep femoral vein thrombosis as a source of embolism, should be looked for.

Investigations

RADIOGRAPHY

A chest radiograph will show a cavity normally with walls at least several millimetres thick, which, as most abscesses follow aspiration, commonly lies posteriorly, either in the apex of the lower lobe or posterior segment of the upper lobe. There is usually a fluid level which may be confirmed by a film taken in lateral decubitus: a lateral view is essential to identify the site of the lesion when planning postural drainage. A large thin-walled cavity (pneumatocele) is very suggestive of a staphylococcal or klebsiella infection.

There is a strong suspicion of foreign body if the abscess is in the right lower lobe, in which case rigid bronchoscopy is mandatory. Inhaled foreign bodies most commonly enter the right lower bronchus because it lies at only a very slight angle to the trachea, in contrast with the left lower bronchus which is directed laterally (*Fig.* 2.3).

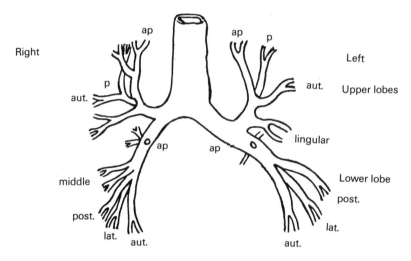

Fig. 2.3 The bronchial tree. The lingular segment of the left upper lobe corresponds to the middle lobe on the right side. The right main bronchus is shorter than the left, which extends laterally at a greater angle than the right lower lobe bronchus, which is more nearly vertical. ap, apical; p, posterior; lat, lateral; ant, anterior.

When a carcinoma is suspected, tomography and, on occasion, bronchography will be helpful, but the latter investigation has been largely replaced by fibreoptic bronchoscopy.

A barium swallow and meal, and pictures of the nasal sinuses, may also be helpful.

LABORATORY

Culture of the sputum and blood, and tests for sensitivity of any pathogens to antibacterial agents, are essential to management.

A white blood count will show a substantial polymorph leucocytosis.

Management

1. Postural drainage, precisely directed according to the site of the abscess, must be carried out several times daily.

2. Antimicrobial treatment must employ multiple agents to cover possible anaerobic organisms (*see Tables* 2.1 and 2.2), pending the results of sputum or blood culture. It usually needs to be prolonged.

3. Surgical excision is only very rarely necessary. Pneumothorax will require underwater seal drainage using a soft, self-retaining, intercostal catheter, while empyema requires regular aspiration.

4. Any contributory associated lesions will also require correction.

Bronchiectasis

Introduction

The word bronchiectasis means dilatation of the bronchi, but has come to be used as a descriptive term for the clinical syndrome, namely, permanent cough with abundant purulent sputum found in some cases.

Occlusion of a bronchus leads to atelectasis of the lung distal to the occlusion, due to absorption of air into the circulation, which continues as before; the collapse is accompanied by dilatation of the bronchi, which becomes permanent if infection is also present, particular for any long period. Extensive cystic change involving a lobe or a whole lung may follow incomplete expansion after birth.

It follows that the disorder, which in the past commonly arose in childhood following pneumonia, pertussis, or primary tuberculosis, occurs much less frequently since the introduction of effective prophylactic measures and antibiotic therapy.

Clinical features

The advanced case is characterized by permanent cough with production of purulent, often offensive, sputum on each occasion; these symptoms are due in no small part to associated purulent bronchitis. The chronic disorder may be punctuated by recurrent attacks of pneumonia, and is often accompanied by airway obstruction. Haemoptysis is frequent. Physical examination usually reveals clubbing of the fingers, with abundant râles over the affected lobe or lobes. Permanent cyanosis and secondary polycythaemia due to ventilation/perfusion imbalance may develop in time, leading after many years to respiratory failure. Amyloidosis in an uncommon sequela.

In milder cases, which are much more frequent, the patient develops a loose productive cough only intermittently, following upper respiratory infections: the exacerbations may be accompanied by minor haemoptysis, but the general health, lung function and expectation of life are unimpaired.

In the absence of cough or sputum, 'dry' bronchiectasis may cause profuse haemoptysis.

Investigations

Chest radiography in mild cases is often normal; in the advanced case it shows cystic changes, or partial but permanent collapse of the affected lobe or lobes, commonly left lower and right middle, corresponding to the usual effects of enlarged hilar nodes in primary tuberculosis, with diffuse cylindrical bronchial dilatation shown on bronchography. The latter is an unpleasant investigation, and rarely necessary: it should be limited to cases where surgery is being considered, as it serves to define the extent of disease precisely. It may show either cylindrical or saccular changes, a matter of no practical importance, and frequently demonstrates enlargement of the mucous glands in the mucosa of bronchi remote from the bronchiectatic area. This emphasizes that the associated bronchitis is widespread, so that relief from surgery will be incomplete.

Culture of grossly purulent sputum often reveals, surprisingly, no pathogens; but *H. influenzae* and *Staph. pyogenes* are often found, as are gram-negative organisms, especially in patients who have had prolonged courses of antibiotic treatment.

The sputum should also be inspected, and measured over each 24 h, as an index of severity and response to treatment.

Management

Surgical removal is only exceptionally indicated, and is limited to the cases where only a single and evidently functionless lobe or segment is involved. Usually the changes are widespread, so that removal would involve an unjustified sacrifice of function.

The basis of management lies in regular postural drainage, twice or thrice daily for up to 20 min, provided that this leads to increased sputum production. The patient should lie head down, the foot of the bed being raised on bricks, with the affected lung uppermost. Percussion by a relative during forced expiration may be helpful and is easily learnt. Only in this way can the airways be protected from obstruction by sputum, which can lead to pneumonia. Postural drainage need only be episodic, e.g. after colds, in the mild case, but needs to be continued permanently in severe cases.

The paranasal sinuses are frequently infected; treatment of the sinusitis may improve the chest symptoms.

Antimicrobial treatment is best reserved for acute exacerbations. In the chronic state a remarkable symbiosis between the host and the bacteria is usual, the patient often maintaining unexpectedly good health in spite of his abundant purulent sputum. Long-term chemotherapy is rarely justified, both on account of side effects and the emergence of an overgrowth or gram-negative or antibiotic-resistant organisms.

Laboratory culture of sputum is usually of limited help in the choice of antibacterial therapy. Co-trimoxazole is the first choice, 2 tablets (960 mg) twice or thrice daily; alternatively, ampicillin 1 g 6-hourly may be given. In severe illness the possibility of klebsiella, pseudomonas or staphylococcal infection should be kept in kind (*see Table* 2.2).

Pleural effusion: empyema

Introduction

The general features of pleural effusions may be conveniently considered here, with particular regard to infective causes; they also occur in a wide variety of other disorders, and are referred to in the appropriate sections (e.g. rheumatoid and autoimmune disease, pulmonary embolism, primary or secondary neoplasm, asbestos-related disease). The diagnosis depends in considerable part on the recognition of associated features, and may remain elusive despite thorough investigation.

Fluid in the pleural cavity may be a transudate, which is characterized by a low protein content, of less than 4 g/l: this is commonly due to heart failure, or may be part of generalized anasarca with low serum protein levels: in either case it is likely to be bilateral. It may be an exudate, with a high protein content (above 4 g/l), due to direct involvement of the pleura in an inflammatory or neoplastic process. If bloodstained it is likely to be due to neoplasm or pulmonary infarction. In empyema the fluid is grossly turbid or frankly purulent.

Clinical features

PHYSICAL SIGNS

If the effusion is large the mediastinum may be displaced to the opposite side, which may be apparent from displacement of the trachea and heart. Over the fluid the percussion note is very dull, and characteristically the dullness rises into the axilla. The breath sounds are absent in a substantial effusion but in the earlier stages when the acini but not bronchi are collapsed, bronchial breath sounds are conveyed to the surface through the fluid, and the signs are indistinguishable from those of consolidation. Bronchial breathing may also be heard at the upper border of a large effusion, for the same reason.

SYMPTOMS

A patient with pneumonia accompanied by pleurisy will experience relief of pain if an effusion develops; this is rarely large enough to lead to increased breathlessness. An effusion associated with pneumonia is usually clear and pale yellow in colour; but if the patient remains febrile and toxic in spite of antibiotic treatment, empyema is likely, with turbid or frankly purulent fluid.

Investigations

The *chest radiograph* shows a uniform dense opacity in the lower zone, which obliterates the costophrenic angle and rises laterally as a crescentic shadow into the axilla (*Fig.* 2.4). If the effusion is total the trachea and heart shadow may be displaced towards the opposite side: if they are central or displaced towards the same side, this suggests collapse of the underlying lung. Fluid localized in the lesser fissure, between the upper and middle

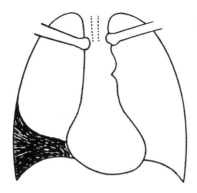

Fig. 2.4 Right pleural effusion.

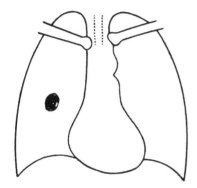

Fig. 2.5 Interlobar effusion mimicking tumour.

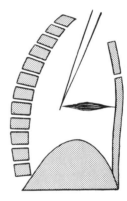

Fig. 2.6 Lateral view showing fluid in lesser fissure.

lobes on the right side, presents a solid, round shadow suggesting a tumour: the lateral view reveals an ovoid shadow in the fissure (*Figs.* 2.5, 2.6).

A polymorpholeucocytosis indicates infection.

Needling of the chest is mandatory to confirm the presence of fluid; it is best carried out in the seventh intercostal space, below the angle of the scapula. A specimen, about 100 ml, is examined for protein content and cytology, and cultured for septic organisms and *M. tuberculosis.* Purulent fluid is likely to be due to infection with *Staph. pyogenes* or *Strep. pyogenes, Strep. pneumoniae* or klebsiella; the sensitivity to antibiotics should be measured.

An empyema due to *E. coli* may complicate a subphrenic abscess: a large clear right-sided effusion, usually sterile, may be due to amoebic hepatitis. The diagnosis, which should be suspected in natives of, or visitors returning from, endemic areas, is confirmed by recovery of *E. histolytica* from the stools, sigmoidoscopy and liver function studies.

PLEURAL BIOPSY

Each time aspiration is carried out, one or more pleural biopsies should be taken. Both procedures may be conveniently done with an Abrams needle, which has a lateral notch which may be felt to catch the pleura as the needle is withdrawn after the aspiration: the biopsy is then taken by turning and advancing the trocar which is hollow and has a sharp cutting edge. Alternatively, after completing aspiration with a standard needle, the biopsy can be taken from the same site using a disposable needle ('Trucut') introduced to the depth at which fluid was first obtained: a pneumatically driven, high speed, rotating (Steele's) drill provides good specimens provided it is sharp and not running eccentrically. Unless the pleura is grossly thickened at a well-defined point, biopsy in the absence of fluid carries the risk of pneumothorax, haemoptysis, or air embolism if, as is almost inevitable, the lung is punctured during the procedure.

Pleural biopsy has the advantage of providing unequivocal histological proof of neoplasm or tuberculosis, but several specimens may be required before a diagnosis can be made.

Bronchoscopy should be carried out to exclude bronchial carcinoma if the above investigations are inconclusive.

Management

Management of pleural effusions is aspiration for the relief of dyspnoea; the amount removed on any one occasion should not greatly exceed 1 litre, as removal of larger amounts may lead to contralateral pulmonary oedema. A serous effusion will absorb leaving little or no functional impairment, but if gross infection or blood is present regular aspiration is required to minimize the degree of residual pleural thickening.

Treatment otherwise is directed to the cause of the effusion, and is dealt with in the appropriate sections.

Tuberculosis

Introduction

Infection by *Mycobacterium tuberculosis* has effects which differ according to the immune status of the host; organs other than the lungs may be involved, particularly lymph nodes, kidney and bone. Unusual extrapulmonary forms of this protean disease are commonly seen in Asiatic subjects.

Tuberculosis in man dates back to prehistory, as shown by typical changes in skeletons of early man. The greatest prevalence in Europe coincided with the overcrowding and poor nutrition of the industrial revolution, since when there has been a steady decline with improved social conditions, greatly accelerated in the last 30 years by the introduction of effective antibiotics. The overall mortality in Britain has declined from over 30000 per annum in the 1940s to less than 1000 per annum in the 1980s.

The disease still exacts a heavy toll in many under developed societies in whom immunity has not yet developed, where acute progressive disease in young people is common. In contrast, in the developed countries it now predominantly affects older people, and tends to follow a chronic course.

Pathology
PRIMARY TUBERCULOSIS

Primary infection occurs following inhalation of *M. tuberculosis* contained in droplets expectorated by an infectious patient. The ensuing primary complex consists of a small granuloma in the lung (Ghon focus) with gross enlargement of the associated lymph nodes as the predominant feature (*Fig. 2.7*). This process leads in a few weeks to tissue immunity, recognizable by the development of a positive skin reaction 48 h after the intradermal injection of old tuberculin.

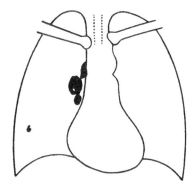

Fig. 2.7 Primary tuberculous complex.

Primary infection may also occur in the tonsil, leading to cervical adenitis (the 'scrofula'), or gastrointestinal tract sometimes leading to tuberculous peritonitis, following ingestion of infected milk. This is now uncommon following eradication of the disease in cattle.

ADULT OR POST PRIMARY TUBERCULOSIS

As a result of tissue immunity, which may also be induced prophylactically by the intradermal injection of attenuated tubercle bacilli (Bacille Calmette-Guérin, BCG), any subsequent infection follows a different pattern. This does not involve the lymph nodes, but leads to a local inflammatory lesion characterized by endarteritis leading to tissue necrosis, and the formation of caseous pus: this provides an ideal culture medium, and is discharged into the draining bronchus and thence expectorated. It may also embolize through the airways to other, usually dependent, parts of the lungs, giving rise to new areas of disease. The bronchus itself is involved in endobronchitis with mucosal oedema: this forms an effective valve mechanism with changes

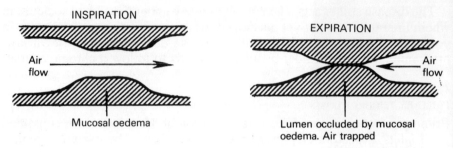

Fig. 2.8 Diagram showing blockage of bronchial lumen by mucosal oedema.

in calibre during respiration (*Fig.* 2.8) leading to trapping of air in the space evacuated by caseous material. The formation of cavities in the lung in this way is highly characteristic of adult tuberculosis.

Clinical features

PRIMARY TUBERCULOSIS

The large majority of primary infections cause no symptoms, pass unnoticed, and are self-healing. The primary complex usually calcifies, and is therefore readily identified on radiography.

COMPLICATIONS OF PRIMARY TUBERCULOSIS

In a few individuals, enlargement of the hilar nodes may progress and lead to atelectasis due to compression of a bronchus; the right middle lobe is frequently involved. In the long term permanent bronchiectasis may persist in the affected area, and may later be secondarily infected by septic organisms. Sometimes a quite extensive radiographic shadow is seen in the lung, which is transient and does not give rise to symptoms: this relates to a hypersensitivity state, and is referred to as epituberculosis.

Similarly, when the pleura is involved during the phase of hypersensitivity, a large pleural effusion may develop, which is associated with initial pleural pain and fever, leading to dyspnoea as the effusion develops. The effusion, untreated, takes several weeks to resolve.

Particularly in subjects with poor resistance, more serious complications may ensue, due primarily to erosion of the caseating lymph node either into a bronchus or into a pulmonary vein. Perforation into a bronchus leads to tuberculous pneumonia, presenting as a toxic progressive febrile illness.

Invasion of the bloodstream leads to a widespread systemic infection, with millet-sized tuberculous foci evenly distributed through the lungs, liver, spleen, kidneys and bone marrow. Miliary tuberculosis, untreated, is uniformly fatal in a matter of weeks, the symptoms being fever, anaemia and wasting: the diagnosis is readily made by chest radiography which shows a characteristic 'snowstorm' appearance. The fundus oculi may show tubercles, allowing an elegant diagnosis by fundoscopy.

Tuberculous meningitis accompanies a high proportion of cases, or may occur without miliary lesions elsewhere. It frequently presents with malaise, fever, and disturbed behaviour before signs of meningeal irritation appear. Prompt diagnosis is essential if long-term neurological sequelae, notably epilepsy and deafness, are to be avoided. It may also complicate advanced lung disease in adults.

When the load of organisms invading the bloodstream is less massive, localized embolic disease occurs in areas with maximum blood flow, namely the kidneys and growing ends of the bone, which will not be further discussed.

POST PRIMARY (ADULT TYPE) TUBERCULOSIS

Adult disease may be due either to reinfection, or reactivation of a latent focus often after an interval of many years. Reactivation is likely in old age, and may be precipitated by concomitant illness or drugs leading to immune failure; the long-term use of steroids is particularly dangerous in this connection.

SYMPTOMS

Persistent cough with purulent sputum, often with haemoptysis, is the usual chest symptom, but non-specific symptoms such as fever, malaise and weight loss are of equal importance. Frequently the patient will minimize his symptoms, attributing the cough to cigarette smoking.

PHYSICAL SIGNS

Chest signs are varied: the disease commonly affects the upper lobes, and persistent post-tussive râles in this situation are highly suggestive. Signs of effusion, consolidation, or collapse leading to deviation of the trachea, may be found, but their place in diagnosis is limited. The presentation may be atypical, with non-specific symptoms accompanied by splenomegaly and lymph node enlargement, especially in non-white subjects.

Investigations

Chest radiography is essential and often diagnostic, the presence of upper zone cavitation with bronchial emboli (*Fig.* 2.9) to other parts of the lung being virtually specific. Tuberculosis may involve the apex of the lower lobe (*Fig.* 2.10), the upper lobes being unaffected. Pneumonic lesions without obvious cavitation do not have any specific radiographic appearance, and tuberculosis must be suspected if the opacities do not resolve normally with simple antibiotic treatment.

Tomography is useful in identifying cavities not visible on the plain film; and also in excluding cavities in chronic fibrotic disease of doubtful activity, when the presence of thin-walled apical emphysematous bullae on the straight film may be deceptive.

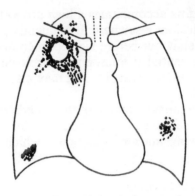

Fig. 2.9 Tuberculous cavity with bronchial embolic spread to lingula and right lower lobe.

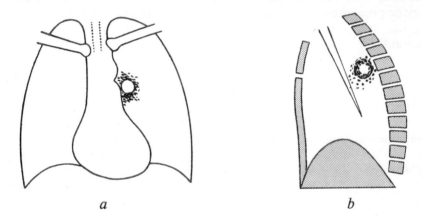

a   *b*

Fig. 2.10 Tuberculous cavity in left lower lobe apex. *a*, AP view; *b*, Lateral view.

BACTERIOLOGY

In underdeveloped communities X-ray facilities may not be available, in which event the diagnosis will rest largely on the finding of acid-fast bacilli in sputum smears stained by the Ziehl–Nielsen technique. With this simple laboratory method valuable progress towards control of this disease in a community can be made. It must be emphasized that a positive sputum smear is found only in patients with a very active lesion communicating with a bronchus; a negative smear does not exclude active tuberculosis.

In developed societies more stringent criteria of activity are applied with the help of radiography, and sputum cultures incubated on enriched (Löwenstein–Jensen) media. The practical difficulty remains that cultures take up to six weeks to grow, which emphasizes the importance of setting up a series of three morning sputum cultures immediately there is a suspicion of tuberculosis, in addition to the routine smear examinations.

Every positive culture should be routinely subcultured onto media containing the relevant amounts of the antibiotics likely to be used. This process takes about another 4 weeks, so that up to 3 months will elapse before information on sensitivities is available as a guide to treatment.

TUBERCULIN TESTING

Tuberculin testing is of relatively little value in diagnosis or assessment, as a positive test indicates only that infection has taken place in the past: it persists after healing is complete. A negative test does not completely exclude active disease, as tissue anergy may develop, particularly in elderly and debilitated subjects; but it may be helpful in the differential diagnosis of sarcoidosis, which is characterized by suppression of type IV tissue reactivity, of which the tuberculin test is an example.

The test is of value in epidemiological surveys, though only in a community in which BCG is not widely used. It identifies individuals who may require protection by BCG.

Technique of tuberculin testing

1. The Mantoux test involves the intradermal injection of 0·1 ml of tuberculin 1/1000 solution (10 tuberculin units). The test is read after 48 h, a positive result showing palpable induration not less than 10 mm in diameter, with erythema which may be more extensive. When an unusual degree of hypersensitivity is present, for example in the presence of a pleural effusion, a severe reaction with ulceration may follow: in such a situation preliminary testing with 1/10000 solution (1 tuberculin unit) should be done. The reaction is suppressed if steroid therapy is being given.

2. The Heaf test is carried out with a multiple puncture gun, spring operated, applied through a film of PPD (Purified Protein Derivative). It is useful when testing large numbers, and particularly in uncooperative subjects such as wriggling infants, when intradermal injection may be difficult. A positive reaction (Grade 3) consists of confluent papules with a raised centre. Grade 1 (isolated papules) and Grade 2 (confluent papules without a raised centre) are doubtfully significant.

3. The tine test involves multiple puncture with a disposable disc with points already coated with old tuberculin. At least two papules of 2 mm diameter indicate a positive result.

The ESR is of only slight value as an indication of progress if serial readings show a fall from the initial high figure.

Management

Admission to hospital is not usually required, unless:

1. It is necessary to impress the patient with the need for strict compliance with the chemotherapy required; or

2. The patient is highly infectious, and has susceptible home contacts (especially children); or

3. Is deemed unlikely to take the simple precautions needed to prevent

droplet spread of infection, before sputum conversion can be expected; or

4. It is judged to be desirable to have the patient under observation for the first 3 weeks of treatment, by which time the majority of untoward side effects from antibacterial therapy will have become manifest. This will depend on the assessment of the reliability of the patient in reporting untoward symptoms; or

5. The patient is toxic and febrile.

The duration of stay in hospital rarely needs to exceed 4 weeks: the patient should return to work without delay, to avoid invalidism.

Bedrest is called for only if general symptoms are severe: in the majority of cases, given adequate chemotherapy, recovery is equally rapid whether the patient is ambulant or on strict rest. An excess of rest may lead to invalidism, or to undesirable weight gain.

CONTROL OF INFECTION

Normally infectiousness persists for only up to about 6 weeks after the start of antibacterial treatment: infection of others is therefore more likely to occur before diagnosis than after it. If the patient can and will cooperate by always coughing into a tissue, the used tissues being collected in a bag and burned, the risk to his contacts is negligible.

ANTIBACTERIAL THERAPY

The mainstay of management lies in effective antibacterial treatment, using initially three agents until information about the sensitivity of the organisms is available: this may take up to 3 months to obtain.

The use of one antibacterial agent alone is to be avoided at all times, as it will inevitably lead to drug resistance. The aim is to ensure the use of two drugs to which the organisms are known to be sensitive; because of the delay in obtaining information about sensitivities, it is usual to give three agents together initially. This covers a situation where unsuspected resistance to one agent is present from the start, as the two remaining ones will effectively be prevented from developing resistance in turn. Primary drug resistance is rare except in countries where single drug therapy is available, usually on the black market.

The recommended duration of antibacterial treatment has been reducing over the years, as successive trials have demonstrated an acceptably low relapse rate with shorter courses than previously. Whereas for cavitating disease 18 months' therapy used to be advised, this has now reduced to 9 months, a trend which may continue.

The standard primary drugs used at present are rifampicin, isoniazide and ethambutol. Streptomycin is not regularly used, but has a definite place when it is felt necessary to ensure that the patient in fact takes his oral drugs, which should be given in a single morning dose when the nurse calls to give the streptomycin injection.

Table 2.4 Chemotherapy of tuberculosis

Agent	Dosage	Principal side effects	Comments
Isoniazid	200–300 mg daily (one morning dose)	Peripheral neuropathy: Acute psychosis Pellegra-like rash	Pyridoxine, 20 mg daily may be given concomitantly as a prophylactic, especially if malnutrition is present
Rifampicin	10 mg/kg bodyweight (one morning dose)	Hepatotoxic: may be transient. Contraindicated if liver damage already present	Monitor with liver function tests
Ethambutol	15–20 mg/kg bodyweight (one morning dose)	Acute retinopathy with bizarre visual disturbances: may leave scotomata but totally reversible if drug stopped at once. Rare	Warn patient to contact doctor and stop drug if eye symptoms occur
Streptomycin	1 g daily i.m. (0·75 g in elderly— over 60)	(1) Allergy: morbilliform rash and fever within 3 weeks of starting. Rarely, CNS demyelination (2) VIII cranial nerve toxicity mostly in elderly. Deafness, irreversible. Unsteadiness, reversible	Desensitize, or cover with steroids, or change drug

Discontinue Physiotherapy—walking exercise Discontinue |

The use of intermittent regimes, all the drugs being given twice or thrice weekly, is being investigated but cannot be confidently recommended as routine practice until after a further period of assessment of relapse rates. Such regimes receive theoretical support from the fact that tubercle bacilli reproduce about once in 48 hours.

Second-line agents, of use when resistance to first-line drugs is present, or when unacceptable side effects have developed, include para-aminosalicylic acid, ethionamide, cycloserine, pyrazinamide, viomycin, capreomycin, and kanamycin.

The dosage and side effects of the principal agents used is shown in *Table* 2.4.

USE OF STEROIDS

Whilst not standard practice, the use of steroids, along with chemotherapy, e.g. prednisolone 15 mg daily, has a striking and prompt beneficial effect on symptoms in toxic and ill patients, especially those with extensive disease. Radiological clearing is quicker, but the results after 12 months are not strikingly different whether steroids are given or not. Theoretically some reduction in residual fibrosis may be expected. Caution is, however, required if there is any suspicion of drug-resistant organisms, in which event the infection could be exacerbated. The steroid should not be continued for more than 3–6 months.

SURGICAL TREATMENT

Surgical removal of residual disease is only very rarely required, usually in unreliable patients with concomitant alcoholism, or other psychiatric or environmental problems.

FOLLOW-UP ARRANGEMENTS

A single follow-up appointment 6 months after completing treatment is all that is necessary: this should include a chest radiograph for reassurance purposes. Repeated clinic attendances do not allow the patient to forget his disease, and are to be condemned. The only exception is when there is doubt about the patient having taken his treatment regularly.

Late complications of pulmonary tuberculosis

1. COR PULMONALE

When the disease is very extensive and chronic the infection will be eliminated but substantial residual fibrosis will remain, which may lead ultimately to cor pulmonale.

2. MYCETOMA

Tuberculosis cavities may heal under treatment without closing. Such persistent spaces are liable, in about 10% of cases, to become infested by *Aspergillus fumigatus,* with the formation of a fungus ball within the cavity (p. 148). The resulting radiological opacity may be erroneously interpreted as an indication of reactivation of the tuberculosis.

3. RENAL TUBERCULOSIS

Particularly if chemotherapy has been·doubtfully adequate, care must be taken to check the urine for pus cells and culture it for *M. tuberculosis:* this is to exclude latent renal tuberculosis, which may be advanced before causing symptoms.

Prevention of tuberculosis

Prevention involves identification and effective treatment of infectious cases. Mass miniature radiography (MMR) was introduced in the 1939–45 war with this in mind, particularly for the protection of submarine crews; it is effective when the whole of a suspect population can be examined, but has proved disappointingly unproductive in civilian conditions when examination is voluntary. Assiduous seeking out of contacts for radiographical examination in the family and work place is much more productive.

INDIVIDUAL PROPHYLAXIS

1. *BCG vaccination*

Tuberculin-negative individuals are susceptible to tuberculosis, and can be protected by BCG, which is a live attenuated strain of tubercle bacillus, a suspension of which is injected intradermally. A papular and sometimes pustular lesion develops at the vaccination site, which clears spontaneously in a few weeks; after about a month the tuberculin test becomes positive indicating tissue hypersensitivity, which is accompanied by a high level of immunity to any subsequent exposure to tuberculosis.

INDICATIONS FOR BCG VACCINATION Vaccination should be offered to tuberculin-negative contacts of known infectious cases, especially babies and children; and to tuberculin-negative adults who are likely to be exposed to infection occupationally, for example nurses. It is currently offered in the UK to all children about to leave school, but with the great decrease in prevalence in the community the need to continue this policy indefinitely is now open to doubt.

COMPLICATIONS OF BCG VACCINATION Rarely, axillary lymph node enlargement may progress to caseation and discharge through the skin; the attenuated bacillus is fully sensitive to antibacterial agents, which may need to be given for a short period in these circumstances. A few cases of disseminated BCG infection have been reported, invariably in subjects with immune incompetence.

2. *Chemoprophylaxis*

Isoniazid alone, given for 12 months immediately after tuberculin skin sensitivity develops, is widely used in the USA in preference to BCG. This method is little used in the UK because of the fear of inducing drug resistance.

Atypical mycobacteria

A small proportion of cases, about 1% in the UK, are due to atypical mycobacteria, which produce abnormal colonies on culture: some species (photochromogens) develop a yellow pigment on exposure to light. All show a high degree of resistance to most antibacterial agents.

The disease is radiologically indistinguishable from tuberculosis due to normal organisms; it tends to run an indolent course, and surgical resection may be required because chemotherapy alone is likely to be ineffective.

The same group of organisms may also cause cervical adenitis, the prevalence being highest in the central and southern United States.

2.3 OBSTRUCTIVE AIRWAY DISEASE

Introduction

Airway obstruction is the functional abnormality common to chronic bronchitis, emphysema, and asthma. It is common practice to use two or more of these terms in conjunction to describe well recognized clinical situations, but the relative degree of emphysema is so difficult to establish in any particular patient that it seems wise to consider bronchitis, emphysema and asthma separately. This avoids oversimplification which may lead to errors in management. Because the diagnosis of emphysema implies to many people that treatment is unlikely to be helpful, it is best not given to the patient unless the evidence is very clear.

Airway obstruction

A number of distinct factors are involved in the genesis of obstruction to the flow of air at different levels in the bronchial tree; all involve narrowing of the airways with increased resistance to flow.

1. *Increase in the tone of smooth muscle* is a factor which remains important, but less so than used to be thought.

2. *Excessive mucus* within the lumen may cause narrowing with audible wheeze, which disappears after expectoration. (Complete obstruction of the bronchus by secretions may lead to atelectasis, with impairment of the ventilation/perfusion ratio because of the continued passage of blood through non-aerated lung.)

3. *Acute oedema,* or

4. *Permanent thickening,* of the bronchial mucosa are clearly important causes of obstruction.

5. *Undue collapsibility of the major bronchi,* resulting in trapping of air distally on expiration, can be demonstrated in some patients at bronchoscopy and by bronchography, as well as by showing an abrupt fall in the expiratory spirogram.

6. *Distortion and narrowing of the peripheral airways* may accompany emphysema, and lead to obstruction which may be recognizable only by sophisticated physiological techniques. Small airway obstruction is also common in smokers, and is to some extent reversible if the habit is given up.

Lung function tests

The most useful overall test for airway obstruction is the FEV_1 (forced expiratory volume in one second): it does nothing to distinguish between the various contributory factors, the relative importance of which vary from patient to patient and from time to time.

It is usefully expressed as a proportion of the FVC (forced vital capacity) which may itself be little changed in the presence of quite substantial obstruction; whereas the FEV_1 drops substantially and with it the FEV_1/FVC ratio. In normal subjects the FEV_1 is from 70% to 80% of the FVC: in severe obstruction it may be as low as 35% (*Figs.* 2.11, 2.12).

This can be conveniently recorded graphically using a simple spirometer such as the Vitalograph. The peak expiratory flow rate (PEFR), measured in litres per second, is a useful measurement, easily obtained with Wright's peak flowmeter; the best of three consecutive readings is accepted.

Both tests require full cooperation in producing the fastest possible expiratory effort. They are useful for measuring the response to bronchodilator drugs, by repeating the test 15 min or longer after inhaling a salbutamol aerosol. Clinical progress, by measurements at least twice daily on a portable machine, may be recorded as a routine matter in the ward or as an outpatient.

Definitions

Chronic bronchitis is defined as a chronic cough with sputum production on most days for at least 3 months in the year, for not less than 2 years. The sputum may be mucoid but is commonly purulent during exacerbations.

This definition involves no consideration of function.

Asthma is a disorder of function rather than a distinct disease; it is characterized by dyspnoea which varies in severity, the airway obstruction being substantially and rapidly reversible either spontaneously or following the use of drugs.

Emphysema describes a pathological lesion, namely enlargement of the air spaces distal to the terminal bronchioles with destruction of the alveolar walls.

Chronic bronchitis

Introduction

Chronic bronchitis was at one time believed to be particularly prevalent in Britain compared with other countries, but it is now known to occur with comparable frequency in many other industrial societies, particularly in cities where atmospheric pollution is a problem.

Mortality

In the UK chronic bronchitis accounts for some 30000 deaths a year, and is about three times commoner in men than in women; it also accounts for a vast loss of working time.

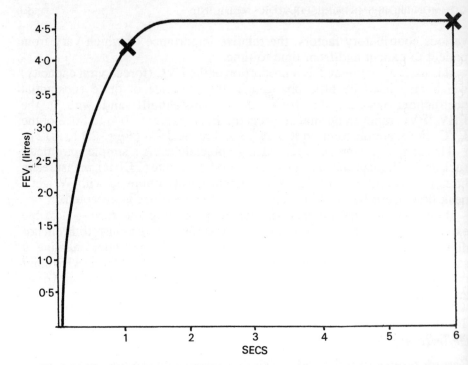

Fig. 2.11 Normal vitalograph, $FEV_1 = 4.1$ litres; $FVC = 4.6$ litres; ratio = 89%.

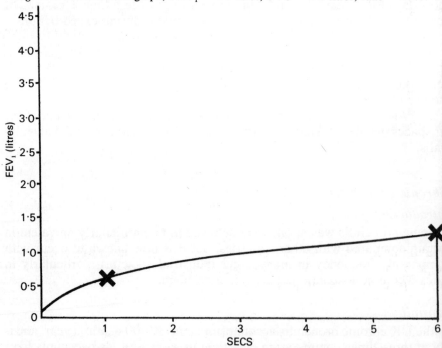

Fig. 2.12 Vitalograph in severe COAD. $FEV_1 = 0.6$ litres; $FVC = 1.4$ litres; ratio = 43%.

Aetiology

Chronic bronchitis is commonest in social grades III to V, and its geographical distribution is directly related to atmospheric pollution; cigarette smoking is of paramount importance in its aetiology and progression. The mortality is directly related to the number of cigarettes smoked, being increased in heavy smokers by a factor of twenty compared with non-smokers.

Whilst both social conditions and atmospheric pollution are the subject of steady improvement in the UK, the level of cigarette smoking shows little change, particularly in the social grades most afflicted by chronic bronchitis.

Pathology

The disorder is characterized by gross hypertrophy of the mucus-secreting cells leading to permanent thickening of the mucous membrane, and with it, increasing airway obstruction; at the same time the function of ciliary clearance is lost. Acute infective episodes may be accompanied by peripheral microabscesses, healing of which leads to distortion of small airways and contributes to the development of emphysema.

Clinical features

SYMPTOMS

The onset of chronic bronchitis is usually insidious, though the symptoms may date from a particular episode of infection. Initially the patient complains only of cough with modest sputum production, without dyspnoea. With the passage of the years he suffers repeated exacerbations, which usually follow an upper respiratory virus infection; they are associated with purulent sputum and wheeze on waking in the mornings, and with progressively longer spells off work. The severity of the illness is effectively assessed by enquiry into the duration of exacerbations, particularly the amount of time taken off work during the previous few years; eventually the patient may be incapacitated for the whole winter, and finally for the whole year.

As the disease progresses he develops symptoms of bronchial hyper-reactivity, with wheeziness on moving into a cold atmosphere or on exposure to previously well tolerated irritants, such as fog or smoke. The sputum becomes viscid and tenacious, and to bring it up the patient may require an hour or more of vigorous coughing after waking. Ultimately he develops chronic respiratory failure, namely hypoxia with retained carbon dioxide due to inadequate gas interchange at alveolar level: this is associated with crippling and permanent effort dyspnoea which engenders great distress even in the performance of simple tasks such as dressing or washing. At this stage he is liable to episodes of acute respiratory failure which require urgent admission to hospital.

PHYSICAL SIGNS

These are usually absent in the early stages; later on the lungs become over-inflated, with reduced breath sounds, mainly expiratory rhonchi, and often basal râles during the exacerbations. Helpful signs of over-inflation include poor respiratory excursion, an increase in the anteroposterior diameter of the chest, overfilling of the jugular veins during expiration, excessive use of the accessory muscles of respiration (scalene and sternomastoid) and reduction of the length of trachea palpable above the suprasternal notch.

In the later stages there are two well-recognized clinical presentations, though the distinction between the two is not always clear cut.

1. The 'blue bloater' has secondary polycythaemia with central cyanosis and engorged conjunctivae; he has poor respiratory drive, and is liable to episodes of respiratory failure with each new infection. These present with hypercapnia, drowsiness, twitching and congestive heart failure: the virtually complete lack of chest wall movement on respiration is very striking. There may be a number of episodes over succeeding months or years before the final illness.

2. The 'pink puffer' is not liable to episodic infective illnesses of this kind; the lungs are grossly overinflated, but respiration is not depressed, and he continues with progressively intense effort dyspnoea until he finally develops heart failure, which is commonly terminal the first time it occurs.

Investigations

Chest radiography is necessary to exclude any associated disorder, particularly bronchial carcinoma which has a common source in cigarette smoking. There are no diagnostic radiological features of chronic bronchitis, severe disease being compatible with normal radiograph. Some patients may show evidence of over-inflation (*see* Emphysema, p. 92). In the later stages cardiomegaly due to cor pulmonale may develop, and may temporarily regress following treatment.

A radiograph of the paranasal sinuses may reveal a treatable focus of infection, and any dental sepsis should also be treated.

A full blood count is required to exclude associated anaemia, whilst a polymorpholeucocytosis suggests a bacterial infection.

The serum proteins should be measured, with electrophoresis to identify a possible congenital deficiency or absence of gammaglobulins (p. 110).

The blood gases should be estimated when the condition is stable to indicate the resting Pco$_2$ as permanent hypercapnia, which maintains respiratory drive, is frequent. During acute exacerbations monitoring is essential as a guide to progress.

Sputum culture is required to estimate sensitivity to antibiotics. *Haemophilus influenzae* and pneumococcus are much the commonest organisms, but it is important to recognize others, especially *Staphylococcus pyogenes* and *Klebsiella pneumoniae,* which are present in a small proportion of cases. Not uncommonly, however, no pathogen is identified. Overgrowth by *E. coli* or *Pseudomonas aeruginosa* following repeated previous antibiotic therapy is a frequent finding in the chronic case.

Lung function tests to measure the degree of obstruction, and its reversibility, should be done as often as necessary as a guide to management, the FEV_1/FVC ratio or PEFR being both useful and simple to estimate. At the initial assessment, more detailed studies should include lung volumes as a guide to the degree of overinflation. Both the total lung capacity (TLC) and residual volume (RV) may be increased; an increase in the RV/TLC ratio suggests concomitant emphysema, but the degree of this can only be estimated reliably at autopsy. The gas transfer factor may also be moderately impaired.

Management of chronic bronchitis

Thought must be given to preventing long-term deterioration, as well as to the immediate relief of symptoms and management of the acute exacerbation.

LONG-TERM MEASURES TO PREVENT DETERIORATION

1. *Smoking.* The paramount requirement is permanent cessation of the cigarette habit, a matter which must be implanted firmly in the mind of the patient as his own responsibility. Motivation to stop may be reinforced by taking time to explain the consequences of smoking, as well as the nature of the addiction, at considerable, even inordinate, length. As withdrawal symptoms are specifically due to decline in the blood level of nicotine rather than other and more dangerous components of cigarette smoke, those severely addicted may get some help during the withdrawal phase by substituting chewing gum containing appropriate amounts of nicotine: but this or similar techniques will not succeed unless motivation is high. In suggestible subjects success occasionally follows acupuncture or hypnosis.

Attempts to achieve motivation by collective activity, for example in anti-smoking clinics, have been on the whole disappointing on account of the high relapse rate.

2. *Focal sepsis,* whether dental or in the upper respiratory tract, may exacerbate bronchitis due to aspiration of infected material, particularly during sleep when the cough reflex is suppressed. It should always be looked for and treated where appropriate.

3. *Prophylactic antibiotic therapy.* Continuous treatment over the winter months with a broad-spectrum antibiotic, for example tetracycline 500 mg b.d., may shorten the individual attacks in some patients, but the overall effect in slowing the decline of lung function has proved disappointing.

4. *Physiotherapy.* Regular expiratory breathing exercises, after instruction by an expert therapist, help to keep the airways clear and reduce the incidence of intercurrent infections.

5. *Simple bronchodilator drug therapy.* In the established case, particularly when some degree of response has been demonstrated, a beta-adrenoceptor stimulant will relieve symptoms and help to maintain effective drainage of the airways. A salbutamol aerosol spray, 2 puffs four times daily, is effective, and less likely to produce side effects (tremor, tachycardia) than the oral preparation. It is most important to be sure the patient understands the technique of inhalation, which should be demonstrated; for those who find this difficult, terbutaline sulphate 250 μg inhaled four times a day in a 'spacer' unit provides a useful alternative.

Many patients experience nocturnal attacks of breathlessness, which may be confused with the paroxysmal nocturnal dyspnoea of left heart failure. The attacks are accompanied by a dip in the FEV_1, and invariably accompanied by wheeze on waking, which is not a feature of cardiac dyspnoea. In this event supplementary treatment with long-acting xanthine derivatives is useful: aminophylline may be given as a suppository at night, or as delayed release tablets, e.g. Phyllocotin 225 mg, 1 or 2 tablets on retiring. If Phyllocotin is not tolerated due to nausea, delayed-release theophylline, e.g. Nuelin SA, 50 mg or Theograd, 350 mg, may be acceptable.

There is a need for an aerosol preparation effective for 8 h, no currently available preparation lasting more than 4–6 h.

6. *Corticosteroids.* Steroid therapy should be used when a substantial improvement in FEV_1 is demonstrable. Subjective improvement alone may be a result of drug-induced euphoria, and lead the patient into long-term side effects with little if any long-term therapeutic advantage; nevertheless relief of specific symptoms, especially nocturnal breathlessness and early morning wheeze should also be taken into account. Responsiveness should be assessed with the help of PEFR readings two or three times daily: these can be measured with a portable machine in hospital or on an outpatient basis; treatment with prednisone at least 15 mg daily should be continued for 2–3 weeks before a decision is made as to long-term therapy; the dose should then be titrated down in stages to the minimal effective level.

7. *Influenza prophylaxis* is a reasonable measure when an epidemic is forecast, and has the merit of being harmless.

8. *Congenital hypogammaglobulinaemia* may be usefully corrected by giving a weekly intramuscular injection: about 1 g of gammaglobulin is the usual dose, but this should be corrected against the serum levels achieved. In an acute situation, infusions of fresh plasma are also helpful.

MANAGEMENT OF EXACERBATIONS

a. Antibiotic treatment. Acute exacerbations of chronic bronchitis normally follow a virus infection of the upper respiratory tract, which is likely to be followed by secondary bacterial infection.

Prompt antibiotic treatment will help to control the bacterial component, and may shorten the illness: it may also prevent further lung damage. It is helpful for the patient to keep a supply of antibiotic at home so that he can start treatment at the onset of symptoms; once started, treatment should continue for 5 days, or longer if purulent sputum persists.

The choice of antibiotic lies between co-trimoxazole, 2 tablets b.d., or ampicillin, 250–500 mg 6-hourly; tetracycline 250 mg q.i.d. is also useful.

b. Bed rest is advisable until the fever has settled and expectoration has started: it should not be prolonged as mobilization will assist clearing the airways of secretions.

c. Extra bronchodilator drugs may be called for.

d. Mucolytic agents may help expectoration in a small proportion of ill patients with viscid sputum: they have little place in long-term management. Acetylcysteine, 2–5 ml of 2% solution given by nebulizer every 6 h, is the most likely to be effective.

e. Unhappily there is no effective expectorant mixture.

MANAGEMENT OF THE SEVERELY ILL PATIENT WITH LIFE-THREATENING RESPIRATORY FAILURE

Arrangements for admission to hospital. Respiratory failure is an acute emergency in which any delay might be fatal. It is therefore reasonable to arrange for patients known to be at risk to admit themselves to hospital at the onset of symptoms. This procedure is facilitated by keeping a list of known patients available in the admissions department.

Clinical features. The large majority of cases of life-threatening acute lung failure occurs in patients with longstanding airway obstruction. A minority relate to neurological syndromes (myasthenia, muscular dystrophy) associated with incompetent ventilation due to muscular weakness; to immobility of the chest wall (ankylosing spondylitis, kyphoscoliosis); or to limitation of movement by gross obesity ('Pickwickian syndrome'). Acute deterioration should always be assumed to be due to infection.

The cardinal symptoms which should alert the patient and his family to seek urgent help are progressive drowsiness and intermittent twitching of the limbs. A detailed account of the degree of prior disability, and of the quality of life, should be obtained from the immediate family at the first opportunity if these are not already known: this information is an essential guide to management. Details of recent drug therapy are essential, and sometimes most reliably obtained by asking a relative to bring the actual drugs along with the patient.

On examination, *the cardinal signs* are extreme depression of chest movement due to failure of respiratory drive, with plethora and cyanosis; there is likely to be supraventricular tachycardia relating to respiratory acidosis, with overfilled jugular veins and dependent oedema. The breath sounds are distant, with inspiratory and expiratory rhonchi and diffuse moist sounds.

Investigations. A chest radiograph is needed to assess possible pneumonia, pneumothorax, or pleural effusion; and in particular the presence of cardiomegaly, vascular congestion and/or Kerley B lines (enlarged basal lymphatics due to heart failure) which would be an indication for diuretic therapy.

Measurement of blood gases, at least initially from an arterial specimen, for levels of $P\text{co}_2$ and $P\text{o}_2$ (respiratory failure is defined by a $P\text{co}_2$ of $>6\cdot3$ kPa and by a $P\text{o}_2$ of <9 kPa). Knowledge of the resting $P\text{co}_2$ level before deterioration is useful; if not available, a high plasma carbonate will suggest compensated acidosis of long standing.

The blood urea and electrolytes may give the clue to renal impairment due to heart failure, and to the dehydration which is so often present.

Sputum and blood cultures should be set up, even though they cannot provide useful information immediately.

An electrocardiograph is mandatory, especially if there is persistent tachycardia or evidence of heart failure.

Management. Management is devoted primarily to the relief of the hypoxia, and with it the hypercapnia. To this end the airways must be cleared of secretion, effective respiratory movement restored and appropriate oxygen therapy given to maintain the patient until the associated infection has been brought under control.

Dehydration is frequently present and requires correction by intravenous fluids. The addition of sodium bicarbonate to the first litre acts as no more than a holding measure towards correction of severe respiratory acidosis, which only follows the re-establishment of effective gas exchange, but it is a useful measure particularly if supraventricular tachycardia has developed.

Right heart failure, if present, is precipitated by pulmonary artery constriction in response to hypoxia, leading to acute pulmonary hypertension: relief will follow correction of the hypoxia, so that diuretics should be given with due moderation; any tendency to dehydration may render the sputum viscid.

Bronchodilator therapy is best given intravenously initially (aminophylline, 250–500 mg by slow intravenous injection over at least 10 min; or salbutamol, 250 μg every 4 h; or terbutaline, 250–500 mg by slow injection every 6 h or 3–20 μg/min by continuous infusion); this should be immediately followed by vigorous physiotherapy to help expectoration, which should be repeated several times a day, together with virtually continuous exhortation to cough by the nursing staff. The patient should be nursed sitting up in bed or in a chair, and any kind of sedation should be avoided.

If the response is uncertain, systemic steroids (hydrocortisone 200 mg i.m. 6-hourly) should be added without hesitation for the duration of the acute phase, and replaced with rapidly reducing oral steroids during recovery, along with oral or aerosol bronchodilators.

Oxygen therapy. In many cases of chronic bronchitis, with the passage of the years the respiratory centre in the midbrain becomes insensitive to the $P\text{CO}_2$ level which controls respiratory drive in health, and instead becomes dependent on low $P\text{O}_2$ levels to maintain its function. It follows that restoring $P\text{O}_2$ from a low level to normal will in these circumstances remove the stimulus to respiration, which will become further depressed, or even cease altogether. Arterial oxygen tension must therefore be increased only gradually. This is done by using a face mask designed on the Venturi principle to deliver 24% oxygen: a fast stream of 100% oxygen is delivered to the face piece through a plastic extension perforated with holes of a size appropriate to allow enough air to be impelled by the oxygen stream to produce the required dilution. Even with this degree of dilution there may sometimes follow an increase in $P\text{CO}_2$; in this event the use of respiratory stimulant drugs (nikethamide, 2 ml of 25% solution by intravenous injection, or doxapram 1–2 mg/min continuously by drip) may be helpful; the blood gases must always be monitored at least once daily in the initial stages. If clinical improvement follows and the $P\text{CO}_2$ reduces, the proportion of oxygen may only then be increased to 28% by using a mask with a larger air intake.

Endotracheal intubation. If in spite of these measures adequate respiratory drive is not achieved, then a decision must be made whether or not to proceed to endotracheal intubation with intermittent positive-pressure respiration (IPPR) provided by a mechanical respirator; this step is taken only when there is reasonable evidence of some factor, usually an infection, which can be effectively reversed during the period of intubation. A decision cannot be made without detailed knowledge of the patient's capacities before the onset of acute lung failure: if there is little prospect of a reasonable quality of life afterwards, intubation is best reconsidered. The decision can be very difficult and it is most important that the immediate relatives are kept fully informed of the position at all stages. Unexpectedly good results are not infrequent, and sometimes several years of useful life may follow before the next critical episode.

Intubation facilitates the extraction of the bronchial secretions by suction, and should be continued until the infection has been brought under control. Once satisfactory improvement in the blood gas tensions have been achieved, the patient must be encouraged to trigger the respirator for himself for a day or more before final extubation. The total period of intubation should not normally exceed about a week because of the risk of ulceration and later stenosis of the trachea.

Tracheostomy has the advantage of reducing the dead space, and may very occasionally be required when more prolonged assisted respiration is necessary, for example in the presence of antibiotic-resistant infection or impaired chest wall movement due to trauma or a neurological lesion.

Antibiotic treatment must always be given even in the absence of infected sputum, on the assumption of an underlying infection. As in other acute situations, the responsible organism and its drug sensitivities can only be identified after unavoidable laboratory delay. Treatment must be planned empirically on a wide-spectrum basis, to cover possible staphylococcus, klebsiella or *E. coli* infection as well as the more usual *H. influenzae* or *Strep. pneumoniae* (*see Table* 2.2); it should continue until the sputum is no longer purulent.

Emphysema

Emphysema is a pathological diagnosis (*see* p. 83), and difficult to distinguish in the clinical situation from the overinflation that follows air trapping. Its presence or absence in chronic bronchitis therefore has no bearing on management; it is a permanent structural change not amenable to therapy.

Brief mention must be made of some varieties of emphysema other than the centrilobular variety, frequently with widespread irregular fibrotic scars, which is so commonly seen in patients with chronic bronchitis.

1. *Panacinar emphysema,* in which the whole of the acinus is involved, is more likely to be present in the breathless patient with overinflated lungs who does not have episodic hypercapnia, i.e. the 'pink puffer'.

2. *Primary emphysema* shows similar features, and is sometimes familial, in which case it is usually associated with deficiency of the enzyme α_1-antitrypsin; this may also be reduced in family members who do not have emphysema. It is likely that deficiency of this enzyme leads to emphysema only in those who smoke. There is no treatment, but stopping smoking is of course imperative, particularly as the course of the illness is relatively rapid with early incapacity from breathlessness, the only symptom. Unaffected family members should be interviewed and advised not to smoke.

3. *Bullous emphysema* may be isolated, or associated with generalized emphysema. It may lead to spontaneous pneumothorax (p. 152). If localized, it may very occasionally be amenable to surgical removal, which is sometimes followed by striking relief of dyspnoea.

Investigations

Chest radiography shows the signs of overinflation, namely low and flat diaphragms, a heart shadow narrowed because of elongation of the heart by the downward displacement of the diaphragms, and enlargement of the retrosternal space as seen on the lateral radiograph: it should be noted that all these radiological signs may be present in asthma and are compatible with normal lungs at autopsy. The additional signs of peripheral deficiency of blood vessel markings, associated with prominent main pulmonary arteries, are strongly suggestive of severe panacinar emphysema: they are an infrequent feature of chronic bronchitis.

Bullous emphysema may be recognized by randomly distributed hairline shadows with patchy avascular areas: there may also be thin-walled cystic spaces.

Lung function tests show airway obstruction not responsive to bronchodilators, with enlarged lungs, and a marked increase in the residual volume.

4. *Compensatory emphysema* is the term used to describe overinflation of part of a lung, usually a lobe, which follows collapse of the adjacent part due to obstruction or compression of the bronchus.

On radiography, the emphysematous lobe is blacker than the rest of the lung fields, with spreading out and thinning of the blood vessels; it serves as a diagnostic pointer to the adjacent collapsed lobe, particularly the left lower lobe which is concealed behind the heart shadow (*Fig.* 2.13).

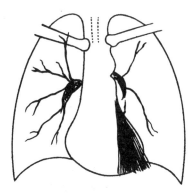

Fig. 2.13 Collapsed left lower lobe, compensatory emphysema of left upper lobe.

Management consists in establishing the cause of the adjacent collapse; most commonly this is a tumour, and less commonly an after-effect of childhood tuberculosis.

5. *Focal emphysema* often accompanies simple coal workers' pneumoconiosis (p. 135) and appears to be an entirely benign condition.

Summary

No lung disorder is more commonly incorrectly diagnosed on inadequate evidence. The presence of the generalized form is difficult to diagnose in life, and in any event has little bearing on management, which remains that of the associated disease. Some localized forms may require further investigation.

Primary emphysema demands investigation of the family.

Asthma frequently relates to a hypersensitivity state, and is therefore appropriately considered in the next chapter.

2.4 IMMUNE DISTURBANCES

This chapter describes a series of lung disorders which have in common some unusual form of immune response. This may be a hypersensitivity state, a system disease in which an autoimmune process is involved, or some other form of unusual host response. Overlapping features between some of these disorders are not infrequent.

Hypersensitivity states

Introduction

Gell and Coombes in 1963 described four types of hypersensitivity; this classification remains a sound basis for consideration of related clinical lung disorders. The types of hypersensitivity are:

Type I. Immediate. This reaction is mediated by IgE (reagin), a non-precipitating antibody, which is attached to the cells of the skin or of mucous membrane. When the appropriate antigen is in contact with cells thus sensitized, there is an immediate 'flare and weal' response with oedema, erythema and infiltration by eosinophils. This reaction is the basis of skin tests for specific allergies and of bronchial challenge tests by inhalation of antigens in solution. It is mediated by a number of locally released agents, including histamine, eosinophil chemotactic factor, and certain prostaglandins.

Type II concerns intravascular cytolytic mechanisms and is not known to be relevant to lung disease,.

Type III is the delayed (Arthus) reaction of which serum sickness is the classic example. Unlike type I it is characterized by the presence of precipitating serum antibodies of the IgG group: when these react with the specific antigen, immune complexes are formed which activate complement, and lead to a local tissue-damaging reaction mediated by leucocytes. There is a delayed reaction to intradermal test solutions, the site becoming substantially itchy and oedematous over an area several centimetres in diameter, but without erythema, or eosinophilia; this occurs 4–6 h after the test, and lasts several hours. It is therefore commonly missed by the clinician as the patient has usually gone home by the time the reaction occurs. He may, however, be asked to report on any delayed reaction himself, or to return after an appropriate interval.

Type IV consists of a cell-mediated oedematous and erythematous reaction to inoculation of antigen into the skin, after a delay of about 48 h. The lesion is granulomatous with lymphocytic infiltration: the classic example is the tuberculin test.

Asthma

Introduction

Asthma is a disorder of function associated with dyspnoea, due to narrowing of the peripheral airways, which is rapidly reversible either by drugs or spontaneously.

It may be extrinsic or intrinsic, though many patients do not fall very precisely into either group.

Extrinsic asthma commonly starts in childhood, and is associated with atopy: this is a tendency to excessive production of IgE, which can usefully be measured in the serum, in response to normal exposure to common antigens. Atopy is present in about 10% of the population, and may also be associated with hay fever, allergic rhinitis and flexural eczema; a positive family history is common.

Intrinsic (late onset) asthma develops later in life, more commonly affects women, is not associated with atopy, and may be less responsive to treatment than extrinsic asthma. It is commonly confused with cardiac dyspnoea.

Prevalence

Asthma is common, affecting about 5% of the population at some time. It accounts for about 1000 premature deaths annually in the UK. An alarming increase in mortality occurred in the 1960s which was due to excessive use at that time of aerosol inhalers containing isoprenaline; it has now subsided.

Autopsy findings

When an asthmatic has died from some other cause, the lungs and bronchi appear normal. If death were due to asthma, the lungs show overinflation and possible terminal pneumonia; the bronchi show plugging by viscid mucus secretion, which is usually loaded with eosinophils, with oedema of the mucous membrane; there is thickening of the basement membrane with an increase in the goblet cells.

The mechanisms controlling bronchial smooth muscle tone are complex and incompletely understood. The following description, though over-simplified, serves to provide a basis for considering the mode of action of some of the drugs used in treatment.

The final chemical pathway for the control of tone in bronchial smooth muscle depends largely on the level of intracellular cyclic adenosine monophosphate (cAMP): an increase leads to bronchodilatation, a decrease to bronchoconstriction.

In atopic (extrinsic) asthma, the excess of IgE, produced by lymphoid tissue, reacts with specific antigen on the surface of the mast cells; this is followed by the release of a number of mediators, including histamine and prostaglandins, from within the cell following disruption of the cell membrane. The simultaneous release of eosinophil chemotactic factor leads to local infiltration with eosinophils, the function of which remains obscure. The mediators react on a variety of receptor sites on the cell membrane of smooth muscle, leading to a reduction in cAMP and bronchoconstriction.

The receptor sites are also under the control of the autonomic nervous system. β-adrenergic receptors when stimulated by sympathetic action lead to an increase in cAMP and bronchodilatation: stimulation of α-adrenergic receptors has the opposite effect. Cholinergic receptors respond to vagal stimulation and also cause bronchoconstriction.

Clinical features

SYMPTOMS

The cardinal symptom is wheezy dyspnoea which is reversible and associated with cough: both the beginning and end of the attack may be remarkably sudden, whilst the attack itself may last from a few minutes to several hours. A severe attack lasting more than 24–48 h, i.e. status asthmaticus, is an indication for admission to hospital.

On the other hand, a relatively mild wheeze may persist for weeks or months. Chronic asthma may be punctuated by increased wheeze and cough on or soon after waking, and not infrequently by nocturnal exacerbations which waken the patient from sleep. These nocturnal attacks, which are often mistaken for left ventricular failure, are accompanied by a sharp dip in FEV_1; a high proportion of deaths from asthma occur at night.

SIGNS

The patient is distressed and preoccupied, the chest overinflated, whilst the accessory muscles of respiration stand out, and the lower chest wall is drawn in during inspiration, which is short and jerky; expiration is prolonged and wheezy, and usually accompanied by overfilling of the jugular veins. The overinflation relates to the fact that expiration is a passive movement, depending largely on the elastic recoil of the lungs, and of insufficient power to overcome the resistance to airflow imposed by the constriction of the peripheral bronchi; this is in contrast to inspiration which is carried out by the powerful contraction of the respiratory muscles, thus drawing air past the constricted airways and trapping it there.

On auscultation wheeze is generalized and continuous, though more marked on expiration; basal crepitations may be abundant, and the heart sounds distant. In a severe attack the breath sounds may be greatly reduced, an indication of obstruction of the peripheral bronchi by mucus, and wheeze may be entirely absent.

Other sinister signs are severe tachypnoea and persistent tachycardia; cyanosis is an indication of substantial hypoxia.

PRECIPITATING FACTORS

These include the following, either separately or in combination:

1. *Infection.* Virus or bacterial infection of the upper respiratory tract are likely aggravating factors.

2. *Exercise* may precipitate asthma, especially in young people. The attack may start during, or a minute or so after, the exercise and continue thereafter; it is thus distinct from the normally expected degree of effort dyspnoea which subsides quickly with rest. The mechanism of its causation is not known; the reaction can in most cases be aborted by the regular prophylactic use of disodium cromoglycate, which it is suggested may act by inhibiting the release of mediators from the mast cells.

3. *Specific allergens* are likely to play a role in atopic subjects, for example pollens in the early summer, or house dust. Sensitivity to animal fur is not unusual, whilst possible occupational allergens should be kept in mind.

4. *Psychological factors.* The importance of these has been exaggerated: anxiety is at least as likely to stem from this unpleasant and sometimes frightening disorder, as to contribute to it, whilst repeated loss of sleep from asthma may lead to further anxiety. Psychoanalytical therapy in the treatment of asthma has proved entirely disappointing. Nevertheless acute stress or frustration can on occasion precipitate an attack in some patients.

Investigations

Chest radiography in the uncomplicated case is normal apart from possible overinflation.

A blood count may show significant eosinophilia.

Physiological testing shows impaired ventilation of obstructive type, with reduced FEV_1, FEV_1/FVC ratio, and peak flow rate. The degree of reversibility of obstruction by drugs is a valuable guide to management.

The total lung capacity and residual volume are increased, according to the degree of overinflation present.

Blood gas estimation shows a low P_{CO_2} due to hyperventilation. Only in the severe attack does hypoxia develop, and ultimately hypercapnia in prolonged status asthmaticus; respiratory failure indicates that the illness is critical.

Skin tests are likely to be positive to several common antigens in atopic subjects; they are therefore of little value in the absence of a positive history. It follows that a carefully taken history is of more use in most cases.

Tests may be carried out for example against pollens, house-dust mite, dog or horse hair, and aspergillus, to confirm a clinical history of allergy. They are best done by pricking the skin through a drop of antigen solution placed on the forearm, along with a control solution; intradermal testing may lead to an anaphylactic reaction. Testing against a wide range of possible allergens such as foodstuffs and the like has no place in management.

Challenge testing by inhalation of aerosols containing antigen may cause severe reactions: it should be used only by clinicians experienced in the technique.

Sputum should be examined for cells and organisms. Purulent sputum may consist of eosinophils only, and may not be an indication of infection.

Management

The patient's lifestyle should be altered as little as possible; confidence must be maintained and normal physical activities continued, with the aid of suitable drug therapy as necessary. In atopic patients steps should be taken to reduce exposure to house dust, particularly in the bedroom, by reducing dust-retaining fabrics, and by the regular use of a vacuum cleaner on the mattress as well as the floor. The use of a duvet instead of blankets may be helpful. Cigarette smoking should cease.

Only occasionally should it be necessary to change occupation, but possible occupational causes must always be looked for. A reasonable proportion of people sensitive to dog or horse hair are able to retain their animals by using prophylactic drugs and avoiding unnecessarily close contact.

Desensitization is only rarely called for, particularly as any benefits are likely to be only temporary. Seasonal asthma due to pollen is an exception, regular winter prophylaxis with increasing doses of allergen providing significant benefit in many cases. Weekly injections given over 10–12 weeks, the final dose timed to coincide with the start of the pollen season, are probably more effective than short courses of delayed release antigenic preparations: protection depends on the production of specific IgG antibody which blocks the allergic response. Desensitization to house-dust mite is of uncertain value because it is short lived, and should not replace measures to control dust.

Drug treatment

The patient should understand the use of his drugs, and be able to manage his asthma by making suitable adjustments to meet changes in his condition. Time must be put aside to explain the mode of action of the drugs advised, whilst detailed instruction in the use of inhaled aerosols is of particular importance.

The choice depends on the pattern of the asthma, and includes a remarkably wide variety of bronchodilators, an indication that none is entirely satisfactory, together with steroid hormones and sodium cromoglycate. In addition, *antibiotics* are indicated for control of acute respiratory infections, usually ampicillin 500 mg b.d. or co-trimoxazole, 2 tablets b.d. for 5 days or until the infection has subsided.

DRUGS TO BE AVOIDED

Sedatives have no place, because their use may be lethal due to suppression of the respiratory centre and abolition of respiratory drive. Similarly, cough suppressants (linctus codeine, methadone, diamorphine) should not be used in asthma because they inhibit a vital function, and will lead to retention of sputum with blocking of bronchi in a situation already hazardous by virtue of impaired ventilation.

Ephedrine sulphate, adrenaline and isoprenaline are traditional remedies now replaced by more effective drugs with less side effects, in particular cardiac side effects. Compounds containing a mixture of theophylline or ephedrine, with a little phenobarbitone, are fortunately losing popularity. Antihistamines are of no value in asthma.

Bronchodilator drugs

A wide range of bronchodilator drugs is available; the clinician should be familiar with the side effects and effectiveness of a few. Finding the correct drug for a particular patient is often a matter of trial and error.

Selective β-adrenergic stimulants

This group of drugs has the advantage over its predecessors of causing only minimal cardiac side effects. Salbutamol (Ventolin) tablets, 2–4 mg three or four times daily, is effective but may cause tremor, tachycardia and headache. The side effects are less frequent if the drug is given by aerosol inhalation, 2 puffs three or four times daily, which is probably the first choice of bronchodilator drug, subject to the technique of inhalation being properly understood. If the patient cannot effect the essential synchronization between a deep inspiration and the puff from the canister, terbutaline sulphate (Bricanyl) in the same dosage may be taken from a 'space inhaler', which includes an extended mouthpiece which facilitates the inhalation.

Salbutamol may be given by intramuscular injection, 500 μg every 4 h, or intravenously, 250 μg every 4 h, in acute exacerbations, and may obviate the use of steroids. When side effects are troublesome, orciprenaline sulphate (Alupent) may be given by mouth (20 mg q.i.d.) or by aerosol inhalation 1–2 puffs up to 6 times daily.

Clearly, selective β-blockade, for example in the treatment of hypertension, will block sympathetic receptors and reduce cAMP levels, so that care is required in using drugs of this group in asthmatics.

XANTHINE DERIVATIVES

Aminophylline, 250–500 mg by slow intravenous injection over 10–15 min is a useful initial measure in severe asthma; as it is an anticholinergic agent it is likely to cause tachycardia and palpitation if given more rapidly. It may also cause vomiting and occasionally syncope. Some patients find it helpful taken as a suppository at night; the long-acting preparation (Phyllocontin tablets, 225 or 450 mg b.d.) is useful particularly in the control of nocturnal asthma, but may cause nausea.

Choline theophyllinate (Choledyl, 100 or 200 mg tablets two or three times daily) has similar side effects. Theocontin (200 mg b.d.) is a delayed release theophylline preparation and a useful alternative to Phyllocontin; it is thought to deactivate the enzyme responsible for the breakdown of cAMP. Ipratropium bromide (Atrovent) as an aerosol inhalation, 1–2 puffs three or four times daily, seems to be particularly well accepted by the elderly.

Drug prophylaxis

DISODIUM CROMOGLYCATE (INTAL)

This drug is believed to act by blocking the release of histamine and other mediators from the mast cells in response to a type I hypersensitivity reaction; its value lies in the prevention of asthma and not in the treatment of attacks. It is particularly valuable in the prophylaxis of exercise-induced asthma in young people, and in some cases of hypersensitivity in atopic subjects. It is inactivated if given by mouth or systemically, and must therefore be inhaled. A capsule containing the dry powder is pierced in a device ('Spinhaler') incorporating a propellor in the mouthpiece; the airstream during inhalation rotates the propellor and dispenses the powder into the inhaled current of air. This technique, too, must be the subject of a practical demonstration in the course of consultation. The patient must understand that this is a prophylactic drug only, and has no bronchodilator effect. It must be used regularly, 20 mg q.i.d. initially: the dose can later be regulated according to the response to thrice or twice daily.

The only side effect is transient wheeze due to irritation of the bronchi. To counteract this, Intal Compound, in which a small dose of isoprenaline is incorporated, is recommended: but more satisfactory penetration of the dust into the bronchial tree is achieved by preceding the inhalation with one or two puffs of salbutamol.

Ketotifen (1 capsule t.i.d.) has a similar action, is taken by mouth, and is claimed to be helpful in facilitating withdrawal of steroids; its usefulness in this respect is not yet established.

Steroid hormones may be given orally, systemically, or topically; the indications and dosage are discussed in the following paragraphs.

Either prednisone or prednisolone are suitable oral preparations; other steroids offer no advantage and mostly have disadvantages, such as excessive protein loss or demineralization of bone. Hydrocortisone is given either intravenously or intramuscularly for status asthmaticus. Topical steroid by inhalation of aerosol (beclomethasone dipropionate, 2 puffs q.i.d.) is highly active so that only small amounts are required; about a quarter of the material reaches the lungs, whilst the rest is swallowed but occasions no systemic effects because of the small dosage. Its action is purely prophylactic. The only troublesome side effect is the occasional development of localized thrush (candidiasis) in the upper respiratory tract. Bronchopulmonary candidiasis is not a feature.

Drug management

This depends on the pattern of the illness, which varies from the occasional mild transient attack through a pattern of more or less severe acute exacerbations to severe and disabling chronic asthma. Any of these may proceed to status asthmaticus, which is a life-threatening medical emergency.

Occasional mild attacks can normally be controlled by the use of a salbutamol aerosol for symptomatic relief, without the need for continued prohylactic therapy.

Acute exacerbations normally follow provocation by infection, seasonal allergens, or non-specific irritants. Bronchodilator drugs alone are less likely to be effective unless given systemically; the incident is most conveniently managed by the use of oral steroids in the short term, starting with prednisolone 10 mg t.i.d. for 2 or 3 days, reducing by 5 mg daily until discontinued at the end of about a week. This method is essential to avoid habituation, a risk which the patient should understand. Monitoring of the response by twice daily measurement of the PEFR is helpful; early morning wheeze is usually the last symptom to disappear. Salbutamol by aerosol and delayed release aminophylline by mouth are suitable concomitant drugs which may be continued after the acute attack is over; an antibiotic is called for if infection is present or is suspected.

Chronic asthma, when the patient has some degree of wheeze through much of the year, calls for prophylactic therapy. This is given either as regular topical steroid therapy, which is highly effective except in the severe case, or as disodium cromoglycate, which is the drug of choice for most exercise-induced and some extrinsic cases. Either may usefully be preceded by an aerosol bronchodilator, which improves access to the airways, and supported by prolonged action bronchodilators if symptoms occur at night.

Only in the severe case is long-term oral steroid therapy called for: the response to prednisone should be assessed, usually in hospital, by regular (three or four times daily) measurement of FEV_1 and FVC; a substantial (at least 25%) increase after starting steroids should be obtained if long-term treatment with its attendant side effects is to be justified. Initially 30–40 mg prednisone should be given daily, the dose then being gradually reduced to the minimal level compatible with reasonable comfort. The process of reduction can be continued as an outpatient: in the later stages 1 mg tablets along with the basic 5 mg are useful in achieving the true minimum dosage, which commonly lies between 5 and 10 mg daily. Alternate-day therapy is said to lead to less long-term side effects, particularly fluid retention, but has the disadvantage that the PEFR commonly drops unacceptably on the day prednisone is withheld.

The patient should understand for himself the management of exacerbations occurring in the course of prophylactic therapy by a suitable but strictly temporary increase in oral steroid.

Management of status asthmaticus

The aim should be always to anticipate this dangerous situation by a prompt increase in oral steroids and attention to the precipitating factor, usually an infection. When severe asthma, not responding to bronchodilator treatment, has been present for more than 24–48 h, the patient is in danger from anoxia and must be admitted to hospital promptly. A useful initial measure before admission is intravenous aminophylline or salbutamol, with 200 mg hydrocortisone by the same route. Sedation of any kind must be meticuously avoided, though every effort must be made to instil confidence into the terrified and often exhausted patient, both with regard to his treatment and to his prospects of recovery.

After admission, an intravenous drip must be put up immediately to allow the administration of drugs, and to make good the dehydration which is invariably present; unless this is done expectoration of mucus plugs will be difficult or impossible.

Blood should be sent for estimation of gas tensions; oxygen by nasal catheter or by a face mask delivering up to 60% oxygen should be given unless there is evidence of hypercapnia, in which case 28% oxygen by Ventimask is safer. Preparations should be put in hand for endotracheal intubation should this be needed.

Hydrocortisone 200 mg 6-hourly intravenously should be continued, and oral prednisolone 60 mg daily started within 24 h; the hydrocortisone should be withdrawn if possible within 2–3 days as it is likely to lead to hypokalaemia and muscle weakness in a patient who is already exhausted. At the same time intravenous aminophylline or salbutamol may be repeated every 3–4 h during the critical phase. Aerosol therapy has little place at this stage, as no useful penetration of the narrowed and obstructed airways can be achieved.

Progress is indicated by reduction in the tachycardia and tachypnoea, by the relief of distress, by the ability to expectorate, and by improved chest wall movement. Auscultation gives little valuable information other than improvement in the breath sounds as the airways are cleared of mucus.

Indications for intubation and intermittent positive-pressure respiration are failure to improve with the above measures, the progressive exhaustion which follows the massive effort required to maintain respiration, persistent cyanosis, and even a minor degree of respiratory failure as shown by the blood gas tensions. IPPR requires sedation and a muscle relaxant, and provides a welcome release from the burden of breathing; it permits direct control of respiration, and, most importantly, it permits the regular aspiration by suction of bronchial secretions. Rarely, as a supplementary measure to clear bronchial plugs, lavage of the bronchial tree through the rigid bronchoscope may be very productive; up to 50 ml of 1% bicarbonate solution are injected under direct vision directly into the main segmental orifices, and followed by suction which frequently removes large numbers of bronchial casts. Intubation should be discontinued as soon as improvement is established; this may be after 24 h or several days. A week is the accepted maximum because of the risk of tracheal ulceration; exceptionally at this point tracheostomy may be called for.

During recovery the patient should be mobilized rapidly and the dose of steroid steadily reduced; he must be given full insight into his future management.

Pulmonary eosinophilia

Introduction

The function of eosinophils is unknown; an increase in the blood eosinophils (an arbitrary level of $500/mm^3$ is accepted as abnormal) is common in extrinsic asthma, and is often a feature of autoimmune pulmonary arteritis (also called polyarteritis nodosa (PAN) pulmonary form), which presents as asthma in a substantial proportion of cases. The concept of a spectrum of disease progressing from simple asthma to fully developed PAN is helpful; intermediate stages include asthma with eosinophilia and pulmonary shadows which may be transient. These lesions may have an autoimmune basis, or may represent a hypersensitivity reaction to an external agent, which in temperate climates is likely to be infestation with *Aspergillus fumigatus,* and in the tropics to filaria, a condition which responds well to treatment with diethylcarbamazine.

The cases of transient pulmonary shadowing with eosinophilia originally described by Loeffler were associated with infestation with the roundworm, *Ascaris lumbricoides,* and were relatively symptom-free. A similar clinical picture may follow reactions to drugs (p. 155).

Investigations

These include serial chest radiographs and differential white blood counts, together with a search for a possible causative agent. The erythrocyte sedimentation rate may be greatly elevated, particularly in autoimmune disease. Examination of the serum proteins may show a substantial increase in gammaglobulin.

Management

Management involves attention to any recognized causal agent—when none is found, oral prednisolone is usually highly effective, as asthma is more likely to be steroid sensitive with a high eosinophil count. An initial dosage of not less than 30 mg daily should be scaled down according to the response, and may need to be continued for many years.

Bronchopulmonary aspergillosis

Introduction

Infestation of the bronchial tree with the fungus *Aspergillus fumigatus* is a relatively common complication of atopic asthma, particularly if bronchiectasis is present. It is associated with both type I and type III hypersensitivity.

Clinical features

Aspergillosis not only leads to exacerbations of asthma by virtue of the reagin-mediated hypersensitivity to the fungus, but also may lead to progressive long-term lung damage as a result of plugging of bronchi by mucus laden with mycelium, which reacts in situ with antibody in the bronchial mucosa; the resulting antigen–antibody complexes are tissue damaging, and characteristically lead to localized bronchiectasis which is proximal in distribution. Expectoration of bronchial casts is a very characteristic feature.

Investigations

The *blood count* shows substantial eosinophilia in the majority of cases. Colonies of fungus are grown only if *sputum culture* is carried out on Sabouraud's medium at 37 °C. Mycelium may be seen on direct microscopy of bronchial casts.

Precipitating antibodies are readily demonstrable in the serum, which may be tested against the patient's own strain of fungus.

Skin testing, by the prick test, using a standard solution of aspergillin, leads to an immediate weal and flare reaction, and, in addition, very commonly to a delayed response 4–6 h later, with itching, and oedema often several centimetres in diameter, but without erythema.

Chest radiography shows transient infiltrates during acute exacerbations; when bronchiectasis is established mucus plugging may show as finger-like opacities extending from the hilum.

Management

Because of its high potential for causing progressive lung damage, the acute attack of asthma with aspergillosis and bronchial plugging requires vigorous treatment, with energetic and precise physiotherapy along with a temporary increase in steroids. The aim is expectoration of bronchial plugs without delay.

In the intractable chronic case, antifungal agents may be used, and sometimes lead to a limited degree of improvement. Amphotericin B is nephrotoxic and should be reserved for the severely ill; it is given by intravenous infusion, 250 μg/kg to 1 mg/kg body weight daily. Natamycin, 25 mg/ml is relatively non-toxic, and administered in a nebulizer, 1 ml/8-hourly, for 2–6 weeks.

The associated chronic asthma is treated on its merits; steroids tends to promote growth of fungus, but nevertheless may be necessary. Cromoglycate is very often effective.

Oral antifungal agents, such as ketaconazole 200 mg daily, are not of proven value but hold some promise.

Summary

Bronchopulmonary aspergillosis should be considered in any severe asthmatic with eosinophilia, especially if there are transient lung opacities on radiography. It is not uncommon, and must be recognized and treated to minimize progressive lung damage.

Extrinsic allergic alveolitis

Introduction

External allergic alveolitis is a type III hypersensitivity response which may follow exposure to a wide variety of inhaled organic antigens, most of which are occupational in origin (*see* Farmer's lung, p. 144). The lung parenchyma is involved, with infiltration by plasma cells, polymorphs and lymphocytes, thickening of the alveolar walls, and in chronic cases granuloma formation and irreversible lung fibrosis. The commonest non-occupational variety is bird fanciers' lung, which commonly relates to pet budgerigars. More than one antigen may be involved in the same individual, e.g. a farmer who keeps a budgerigar.

Clinical features

There may be an immediate non-specific reaction to dust exposure with cough and wheeziness, but the typical symptoms occur some 4–6 h after exposure, and include malaise, aches in the limbs, cough and tightness in the chest. The main symptom with regular exposure is constant effort dyspnoea, which disappears after removal from the antigen; thus spontaneous relief after admission to hospital is a strong pointer to the diagnosis. In chronic cases with established fibrosis the dyspnoea is of course permanent.

Physical signs

In the acute stage there may be obstruction of the pulmonary vascular bed with tachypnoea, cyanosis, and grossly overfilled jugular veins; auscultation reveals abundant basal râles with diffuse fine rhonchi. In the chronic case the râles persist and finger clubbing may develop.

Investigations

Precipitating antibodies are demonstrable in the serum; they may be present, however, in symptom-free individuals who have been exposed to the dust but have developed no obvious lung reaction.

Lung function tests show a restrictive impairment of ventilation, along with impairment of the gas transfer factor, which is a useful guide to the effectiveness of treatment if repeated at intervals.

The *chest radiograph* in the acute stages shows widespread soft, nodular shadowing which may be confluent, and which clears completely with recovery; chronic cases show linear shadowing sometimes with microcystic changes, which may predominantly affect the upper zones.

Management

Recognition of, and removal from, the responsible antigen effects complete relief in the early case: if symptoms are severe steroids are highly effective, and should be continued only to the point of maximal clinical and physiological improvement. Established fibrosis does not respond to any form of treatment.

Systemic diseases (including the collagenoses and autoimmune disease)
Fibrosing alveolitis

The principal pathological features are thickening of the alveolar membrane, desquamation of macrophages into the alveoli and progressive interstitial fibrosis with ultimately microcystic changes. It may be associated with rheumatoid arthropathy, commonly, or chronic active hepatitis, rarely. Identical lung changes may be present in scleroderma (systemic sclerosis). Although immunofluorescent staining of the lung sections shows antigen–antibody complexes, organ-specific antibodies are not present in the serum. The relationship with other collagen or immune disorders is ill-defined and the aetiology usually obscure: the prefix 'cryptogenic' makes the position clear.

The eponym, Hamman–Rich disease, should be reserved for rapidly progressive fibrosis fatal in less than a year, as described by those authors.

Clinical features

The onset is commonly in middle life. The leading *symptom* is progressive effort dyspnoea; the course is very variable, but progression to a fatal outcome in less than 5 years is frequent. There is an increased incidence of bronchial carcinoma as a terminal complication.

The *physical signs* are widespread showers of late inspiratory crepitations extending from the lung bases to the interscapular region; these are more widespread initially than the radiographic changes. Finger clubbing is usual; the classic changes of rheumatoid arthritis are present in upwards of 10% of cases.

Investigations

The *chest radiograph* shows micronodular and linear shadowing, mainly in the lower zones; late in the illness microcystic changes develop (*Fig.* 2.14).

Lung function tests show small lungs with restriction of ventilation, substantial impairment of the gas transfer factor, and hypocapnia due to hyperventilation. Hypoxia is a late development.

The *ESR* is commonly raised, along with the serum gammaglobulins. The *serum rheumatoid factor* is positive in half the cases, many with no evidence of arthritis. Antinuclear antibody and other non-specific antibodies may also be present.

Lung biopsy may, very rarely, be advisable to confirm the diagnosis and

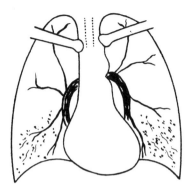

Fig. 2.14 Fibrosing alveolitis.

assess treatability: this should be done by formal, though limited, thoracotomy, which provides a better specimen, and is safer than needle biopsy. Washings obtained at bronchoscopy may also give guidance as to steroid therapy, which is more likely to be effective if the cellularity is high.

Management
The differential diagnosis is wide, including extrinsic alveolitis, bronchiectasis, and heart failure. A clinical trial of steroids (prednisolone 40 mg daily) is justified, preferably monitored by serial gas transfer tests as well as radiographs. When improvement follows, which happens only in a minority, the steroid requirement may be reduced by giving immunosuppressive drugs, e.g. azathioprine (Imuran) 50–100 mg daily, in addition. In the late stages portable oxygen therapy may facilitate the performance of daily necessary tasks.

Rheumatoid lung disease

This presents in several ways:
1. *A pleural effusion* may considerably antedate the arthropathy; it is not accompanied by constitutional disturbance, but may be preceded or followed often for several months by dry pleurisy, of which the patient is aware. Both serum and pleural fluid are positive for rheumatoid factor, which should be looked for in all undiagnosed pleural effusions. Treatment is not normally required.
2. *Fibrosing alveolitis.* A proportion of patients with seropositive rheumatoid arthritis have lung lesions indistinguishable, clinically or pathologically, from fibrosing alveolitis. This form of rheumatoid lung disease also requires a trial of steroid therapy, starting with a substantial dose (e.g. 40 mg daily) of prednisolone to assess responsiveness.

3. *Nodular rheumatoid lung disease* may present with one, or more often several, well defined and usually rounded lesions from 0·5 cm to several centimetres in diameter (*Fig.* 2.15). They may cavitate, and vary in size spontaneously; they are unaffected by treatment, and ultimately may progress to malignant lymphoma with hepatosplenomegaly. The nodules may antedate the arthropathy and lead to a mistaken diagnosis of malignant disease unless the serum is examined for rheumatoid factor.

4. *Caplan's syndrome.* Lung nodules complicating coal workers' pneumoconiosis, in the presence of rheumatoid arthritis, is referred to on p. 135.

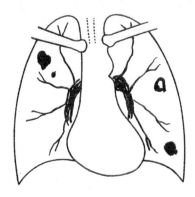

Fig. 2.15 Nodular rheumatoid lesions.

Autoimmune polyarteritis

Introduction

Polyarteritis nodosa is a multisystem collagen disorder, protean in its manifestations, as the endarteritis may lead to ischaemic damage and infarction in any organ. Muscle pain and constitutional disturbance, together with hypertension and renal impairment, are among the commoner findings, but in a high proportion of cases the lungs alone are involved initially. Particularly with steroid treatment, the disease may not progress to involve other organs.

Pathologically there is dense round cell and polymorph infiltration of the vessel walls, with endothelial thickening and, ultimately, thrombosis.

Clinical features

The clinical features of the pulmonary form of polyarteritis include malaise, fever, cough, tightness in the chest, tachypnoea, and pleurisy; physical signs are not usually helpful, except in those patients who present initially with asthma, with eosinophilia. The possibility of a drug hypersensitivity reaction should be kept in mind. In the generalized form of the disease any organ may be involved, and the clinical picture is correspondingly complex; death is commonly due to renal failure.

Investigations

The *blood count* shows a substantial polymorphonuclear leucocytosis, often with a high proportion of eosinophils. The *ESR* is substantially raised, as are the serum gammaglobulins. There is no diagnostic serological test.

The *chest radiograph* shows fluffy shadows, usually bilateral, which are due to localized oedema, and sometimes infarction relating to arterial or arteriolar occlusions. The appearance is not specific, but the spontaneous changes both in size and location of the lesions are highly characteristic; over the course of a few days some may disappear as others appear elsewhere.

Detailed renal function studies are necessary. *Muscle biopsy* is usually only helpful if muscular tenderness or palpable nodularity is present.

Management

The response to steroids is immediate and striking, not least to the patient whose symptoms may vanish in a matter of hours after starting treatment. The radiological shadows clear substantially in the course of a few days. Steroid therapy may therefore be useful as a diagnostic test, but must not be started before all the necessary investigations are set up, because any biochemical changes will be rapidly masked. Once started, treatment needs to continue for many years; initially at least 40 mg prednisolone daily should be given, but this can be reduced in stages to a maintenance dose which will vary from patient to patient. After some months an immunosuppressive drug (e.g. azathioprine) can be introduced to facilitate reduction of the steroids. Therapy may be stopped after an arbitrary period of 5 years or more, but the patient must be carefully observed for evidence of relapse for some years after this.

Systemic lupus erythematosus (SLE)

SLE is an autoimmune disease; the very similar features due to drug hypersensitivity have already been referred to (p. 103).

The characteristic *clinical features* include a facial rash of butterfly distribution, renal impairment, small joint arthropathy and polyserositis involving both pleura and pericardium. The salient feature in the chest therefore is pleurisy.

Investigations

The *chest radiograph* may show small basal pleural effusions, with an enlarged heart shadow; the ECG usually confirms the presence of pericarditis. Patchy irregular lung shadows may also be present.

The *blood count* shows a leucopenia, usually less than 5000 total white count, with a high ESR. Smears should be examined repeatedly for LE cells (lymphocytes swollen with dark-staining antigen–antibody complex) which if present are diagnostic.

Antinuclear and anti-DNA antibody is usually present in the serum to a high titre.

Management

Management is along the same lines as for polyarteritis nodosa, but the response to steroids is by no means as immediate. Permanent remission may sometimes occur after several years of treatment; the degree of aggressiveness of the disease varies considerably.

Systemic sclerosis (sclerodema)

This presents with tightening of the skin of the fingers and face, leading to pinching of the features, and subungal telangiectases. There is usually a long prior history of Raynaud's phenomenon. The oesophagus may be narrowed with an incompetent cardia, leading to aspiration pneumonia as a secondary effect on the lungs; the other, and frequent, pulmonary complication is diffuse fibrosis, indistinguishable from fibrosing alveolitis.

Management

Steroids tend to have disappointingly little effect, but progression may be delayed by the use of immunosuppressive drugs.

Immune failure

1. Agammaglobulinaemia

This is due to congenital reduction or absence of circulating gammaglobulin, leading to a failure of antibody response when infection occurs. It should be looked for in any patient with a long history, usually from childhood, of recurrent severe chest infections responding poorly to treatment. The patient develops severe chronic bronchitis, often with bronchiectasis, with airway obstruction and, ultimately, cor pulmonale. The prognosis may be greatly improved by giving regular injections of gammaglobulin, usually 1 g weekly, but the dose should be adjusted according to the serum level achieved; antibiotic-resistant organisms pose great problems.

2. Due to immunosuppressive or cytotoxic therapy

Immune failure due to immunosuppressive or cytotoxic therapy in the treatment of transplants, malignant disease, leukaemia, or lymphoma, may be followed by infection by opportunist organisms, e.g. *Pneumocystis carinii, Aspergillus fumigatus,* which may be difficult or impossible to eradicate.

Sarcoidosis

Introduction

Historically the first manifestation of sarcoidosis to be recognized clinically was the chronic violaceous skin lesion (lupus pernio). The papular lesions vary in size, and cause no symptoms, but may pose a cosmetic problem. The histology shows a granuloma with large epitheloid cells with occasional giant cells, together with peripheral lymphocytic infiltration; fibrosis is variable and caseation absent. This diagnostic appearance may be present in almost any organ, those commonly affected being the reticulo-endothelial system, lungs, skin, uveal tract, and kidneys; the heart and central nervous system are less often involved. The diagnosis should be positively established by biopsy as soon as possible, particularly in chronic cases, in view of the protean nature of the disease which can otherwise lead to difficulties in management.

The cause of sarcoidosis is unknown; it is more commonly seen in advanced than in underdeveloped societies, and there are considerable racial variations in prevalence. It is much commoner for example in American negroes than whites, and in Irish immigrants to the UK than in English residents. Several members of one family may be involved; simultaneous onset in siblings has been recorded, which suggests the possibility of an infective agent, but none has been identified. On the other hand, industrial exposure to beryllium, used in the manufacture of strip lighting, may lead to a disorder clinically indistinguishable from chronic sarcoidosis; the beryllium salt is recoverable from the lesions.

Sarcoidosis appears to be an abnormal immune response to a variety of unidentified causes and is, curiously, associated with suppression of type IV delayed hypersensitivity to tuberculin or other agents. The characteristically negative Mantoux test was thought to suggest a relationship to tuberculosis, but this view is no longer widely held as the suppression of hypersensitivity is non-specific.

Clinical features

1. *Acute manifestations*
The commonest acute presentation is bilateral hilar lymph node enlargement, often associated with erythema nodosum, which in itself causes no symptoms, and sometimes with transient polyarthropathy affecting the larger joints, parotid enlargement and anterior uveitis.

These changes usually settle without treatment; the clinical features are sufficiently characteristic for a clinical diagnosis to be made with confidence in the majority, without recourse to biopsy.

2. *Chronic manifestations* include hypercalcaemia and hypercalciuria, which may lead ultimately to renal failure; chronic iridocyclitis, which may cause severe visual loss or blindness; central nervous system changes including VIIIth nerve palsy, and epilepsy; skin lesions and bone cysts (affecting the terminal phalanges) which constitute clear indications of chronicity; and infiltration and later fibrosis of the lungs. Infiltration may be very extensive without causing any dyspnoea at all, which is the converse of the situation in fibrosing alveolitis. Only a small proportion goes on to

develop disabling lung fibrosis and ultimately cor pulmonale. Chronic disease commonly requires treatment to anticipate ultimate organ failure.

SARCOIDOSIS OF THE HEART

Chronic sarcoidosis may involve the myocardium and the conducting tissues; it is being increasingly recognized as a cause of sudden death in previously symptomless young people; but it more commonly presents with recurrent dysrhythmia. The prevalence of this manifestation of sarcoidosis is unknown as the diagnosis is likely to be missed unless other features of sarcoidosis are also present. It should be suspected particularly in younger people with persistent dysrhythmias, and is of particular importance if there is an occupational hazard, for example in the case of airline pilots.

Investigations

The Mantoux test is commonly negative, even using 1/100 tuberculin. The *Kveim test* is carried out by an intradermal injection of an extract of human sarcoid spleen; the site is marked and biopsied 4–6 weeks later; positive cases show a typical sarcoid granuloma with giant cells. The test is claimed by some to be a non-specific reaction common to many forms of adenopathy; it appears to be reliable, however, provided the correct specific antigen is used.

The serum gammaglobulins are raised in about half the cases; the ESR is raised in the acute stage.

BIOPSY

The Kveim test is unnecessary if a positive biopsy of liver, skin, or a lymph node is obtained.

RADIOLOGICAL CHANGES

Acute. In the chest film bilateral hilar lymphadenopathy is usually symmetrical (*Fig. 2.16*), the nodes tending to stand clearer of the hilum than is the case with many other forms of lymphadenopathy. It may occur without erythema nodosum, but the diagnosis may nevertheless be clear from radiological features, particularly as spontaneous regression is the rule.

About 1 case in 5 of nodal enlargement also shows scattered infiltrates in the lung fields at the time of diagnosis, or developing within a few months of the onset.

Chronic. A minority show initial widespread chronic disease with linear as well as nodular shadowing indicating established fibrosis; this may be associated with minor cystic changes, up to 1–2 cm in diameter, and tends to affect the midzones.

Cystic changes in the terminal phalanges are uncommon and a feature of very chronic disease; routine diagnostic radiography of the hands is not justified unless there is already evidence of chronic disease.

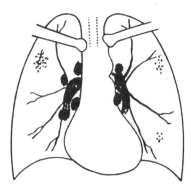

Fig. 2.16 Sarcoidosis.

Lung function tests are normal in acute disease. When lung infiltrations are substantial there is a relatively modest reduction of the gas transfer factor, which may be monitored as a guide to the effectiveness of therapy; there may be restrictive impairment of ventilation in extensive disease, but airway obstruction is not a feature.

Electrocardiography may show conduction defects when the heart is involved; scanning of the heart may demonstrate deposits in the myocardium.

Management

The acute manifestations settle down without treatment; erythema nodosum in a few weeks, hilar adenopathy in a few months. Late recurrence is rare, but occasional review for a couple of years is usual.

When pulmonary infiltrates are present at diagnosis they should be observed for about 6 months: about a third will have regressed by this time. If they are static or progressive, treatment (*see below*) will be required to prevent progression to lung failure or cor pulmonale, but this occurs in only a small proportion, less than 10% of cases with infiltrations. Treatment is also required for those few patients who present initially with widespread chronic disease, without hilar adenopathy.

Hypercalcaemia is an indication for treatment, to anticipate ultimate renal failure; it is usually controlled by a modest dose of prednisone.

Chronic iridocyclitis requires local steroid treatment indefinitely, to prevent progression, supported by oral therapy in severe cases.

Skin lesions may also require local steroid, hydrocortisone as a cream or by local injection, if they are cosmetically troublesome.

The treatment of chronic lung changes is with oral steroids, prednisolone 30 mg initially, and reducing, according to the radiological and physiological response, usually to 10 mg daily or less. Once started steroids have to be continued for some years, and possibly indefinitely, as the disease is liable to relapse acutely on withdrawal of treatment.

Other drugs are relatively ineffective and rarely used, e.g. chloroquine
sulphate, 250 mg once or twice daily, or anti-inflammatory drugs
Permanent pace-making is mandatory for cardiac dysrhymias.

2.5 VASCULAR DISORDERS

Pulmonary embolism and infarction

Introduction
Obstruction of the pulmonary arteries by clots presents in a variety of ways
varying in degree from the immediately fatal massive embolism to repeated
silent minor infarcts, which lead ultimately to pulmonary hypertension as the
vascular bed becomes progressively obstructed.

The term 'embolism' should be reserved for cases in which there is good
evidence of a source, most commonly in the leg or pelvic veins, but sometimes
in the right side of the heart. When there is no such evidence, it is more accurate
to refer to infarction, which does not in itself imply any particular causation
Infarction is common when the lung is already congested, and may relate to
endocrine causes, intimal damage, or platelet abnormalities.

It follows that there is a variety of clinical presentations.

1. Massive pulmonary embolism

Clinical Features
Massive embolism occurs most frequently following prolonged bed rest and
characteristically about 10 days after major surgery. Its incidence has been
greatly reduced in recent decades, by reason of much earlier mobilization
and in some circumstances by the use of prophylactic anticoagulant therapy
The source lies in the deep femoral or pelvic veins, where lengthy and friable
clots may build up remarkably quickly, with little adherence to the venous
intima; local signs may be remarkably few. The thigh or leg may or may not
be oedematous, and though the deep femoral vein is usually palpable, it may
not be; the only evidence of thrombosis in the pelvic veins may be a mild
fever and leucocytosis. When a substantial clot passes through the heart into
a pulmonary artery, and is large enough to obliterate a major branch, the
principal feature is the dramatically sudden onset of shock, often with
transient loss of consciousness. Obstruction of more than one major branch
of the pulmonary arterial tree is likely to be fatal; in contrast, ligation of a
main pulmonary artery during pneumonectomy is uneventful, so that in
embolism an extra factor is involved, probably reflex constriction of the
remainder of the pulmonary arteries. The result is an abrupt and severe fall in
cardiac output.

If the patient survives the immediate impact, examination reveals severe
distress, with marked tachypnoea, sweating, pallor and cyanosis which does

not respond to oxygen therapy; the periphery is cold and pale, the blood pressure low or unrecordable, the pulse rapid and thready, the neck veins distended, and an extra heart sound is usually present. There may be crushing central chest pain.

Investigations

The condition must be differentiated from cardiac infarction, severe internal haemorrhage, gram-negative septicaemia, acute pancreatitis, dissecting aneurysm, and cardiac tamponade due to haemopericardium following rupture of a cardiac infarct.

Investigations include an *ECG*, which may show acute right ventricular strain (T inversion in the right chest leads with right bundle-branch block— S_1Q_3 pattern) or may be normal; a *chest radiograph*, which may show peripheral ischaemia, but is often unhelpful; and when facilities are available, pulmonary arteriography provides definitive information, and is the most useful single investigation. Blood should be taken for culture, and for serum amylase and transaminase levels.

Management

No drug is likely to help the immediate situation. Oxygen therapy should be given, followed by *fibrinolytic therapy* in the form of streptokinase, 600000 u intravenously by infusion over 30 min, followed by 100000 u hourly for several days. Anticoagulant therapy is indicated, to anticipate further embolism, but must on no account be started until the fibrinolytic treatment has been completed on account of the risk of haemorrhage.

Embolectomy may be successful, but is rarely performed because facilities and the necessary expertise are not usually immediately to hand; furthermore, fibrinolytic therapy appears to give comparable results.

The emphasis, in the face of an expected mortality of about 50%, must lie in *preventive* measures, of which early postoperative mobilization is the most important, along with a frequent cycle of leg exercises whilst the patient is still in bed. Treatment with routine *prophylactic anticoagulants,* started immediately after operation, has produced a dramatic drop in mortality, particularly in the treatment of fracture of the femur.

Anticoagulant treatment should be started on even slight suspicion of pelvic or deep femoral vein thrombosis during the postoperative period— slight unexplained fever and leucocytosis, without any local signs at all, is sufficient indication. Additional tests for venous thrombosis (ultrasonic probes, ^{125}I fibrinogen isotope uptake) are only occasionally helpful.

2. *Minor pulmonary embolism and infarction*

Smaller emboli occur more frequently, and may arise from obvious thrombophlebitis in the leg veins, where the local inflammatory response, recognizable by local erythema and tenderness, renders the clot more adherent to the venous intima; massive embolus is therefore much less likely. Minor embolism may also occasionally stem from mural endocardial thrombus after septal cardiac infarction.

Infarction may be due to local thrombosis associated with increased blood coagulability, which may be related to the use of contraceptive hormones and may be exacerbated by smoking; in either case the platelet stickiness is likely to be increased. Infarcts are found at autopsy in chronic obstructive airway disease with much greater frequency than they are recognized in life.

Clinical features

The symptoms are referable mainly to the chest, without the profound collapse characteristic of massive embolism. The classic triad of symptoms are pleuritic pain with dyspnoea followed by minor fresh haemoptysis. The clue to the diagnosis of embolism lies in the very sudden onset of pain, which can usually be accurately remembered and related to what the patient was doing at the time; it varies in degree, but is usually troublesome. Infarction, particularly when not due to embolism, is frequently misdiagnosed as an infection. On physical examination there is mild fever, often but not always rapid breathing, with showers of râles over the affected area. After a day or two the signs of a small effusion may develop, which is usually slightly haemorrhagic.

Pulmonary infarcts are liable to secondary infection, either by septic organisms or fungus infestation with *Aspergillus fumigatus*. This may lead to liquefaction of the infarct and abscess formation, with associated abundant infected sputum.

Investigations

The *chest radiograph* shows a non-specific ill-defined opacity which is not usually recognizably wedge-shaped (*Fig.* 2.17). In the early stages elevation of the diaphragm is usual, and a positive diagnostic feature. After a few days an effusion may develop, along with linear shadowing which represents pleural invagination at the site of the infarct, and which may take several weeks or months to clear. These linear shadows may be bilateral, and are usually seen just above the diaphragm or in the costophrenic angle (*Fig.* 2.18). They require to be distinguished from 'plate atelectases' which look similar, but are not associated with other features of embolism, and tend to occur when the diaphragm is raised for other reasons (e.g. pregnancy, ascites); they do not require treatment and disappear when the diaphragm returns to normal. They are a feature of acute cholecystitis.

A *scintiscan of lung* may show unsuspected multiple defects, but similar changes may also be seen in obstructive airway disease.

Blood examination shows a moderate polymorphonuclear leucocytosis; fibrinogen breakdown products are increased initially and may help in the diagnosis from pneumonia.

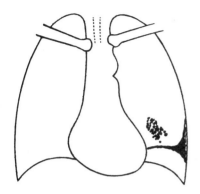
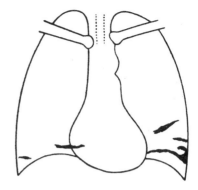

Fig. 2.17 Minor pulmonary embolism.

Fig. 2.18 Minor embolism during resolution, showing invaginations of pleura.

The *ECG* may show transient T wave inversion over the right chest leads.

The *platelet stickiness* should be measured, if possible before starting treatment.

Management

The diagnosis is not always straightforward, and even when suspected may be difficult to confirm. The basis of management is to give short-term anticoagulants, up to 3 months, whilst taking steps to treat the source of embolism, or to find, and when possible remove, other causes of infarction, in particular smoking or contraceptive hormones. Recurring incidents are not infrequent, often without obvious cause, and may be an indication for long-term anticoagulant treatment, particularly if the platelet adhesiveness is increased. If an infarct becomes infected, antibacterial therapy is indicated, as for lung abscess (*see* p. 64).

Microembolism

Clinical features

Microembolism may occur without causing any immediate symptoms; eventually effort dyspnoea ensues as pulmonary hypertension develops because of progressive obliteration of the pulmonary vasculature. This is recognized on clinical examination by the presence of a left parasternal heave due to the enlarged right ventricle, with a loud and often reduplicated pulmonary second sound. Microembolism may follow pregnancy or the use of contraceptive hormones, or have no recognizable cause; it is impossible to distinguish from primary pulmonary hypertension, a rare disorder of unknown aetiology. Rarely, the microemboli consist of clumps of malignant cells, usually stemming from carcinoma of the breast or ovary.

Investigations

Cardiographically the right chest leads show an rR pattern with T wave inversion, and the left chest leads show deep S waves.

Chest radiography is unhelpful.

Management

Long-term anticoagulants are indicated as offering the best chance of delaying progression of a disorder which may be fatal after only a few years; a possible but unproven alternative is to use dipyridamole (Persantin) 100–200 mg q.i.d. In the later stages heart failure treatment is indicated, but is unlikely to be very effective.

Pulmonary oedema

Introduction

Under physiological conditions the interstitial space in the lungs, between the alveolar cells and the small blood vessels, is kept free of any excess of fluid by the osmotic gradient exerted by the plasma proteins, and by centripetal lymphatic drainage. The space is continuous from the lung periphery to the interstitial tissue surrounding the large blood vessels and airways. Interference with fluid clearance is commonly due to an increase in pulmonary capillary pressure because of impaired contraction of the left ventricle, leading to interstitial oedema; this in turn leads to compression of the small airways and small blood vessels, and consequent impairment of both ventilation and perfusion. The resulting local anoxia leads to vasoconstriction and redirection of the blood supply to unaffected areas. It may also interfere with the production of surfactant, a lipid substance which normally counteracts surface tension and maintains distensibility of the lung; a deficiency of it leads to increasing stiffness and loss of compliance. The accumulated interstitial fluid causes reflex stimulation of the respiratory centre and tachypnoea: it is mediated by vagal nerve endings.

Severe interstitial oedema may be followed by leakage of fluid directly into the alveoli after inadequate lymphatic clearance.

Interstitial oedema also occurs in some other situations, for example after head injury or cerebral haemorrhage, probably mediated by a reflex mechanism; or as part of general anasarca when intracapillary osmotic pressure is impaired following reduction in the plasma proteins for any reason.

Fluid may also leak into the alveoli directly as a result of damage to the alveolar cell membrane following inhalation of toxic gases such as chlorine.

Clinical findings

Dyspnoea is the *cardinal symptom,* the pattern depending on the degree of oedema. Initially it occurs only after effort, and after lying flat in bed which leads to distressing paroxysms of nocturnal dyspnoea; it may be difficult to distinguish from nocturnal asthma, but unlike asthma morning wheeze on waking is not a feature. As the condition progresses non-productive cough, either at night or on effort, is usual, together with breathlessness sitting up at rest. Finally as alveolar fluid increases and passes into the larger airways, extreme dyspnoea, cyanosis, abundant frothy and often bloodstained watery sputum develop, with terror of impending death; acute pulmonary oedema is of course a life-threatening medical emergency. Cheyne–Stokes respiration, with intermittent apnoea, may be a feature from the relatively early stages.

On auscultation, rattling of oedema fluid in the larger airways is audible in the severe cases without the help of a stethoscope; diffuse expiratory rhonchi, due to compression of the small airways by interstitial fluid, may be indistinguishable from those of asthma. In the early case the characteristic sign is showers of late inspiratory crepitations as the compressed small airways snap open; the crepitations give way later to coarse mid-inspiratory râles.

The cause of the oedema is usually left ventricular failure; cardiac signs may not be easy to elicit because of the noises in the lungs, but a fourth heart sound is the most useful single piece of evidence, and may disappear in a few hours after effective treatment has been initiated. The signs of congestive heart failure (overfilled neck veins, hepatomegaly, dependent oedema) may be inconspicuous or absent.

Investigations

The *chest radiograph* may show both vascular and lung changes. The heart is commonly enlarged, and the mid-lung blood vessels prominent, especially in the upper zones due to diversion of the blood flow thither from the stiff and oedematous lower lobes. The lungs may appear normal in early cases, but with established oedema dilated lymphatics, seen as horizontal linear opacities in the costophrenic angles, are a common and diagnostically specific sign. In acute severe oedema, and particularly in the fluid retention of acute renal failure, large ill-defined opacities may fill most of both lung fields ('butterfly' shadows); or they may be of more patchy distribution. There may be associated soft generalized nodular shadowing.

As pulmonary oedema is often precipitated by acute renal failure, renal function must be carefully watched.

Lung function tests show restricted ventilation with impaired gas transfer; due to hyperventilation the $P\text{CO}_2$ is often reduced, along with the $P\text{O}_2$.

Management

Morphine sulphate 10–20 mg by subcutaneous or intramuscular injection should be given as soon as the diagnosis of pulmonary oedema due to cardiac or renal failure has been established; it has a dramatic effect in reducing fear and restlessness and therefore the demand for oxygen but it must be remembered that it also reduces respiratory drive and is not to be given in the presence of respiratory failure.

Oxygen should be given by spectacles with nasal catheters, or by a mask designed to deliver up to 60% oxygen; if there is any question of hypercapnic lung failure, the percentage of oxygen should not initially exceed 28% unless the trachea has already been intubated. The prolonged use of high concentrations of oxygen may lead to toxic damage at alveolar level, with patchy lung collapse and progressive deterioration which can be fatal unless the development of oxygen toxicity is recognized.

Diuretic therapy is given immediately as intravenous frusemide, not less than 80 mg repeated at least 12-hourly in the initial stages; this is gradually reduced during convalescence.

Digitalis is indicated, particularly if atrial fibrillation is present.

In the acute emergency, tourniquets (sphygmomanometer cuffs inflated above diastolic blood pressure) applied to all four limbs may be life saving in the short term, pending further measures; removal of a pint of blood by venesection is similarly effective.

Intermittent positive-pressure respiration (IPPR) after tracheal intubation may be sometimes called for to enable safe administration of high concentrations of oxygen, to facilitate aspiration of bronchial secretions by suction, and to relieve exhaustion.

Some miscellaneous vascular disorders

Angiitis may be due to hypersensitivity to a drug, or to autoimmune disease (*see* p. 108); in either event it clears dramatically with steroids.

Idiopathic haemosiderosis follow the deposit of haemosiderin in the alveoli, resulting from episodes of microscopic angiitis; this produces dense nodulation on the radiograph, and haemosiderin-laden macrophages are found in the sputum. The condition leads to death from lung failure usually before adult life is reached.

Similar lung changes are sometimes seen as a complication of mitral stenosis, and may be reversible if the stenosis is relieved.

Congenital arteriovenous aneurysm in the lung may be multiple, and is often associated with similar lesions in the liver and buccal mucosa. It presents radiologically as a dense lobulated shadow or shadows, continuous with a major branch of a pulmonary artery and well demonstrated on tomography; it may nevertheless be confused with bronchial carcinoma. On auscultation a localized bruit may be heard over the lesion. Arteriovenous aneurysm may lead eventually to haemodynamic problems due to the shunt and may also develop bacterial endarteritis.

Surgical removal is difficult because multiple lesions are usually present.

2.6 CARCINOMA OF THE BRONCHUS

Introduction

Incidence

The incidence of bronchial carcinoma has increased relentlessly over the last five decades. Currently it accounts for over 30 000 deaths per annum in England and Wales, compared with 1000 per annum in the second decade of the century. It is over five times commoner in men but the incidence in women is rising steadily; in men the rate of increase has declined somewhat, the older age group being proportionately more affected. Lung cancer accounts for nearly half of all male cancer deaths and has replaced tuberculosis as a major killing disease.

Aetiology

Smoking

The evidence incriminating cigarette smoking as the major cause is overwhelming, the increase in risk being directly proportional to the number of cigarettes smoked. The chance of developing lung cancer is forty times greater for an individual who smokes forty cigarettes a day than it is for a non-smoker. The lower but steadily increasing incidence in women relates directly to the later adoption by women of the cigarette habit.

In countries where cigarette smoking is not practised, or has only recently been introduced, bronchial carcinoma remains a rare disease.

Pipe and cigar smoking carries only a small increase in risk, whilst smoking filter-tipped cigarettes reduces it a little. The type of tobacco smoked is evidently important: that cured in the sun over prolonged periods, as in Turkey and France, is less carcinogenic than tobacco cured quickly in sheds, as in Virginia and Zimbabwe; the difference is related to the fact that glycolysis is incomplete in artificially cured tobaccos, which therefore have a higher content of sugars.

Efforts to produce a substitute that will satisfy smokers have proved unsuccessful, though the use of chewing gum-containing nicotine, which is the chief factor in maintaining addiction, may help some patients by relieving the immediate withdrawal symptoms; the addict must, however, be highly motivated.

Once smoking has ceased the likelihood of developing lung cancer gradually declines, and returns to the non-smoker's level of risk after somewhat more than 10 years.

Climate

The risk of bronchial carcinoma in European smokers who emigrate to Australasia is diminished, which suggests that climate may be a factor.

Pollution

Atmospheric pollution is thought to play some part as urban dwellers have a somewhat higher incidence than country people which is not accounted for by differences in smoking. Diesel fumes are sometimes held to be important, but no increase has been demonstrated in workers especially exposed to them. Overall, atmospheric pollution plays an unimportant part in aetiology compared with smoking.

Industrial exposure may be important, especially the mining of radioactive ores (cobalt, uranium), whilst haematite mining and exposure to chromates, arsenic and nickel fumes have all been incriminated. Asbestosis and cigarette smoking together carries a prodigiously high risk, suggesting a synergistic effect.

Pathology

Tumour types

The proportion of the different types of tumour varies with the source of the series being reported, due to factors of selection. The position is complicated further by difficulty in classifying some tumours, which may show varying cell types in different areas. Malignant change usually originates in the lung periphery, and the clinical presentation varies with the subsequent pattern of evolution of the tumour.

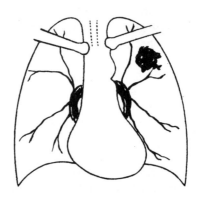

Fig. 2.19 Squamous carcinoma.

Squamous carcinoma accounts for more than a third of all cases, and is characterized by a substantial primary lesion in the lung, with relatively little lymph node involvement (*Fig.* 2.19). These tumours are therefore the most frequently operable, but the late results remain disappointing because of the frequent presence of occult small metastases, which only become manifest after surgery.

Undifferentiated carcinomas account for over half the cases in most series, and may be large or small ('oat') celled. They often have a small

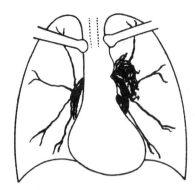

Fig. 2.20 Undifferentiated carcinoma.

primary lung lesion with early and gross hilar node involvement (*Fig.* 2.20), as well as distal metastases, and tend to grow rapidly. The small-cell variety is remarkable for inappropriate hormone production in a proportion of cases.

Adenocarcinoma accounts for less than a tenth of cases and is the tumour found in non-smokers in the very large majority.

Mode of spread
Within the lung, spread is by the peribronchial lymphatics to the hilar nodes; the lymphatic drainage is from left to right, so that a primary in the left lung will readily lead to involvement of the right hilar nodes and the nodes in the right supraclavicular angle. Distal metastasis occurs by the bloodstream, most commonly to the liver, adrenals, brain, bone (usually rib or vertebra) and kidney. The tumour may also involve adjacent structures (chest wall, pericardium, mediastinal structures) by direct invasion.

Clinical features
Thoracic manifestations
1. SYMPTOMS

There are no diagnostic chest symptoms, but persistent, often unproductive, cough and repeated haemoptysis are both common. The frequent association with chronic bronchitis must be kept in mind. Recent dyspnoea on effort may accompany a pleural effusion or collapse of a substantial volume of lung due to bronchial obstruction. Pleuritic pain will accompany involvement of the pleura by tumour or by associated inflammatory change, whilst pain of a more persistent kind follows infiltration of the chest wall (*see also* Superior vena cava obstruction, *below*). Whilst an attack of pneumonia which has not resolved after a month is particularly suspect, this very common disease must be considered in any patient with unexplained ill health, particularly a smoker in or after middle age.

2. PHYSICAL SIGNS

Physical signs in the lungs are frequently completely absent even in the presence of a substantial tumour, and almost invariably so in the presence of an early one. Localized reduction of breath sounds, in the absence of any other signs, is a very useful early finding in some cases; impaired percussion note with tubular breathing will accompany lobar consolidation or an early pleural effusion, which may not be distinguishable. A larger effusion will lead to stony dullness and absent breath sounds, sometimes with tubular breathing at its upper border, and possibly deviation of the mediastinum to the opposite side. Collapse of a lobe or lung due to bronchial obstruction may be recognized by shift of the trachea and mediastinum to the same side. By and large, signs are normally found only when the disease is advanced.

Obstruction of the superior vena cava is characterized by dilated veins on the anterior chest wall and upper limbs, and of small veins just above the costal margin, together with gross distension of the external jugular veins, often with congestion and oedema of the face and neck. This is liable to occur either with a primary tumour in the right upper lobe, or due to metastatic enlargement of the right hilar lymph nodes, in particular the paratracheal node. The accompanying sensations of dizziness, headache and pressure inside the head, are particularly distressing.

Extrathoracic manifestations

Loss of weight is a usual but not invariable symptom, along with fatigue. *Metastatic lesions* are the presenting feature in a substantial proportion, and include hepatomegaly, hard, enlarged supraclavicular or axillary lymph nodes, localized tenderness over ribs or vertebrae, signs of cerebral tumour and secondary nodules in the skin. Metastatic destruction of the adrenals may lead to many of the features of Addison's disease.

Non-metastatic manifestations

1. NEUROLOGICAL CHANGES

These include:

a. Thoracic inlet tumour (also called Pancoast tumour). A tumour in the lung apex may involve the lower end of the brachial plexus by direct infiltration, leading to wasting and weakness of the small muscles of the hand, which may be the presenting feature of the illness. This is accompanied, or followed, by pain in the upper arm and shoulder and down the ulnar side of the arm, where there may be some sensory impairment. The pain may be intense and intractable.

b. Involvement of the adjacent sympathetic ganglia leads to *Horner's syndrome* (ptosis, enophthalmos, constricted pupil).

c. Left recurrent laryngeal nerve palsy due to entrapment of the nerve in the hilar nodes leads to permanent hoarseness, which may be compensated to a variable degree; it is a frequent presenting symptom of bronchial carcinoma, so that laryngoscopy is indicated whenever phonation is lost for more than 2–3 weeks.

d. Phrenic nerve paralysis is also common; it is usually due to carcinoma involving the phrenic nerve in its course through the mediastinum, but it may, rarely, be due to simple pneumonia. It always calls for investigation: it commonly presents with radiological evidence of a raised diaphragm, which on screening is seen to rise on sniffing (paradoxical movement). The raised diaphragm seen with pulmonary embolism or infarction does not show paradoxical movement. Both conditions must be differentiated from congenital eventration, characterized by thinning and very marked elevation of the diaphragm which in this condition consists of fibrous tissue with little or no muscle.

e. Diffuse degeneration of the cerebellum, and sometimes of the cerebral cortex, may be the presenting feature; the symptoms may be relieved following removal of the primary tumour. Metastases should be excluded by CAT scanning.

f. Peripheral neuritis is often of bizarre and scattered, rather than symmetrical, distribution ('mononeuritis multiplex').

g. Polymyositis, with or without a violaceous skin eruption (dermatomyositis) leads to weakness, wasting and sometimes tenderness of the proximal muscles, and is difficult to distinguish clinically from the autoimmune variety not accompanied by carcinoma.

2. FINGER CLUBBING

This is the commonest non-metastatic manifestation. An uncommon extension of this condition is hypertrophic pulmonary osteoarthropathy, a painful and tender affection of the wrists and ankles; the diagnosis is confirmed by radiological demonstration of new bone formation in the periosteum. Interestingly, the pain may be relieved either by removal of the tumour, or by vagotomy alone if the tumour proves to be inoperable.

3. ENDOCRINE DISTURBANCES

These are uncommon. They include, most frequently, inappropriate secretion of antidiuretic hormone (ADH), the resulting hyponatraemia often leading to confusion or stupor; whilst inappropriate secretion of ACTH may lead to the classic features of Cushing's syndrome (plethora, fluid retention, systemic hypertension, subcutaneous striae). Both these syndromes occur most frequently with oat-cell tumours.

Gynaecomastia is always an indication to search for associated bronchial carcinoma.

4. THROMBOPHLEBITIS MIGRANS

As with carcinomas elsewhere, repeated attacks of superficial peripheral venous thrombosis may be the presenting symptom.

Investigations

Plain radiographs

A good quality posteroanterior chest radiograph, well centred and with adequate contrast, is the mainstay of diagnosis. It should be supplemented by the appropriate lateral view whenever an abnormality is revealed, as this frequently serves to localize the lesion precisely, and may also confirm or refute involvement of the pleura and chest wall when assessing operability. In addition, an *overpenetrated film* will help to demonstrate a collapsed left lower lobe, which presents as a triangular shadow concealed behind the heart (*see Fig.* 2.13); it will also assist in the recognition of metastatic lesions in ribs or vertebrae.

The radiological appearances vary considerably, depending on the situation and effects of the primary tumour on the lung, as well as on the presence of enlarged hilar nodes, or other complications such as phrenic paralysis, bony metastasis, or a pleural effusion which may effectively mask the tumour.

When the tumour lies peripherally, it presents usually as a somewhat rounded shadow, characteristically with rather irregular margins, often with spiky extensions into the surrounding lung tissue; a clear-cut margin suggests a slowly growing tumour. Cavitation within the mass due to ischaemic necrosis is common, and may present a problem in diagnosis from simple abscess, tuberculous cavity, or nodular rheumatoid disease, particularly if there is no apparent hilar node enlargement. Visibly enlarged associated hilar nodes favour the diagnosis of carcinoma; the appearance may suggest a primary tuberculous complex, which is however very unusual in adults of Caucasian stock.

By contrast, a more centrally placed tumour may lie within or adjacent to a bronchus, and lead to collapse of the lung, lobe, or segment distal to the obstruction by absorption of air into the bloodstream. The possibility of other causes of bronchial obstruction, for example inhaled foreign body, must of course be kept in mind, but carcinoma is much the most likely particularly in or beyond middle age. The exception is middle lobe collapse which is more commonly an after-effect of primary tuberculosis (q.v.), but which may cause considerable diagnostic difficulty even though carcinoma of the middle lobe is in fact very rare.

On occasion, squamous carcinoma may present as upper lobe infiltration indistinguishable from tuberculosis, with none of the usual radiological features of a tumour (*Fig.* 2.21). In such a case diagnosis is likely to depend on progression of the lesion in spite of antituberculous treatment; localized chest pain is a useful clue. The right upper lobe is more commonly affected.

Occasionally bronchial carcinoma may present with signs of cerebral metastasis with a perfectly normal chest film; a small primary may lie undetected in a bronchus, or behind the heart shadow.

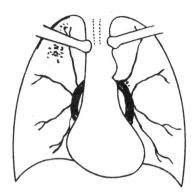

Fig. 2.21 Squamous carcinoma of right upper lobe mimicking tuberculous infiltration.

Additional radiographic techniques

Tomography, in both PA and lateral views, is of great value in defining structures at the hilum, including lymph nodes and bronchi, and must not be omitted in cases of doubtfully prominent hilar shadowing. It is also of use in studying the detailed structure of the lung lesion, and in estimating chest wall involvement if surgery is being considered.

Bronchography may demonstrate bronchial obstruction where other techniques have failed, but it is unpleasant for the patient, time-consuming, and rarely justified if flexible bronchoscopy is available.

Ultrasound scanning of the liver is non-invasive and is a mandatory preoperative measure to help to exclude metastases.

Bronchoscopy

Direct inspection of the bronchial tree is an invaluable technique for confirming the diagnosis visually, for obtaining biopsy material, and for assessing operability. It is therefore a routine procedure when carcinoma is suspected, and gives useful information in a high proportion of cases.

Rigid bronchoscopy should be performed under general anaesthesia, which with the use of muscle relaxants, and the supply of oxygen through the bronchoscope using a high pressure venturi system, allows abundant time for the examination. It has the disadvantages that vision is limited to the main segmental divisions, and relies on telescopes for inspection of the upper lobes and lower lobe apices, where biopsy is difficult or impossible. It has the advantages that secretions are more easily cleared by suction, larger biopsies are obtainable, and hardness and impairment of mobility, as indications of peribronchial node involvement, are readily assessed.

Fibreoptic bronchoscopy has the advantage that it may be done under local anaesthesia on an outpatient basis; it allows considerably deeper penetration into the bronchial tree, with greatly improved visualization of the upper lobes from which biopsies may readily be taken. Its disadvantages include difficulty in clearing secretions and the small size of the biopsies obtained. However, bronchial brushings or lavage through the fibrescope may give useful cytological information, whilst a photographic record of the visual appearances is easily obtained.

Other methods of cytological diagnosis

These include:

   a. Direct biopsy of accessible lymph nodes, especially the scalene node.

   b. Pleural biopsy, which should be done on each occasion that a pleural effusion is aspirated.

   c. Cytology of the pleural fluid.

   d. Sputum cytology should only be done in laboratories provided with a large enough work load to occupy a specialist technician. It hardly needs to be stated that a false positive report may be disastrous to the patient's morale, as well as leading to possibly serious clinical mismanagement.

   If the history suggests the possibility of lipid pneumonia (*see* p. 152) the presence of fat droplets after special staining will confirm this diagnosis.

   e. Direct aspiration needle biopsy of pleural or pulmonary lesions occasionally has a place but carries the risk of pneumothorax, haemorrhage or an embolism. Thoracotomy is therefore safer, and usually to be preferred.

   f. Mediastinoscopy, using blunt dissection downwards from the suprasternal notch, may give useful diagnostic information, but is hazardous; its use is limited to a few special centres.

   g. Liver biopsy, by contrast, is safe and may provide proof of inoperability as well as the histological diagnosis when metastases are present.

Physiological tests

The use of these is limited to assessment of function when considering resection surgery: this is of particular importance as so many patients with carcinoma also have smoking-induced obstructive airway disease.

Thoracotomy

When doubt persists, formal thoracotomy is indicated if the lesion appears operable; frozen sections may be helpful in deciding whether to proceed to resection.

Management

The prognosis without treatment is gloomy, the expectation of life being limited to no more than 2 years from diagnosis in the majority of patients. Very exceptionally, however, survival over many years in proved but untreated cases has been observed. Unhappily the effect of treatment on survival is negligible except in small groups of selected cases; the duration of life depends primarily on the intrinsic rate of growth of the tumour. Thus in the majority of patients management is perforce directed towards maintaining the quality of life, rather than to increasing the length of it.

Some help in estimating life expectancy derives from the duration of symptoms before diagnosis: obviously a long history suggests a slowly growing tumour, and a short history one that is growing rapidly. Although one would expect slow growth in a well-differentiated squamous carcinoma, and rapid growth in an undifferentiated tumour, the correlation between survival time and cell type is in fact surprisingly inconsistent.

Surgical treatment

Radical removal of the primary tumour with its associated lymph nodes, before distal metastasis has occurred, offers the best chance of survival, but is only rarely successful. Of all cases diagnosed, at best about one-fifth will be judged suitable for attempted removal, and of these a half will be found inoperable at thoracotomy. Of those in whom resection is completed, only a fifth will survive 5 years, because the majority have occult metastases at the time of operation. Even these figures are optimistic in the light of experience in recent years, because the disease is tending to affect older patients, who because of obstructive airway disease have insufficient cardiorespiratory reserve to permit surgery.

At best a lobectomy, and more often a pneumonectomy will be required, so that in the presence of any significant degree of obstructive airway disease the risk of respiratory crippling is substantial. Preoperative assessment must include lung function tests, bronchoscopy and tomography to assess lymph node or chest wall involvement, liver scanning and ideally CAT scanning of the brain in a search for hidden metastases.

Palliative surgery has little place, and is largely limited to very rare instances of intractable pain, when neurosurgical procedures such as tractotomy or nerve block may be helpful.

Radiotherapy

Radical radiotherapy is limited to isolated tumours, in general no larger than a 3 cm cube, without hilar node involvement. The results in these circumstances may be very satisfactory, particularly in elderly subjects in whom a useful prolongation of life may follow. The treatment may, however, lead to loss of function comparable with that following surgical resection, due to radiation fibrosis and obliteration of pulmonary blood flow.

Palliative radiotherapy is firmly indicated in only two circumstances: for the relief of the highly distressing symptoms of superior vena caval obstruction, and for the frequently intractable pain of bony metastasis, particularly when one or more vertebrae are involved.

Cytotoxic drugs

Chemotherapy has little effect in prolonging life, with the single exception of undifferentiated small-cell carcinoma. This tumour is usually sensitive to combinations of cytotoxic agents, which are given in repeated courses with, however, diminishing effectiveness. The price paid for the extra months of life is high, both in terms of side effects (vomiting, loss of hair, bone marrow suppression) and of the time required to be spent in hospital, so that combined chemotherapy, whilst offering some prospects of future improvement, is currently a matter for research rather than routine treatment.

In practical terms, cyclophosphamide alone given intravenously can be useful in achieving relief of symptoms for at best a few months. Its use should usually be restricted to treating histologically proved undifferentiated tumours, in particular small-cell carcinoma; if histological proof has not been obtained, a rapidly growing lesion, for example one seen to be increasing in size over a period of weeks, may be an acceptable indication for treatment when symptoms are substantial. It should not be used in slow growing or well-differentiated tumours, as the side effects will greatly outweigh any possible advantages.

The timing of treatment is important, because normally it can be used effectively only once, and should therefore relate to the presence of symptoms. In particular the relief of the headache and vomiting of cerebral metastasis can be very worth while, leaving scope for the use of dexamethasone when the symptoms later return. Cyclophosphamide is given intravenously, after an initial test dose of 100 mg, at a dose of 500 mg daily until the white blood count total drops below 5000 cells/mm^3, which is usually after 10 or more days. It should then be discontinued; a second course given on later relapse is likely to be less effective than the first and is rarely called for. Maintenance treatment with oral cyclophosphamide is more likely to lead to immune failure with exacerbation of symptoms, due to spread of the tumour, than to contribute to the patient's welfare; it should not be used.

Side effects include nausea, and sometimes vomiting. Depression of the white cell count, which should be measured daily during treatment, usually recovers quickly once it has stopped. Subsequently, loss of hair, due to suppression of the hair follicles, is to be expected; the patient should be warned of this possibility in advance.

Cyclophosphamide can usefully be combined with prednisolone 15 mg daily, which acts in a non-specific though impressive manner in improving the patient's well-being; it may also replace impaired steroid production when adrenal metastases are present, and can usefully be continued after the course of cyclophosphamide has been completed.

Other symptomatic measures

An antibiotic may be required for lung infection, distal to bronchial obstruction by tumour. Dexamethasone in full dosage (up to 8 or 12 mg daily) may help the symptoms of cerebral metastatic involvement. The remaining drugs likely to be required are those required for relief of pain, and to secure sleep in the presence of intractable cough. Sedative linctuses (e.g. linct codeine 5 ml every 4–6 h) may at first be adequate, but there should be no hesitation in advising diamorphine linctus 5 ml as required, as the problem of addiction is not relevant. This is effective in relief of pain and cough, is given by mouth, and does less to impair mental clarity than the commonly used Brompton cocktail (morphine sulphate 15 mg, cocaine hydrochloride 10 mg, gin and honey 1 drachm, water to ½ fluid ounce) which may lead to confusion and stupor. In a minority of patients with severe pain, relief may only be afforded by injections of morphine hydrochloride, in as big and frequent a dose as the symptoms demand.

General supportive measures
The patient's next of kin must be given the diagnosis, and likely prognosis; the decision whether or not to inform the patient also can usefully be discussed with the next of kin. If the patient asks directly for the diagnosis he is of course entitled to be given it, in which case it is helpful to link the disclosure with the prospect of some form of active treatment. So long however as he remains free of symptoms it is reasonable to withhold the diagnosis for as long as possible.

2.7 OCCUPATIONAL LUNG DISORDERS

Introduction
The identification of a lung disorder due to some specific organic or inorganic dust, some fume or vapour, inhaled in the course of work, is an interesting and sometimes difficult exercise. New causes of occupational lung disease continue to be recognized, and in an industrial society are likely to go on presenting themselves.

The study of occupational lung disease is greatly complicated by the fact that a high proportion of the work-force is affected by chronic bronchitis, and by the addiction to cigarettes which nearly always accompanies it. Furthermore many physicians do not have the necessary detailed knowledge of, or access to, the industrial processes concerned. There is a clear case for the monitoring of men in potentially hazardous occupations by regular physical and radiological examination and lung function tests to a much greater extent than is currently practised.

The management of the physical and psychological problems that affect the patient may also be difficult. Thus when a patient with simple chronic bronchitis is encouraged to apply for compensation for an industrial disease which he does not have, considerable skill and tact may be required of the clinician to prevent the development of a compensation neurosis, which could lead to permanent invalidism and be a far greater disaster for the patient than an organic occupational disorder.

Industrial history

Recording an accurate industrial history is important not only to the diagnosis and management, but with regard to the question of compensation which may arise at a later date. Failure to take a work history is unfortunately common; the laborious recording of the minutiae of symptoms without so much as a mention of the patient's occupation may well lead to a completely erroneous assessment of the illness. All case histories should therefore include the question: 'What did you do when you left school?' and note later jobs, with approximate dates, in chronological order.

Lung disorders due to hazards at work are numerous, and the issues sometimes complex; they must be considered both in relation to the nature of the offending agent and to the type of host response. Clear evidence of a direct dose relationship is uncommon, whilst the individual reactions are varied, often incompletely understood, and show considerable differences in degree.

Causative agents fall into three main groups:
1. Mineral and inorganic dusts
2. Organic dusts
3. Gases and fumes.

Pathogenesis

The lungs are normally protected from dust by the filtering of air through the nose; by mucociliary clearance, the mucosa of the upper respiratory tract and of the trachea and bronchi being lined with ciliated epithelium which propels any foreign material towards the exterior, and by macrophage activity in the lung periphery. When the dust load is too large, or ciliary function is impaired as in chronic bronchitis, dust is able to pass through the bronchial tree to the lung periphery, provided always that the particle size is small enough.

It is well recognized that camels in the desert do not get silicosis, even though the grains of sand are chemically identical with the particles given off from the making of a metal casting, which lead to silicosis in foundry workers. The difference lies in the size of the particles.

The nasal filter effectively prevents access of particles 20 μm or more in diameter to the bronchial tree: particles of 3 μm or less may pass the respiratory bronchioles to the alveoli, where they are ingested by alveolar macrophages and transported back to the ciliated epithelium at the terminal bronchiole level, and thence to the exterior. Some types of particle, for example silica, are toxic to macrophages, which, after ingestion, are unable to remove them from the alveoli; they therefore remain in situ and give rise to a fibrotic reaction.

The large majority of particles less than 20 μm and greater than 3 μm in diameter are removed by the ciliary blanket lining the bronchial tree.

Modes of response

When dust (e.g. isocyanate) or vapour reaches the bronchial tree it may provoke an asthmatic response (type I reaction); when it penetrates to the respiratory bronchioles and alveoli it may lead to acute pulmonary oedema (chlorine, sulphur dioxide, ammonia), peripheral granulomatous disease (beryllium), or extrinsic allergic alveolitis (type III (Arthus) reaction), e.g. farmer's lung, bagassosis, mushroom grower's disease. After a delay of many years malignant change may supervene in the lung (e.g. asbestosis). Fibre particles of the appropriate length and flexibility may pass through the alveoli into the pleura (e.g. asbestos, especially blue asbestos) and there cause a fibrous reaction (pleural plaques or diffuse pleural thickening); or many years later a malignant mesothelioma.

The only industrial agent currently known to cause lung fibrosis after ingestion is paraquat, which affects both lungs and kidneys via the bloodstream after absorption from the gastrointestinal tract.

The clinical features of occupational lung disease

Symptoms may be limited to dyspnoea on effort, which may become disabling with the passage of time, particularly if an inhaled mineral is causing progressive fibrosis in the lung. Alternatively, wheeze and tightness in the chest may occur shortly after inhalation (e.g. byssinosis), or after a delay of several hours in a type III reaction, such as farmer's lung, which also causes fever and malaise.

Physical signs are frequently absent, and when present have no specific features. The showers of fine inspiratory râles found in asbestosis do not differ from those heard in fibrosing alveolitis of other aetiology; the wheeze of an asthmatic reaction sounds like asthma from any other cause.

Investigations

Essential investigations in all cases include chest radiography and lung function studies, though the history may be more important than either. When an allergic or immunological disturbance is likely the appropriate biochemical and serological tests are called for.

Management

Once the cause of the disorder has been established, a decision will have to be made as to whether further exposure must be avoided; against this must be set the possible financial disadvantage which would so often follow a change of occupation. If the patient is to remain in his job, means of protection must be devised and put into effect.

Drug treatment has little place, save in the management of the acute phases of allergic or immunological responses, and of course of any coincidental troubles such as chronic bronchitis. Compensation neurosis can be far more disabling than occupational lung disease, so that every possible step must be taken to avoid it.

If there is any question of carcinogenic effects the problem of cigarette addiction will require particular attention, in view of the possibility of synergism between retained dust and cigarette smoke.

There follow some of the commoner examples from the three main aetiological groups; the list is in no way comprehensive.

Mineral and inorganic dusts
Silicosis
Introduction

In the mid-nineteenth century acute silicosis or 'knife-grinder's lung' was responsible for premature death on a very wide scale in Sheffield; it was common, too, in pottery workers. It is now relatively uncommon following the recognition of the need to suppress or eliminate fine silica dust, but is still seen in more chronic form, in foundry workers, sand blasters, slate quarry workers, and in stone masons working in sandstone, though not of course in limestone.

Clinical features

The characteristic radiological changes of uncomplicated silicosis, commonly revealed on a routine radiograph, may persist for many years, or for a life-time, before the development of effort dyspnoea, which is usually the only symptom, and which may become disabling. There are no abnormal physical signs.

In the face of very heavy dust exposure, the disease may pursue a fulminating course with rapidly progressive lung fibrosis leading to death in less than five years; happily these conditions are not now seen in the UK as a result of appropriate legislation.

Complications

There is no proven increase in bronchial carcinoma. Tuberculosis was once a frequent complication, but is now uncommon following the decline in sources of infection.

As in coal worker's pneumoconiosis (*see* p. 135), progressive massive fibrosis may develop; Caplan's nodes may occur in subjects with rheumatoid arthritis, or with a positive circulating rheumatoid factor without clinical arthritis.

Investigations

The radiographic appearance of widespread discrete nodules 2–5 mm in diameter is diagnostic, taken in conjunction with a history of dust exposure over a period of years. The nodulation is denser in the midzones, and may become confluent with the passage of time; it may be associated with calcification of the hilar nodes.

Lung function tests show impaired gas transfer, with impaired ventilation of restrictive type in the later stages.

Management

Prevention is effected by suppression of dust and the use of an efficient respirator; unless the respirator is comfortable during heavy physical work it will not be worn consistently. Inhalation of aluminium powder is claimed to prevent silicosis, but any such advantage is outweighed by more or less severe lung damage which may be caused by the aluminium itself.

Once the disease is established, the silica will remain in situ at alveolar level due to its toxic effect on macrophages; this will lead to a continuing fibrotic reaction, even after removal from exposure, but there is evidence that the process is slowed down by a change in occupation. Any resulting disability is eligible for industrial compensation.

There is no *drug treatment* unless tuberculosis is present; this responds to antibacterial treatment though rather more slowly than normally.

Coal worker's pneumoconiosis

Introduction

Coal worker's pneumoconiosis follows the inspiration of respirable coal dust, which consists mainly of carbon particles up to 7 μm in diameter—with a variable but small amount of silica, e.g. about 2% in South Wales. The silica, however, plays little or no part in the genesis of the lung lesion, which is a non-specific reaction to the carbon; the simple form is characterized by mild fibrosis with some degree of centrilobular emphysema. In a small proportion the lesion is complicated either by progressive massive fibrosis or by rheumatoid nodules; the incidence of bronchial carcinoma tends to be low, possible due to restrictions in smoking underground.

Simple pneumoconiosis

Clinical features

Simple pneumoconiosis causes *no symptoms* and no measurable physiological changes: the lesions do not progress after exposure to the dust has ceased. It follows that if symptoms are present in a man with simple pneumoconiosis, they are due to some other disorder. The expectation of life is normal, the importance of the lesion being mainly in the potential development of progressive massive fibrosis (PMF).

Investigation

The diagnosis is made on the radiological appearance—small diffuse nodules are present which represent accumulations of coal dust in the parenchyma, with their attendant mild fibrotic reaction. The extent of the lesions is categorized according to the profusion and size of the lesions, assessed by comparison with standard films published by the International Labour Office.

Management

The discovery of simple pneumoconiosis does not necessarily involve leaving the industry, but a change to a less dusty environment is commonly advised.

Complicated pneumoconiosis

A. *Progressive massive fibrosis* is an obscure immune response to coal dust, which was at one time believed, incorrectly, to be an unusual manifestation of tuberculosis.

Clinical features

As this lesion progresses, the patient develops progressive effort dyspnoea with cough and mucoid, or sometimes black, sputum. The expectation of life is reduced, particularly if there is associated bronchitis and emphysema; but in the earlier stages there may be no symptoms for a number of years. Clubbing is not a feature.

Investigations

Chest radiographs show extensive confluent shadows, usually in the upper lobes, which are seen to be adjacent to the greater fissures on the lateral picture; these are due to massive areas of fibrosis containing carbon, which may undergo aseptic necrosis with cavitation and melanoptysis.

The differential diagnosis from bronchial carcinoma or cavitating tuberculosis may be difficult.

Lung function tests show progressive impairment of ventilation of restrictive type, with variable impairment of gas transfer.

Sputum should always be cultured for tuberculosis.

Management

There is no specific treatment; the patient is eligible for compensation.

B. *Caplan's syndrome* occurs in coal workers with rheumatoid arthritis, or sometimes with circulating rheumatoid factor without arthropathy.

Clinical features

The clinical features are those of the arthritis; pulmonary symptoms are remarkably few bearing in mind the sometimes very extensive radiological changes.

Investigations

Chest radiographs show multiple rounded opacities of varying size, often with limited or even no evidence of simple pneumoconiosis; these represent rheumatoid granulomatous lesions, and may be mistaken for metastatic carcinoma.

Management
There is no specific treatment. Some long-term survivors may go on to develop leucopenia and ultimately malignant lymphoma.

Berylliosis

Beryllium is used in the manufacture of strip lights: its introduction in the 1939–45 war led to a substantial number of cases of rapidly progressive and fatal lung fibrosis. Further investigation revealed a disease histologically and clinically indistinguishable from pulmonary sarcoidosis, save that the granulomas contained demonstrable beryllium particles, and that the disease tended in a proportion of cases to be more rapidly progressive and less responsive to steroids. Since measures were taken to control the dust new cases are rarely seen.

Stannosis

Stannosis is a benign pneumoconiosis affecting those handling tin ore in the mines or subsequently: it is characterized by extremely dense nodulation on the radiograph, in keeping with the high atomic weight of the dust. It causes no disability.

Haemosiderosis

Haemosiderosis due to inhalation of iron oxides, is found in haematite miners. The nodulation is radiologically dense, often with involvement of the hilar lymph nodes.

It causes no disability: an excess of carcinoma found in Cumbrian miners was thought to be due to a coincidental excess of radiation in the atmosphere in the mines, namely radon (*see also* Welder's lung, p. 147).

Asbestos

Introduction
Asbestos ($\dot{\alpha}+\sigma\beta\varepsilon\sigma\tau\acute{o}\varsigma$, incombustible) has been recognized as a fire-resistant material since classical times. It is a mixture of silicates occurring as a variety of natural fibres, widely used as a cementing agent. Over the last century its commercial use has increased dramatically; the gross amount mined worldwide is currently in the order of 5 000 000 tons and continues to increase. The various disorders recognized to be due to inhalation of asbestos are outlined in *Fig.* 2.22 in relation to world production over the last century. The diamond-shaped figure to the left shows the increasing prevalence of pulmonary asbestosis, mainly in the textile industry, from the beginning of the century until the mid 1930s, when regulations to reduce dust exposure were introduced. The inverted V shows the increased prevalence,

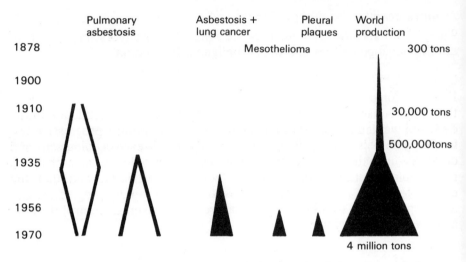

Fig. 2.22 Diagrammatic representation of the growth of the asbestos industry related to the prevalence of associated lesions. (With acknowledgements to Dr J. C. Gilson.)

mainly amongst insulation and building workers, since 1935. Bronchial carcinoma complicating asbestosis has been increasingly recognized since this association was first reported in the early 1930s. Pleural disease due to asbestos has only been recognized since the late 1950s following on the vast increase in asbestos usage since just before the second World War.

Its effects on health vary with the amount of dust inhaled and on the type of fibre. The commonest variety is chrysotile (white asbestos), the fibres being relatively long and flexible, and more amenable to mucociliary clearance than the more dangerous amphiboles, which have shorter and straighter fibres more readily inhaled to the lung periphery. Amphiboles include amosite, anthophyllite, and crocidolite or blue asbestos: the latter has been particularly incriminated in the genesis of malignant disease, and has ceased to be used in most western countries.

Asbestos is widely used as an insulation material, either for lagging pipes with asbestos cloth and cement, or sprayed onto walls or partitions to make them fireproof. It is a major component of hardboards, roof tilings, and composite cements used in the building industry: no effective substitute in the manufacture of brake linings has been found. Laggers, plumbers, joiners, construction workers, and motor mechanics are among the many trades exposed to risk. In some industries, notably shipbuilding, its widespread use has in the past led to extensive environmental contamination, with resulting exposure of workers in a wide range of trades. Family members may be significantly exposed as a result of dust brought home on clothing.

Once asbestos has been bound in a composite material, for example in roofing, it carries no risk; it should be left where it is, or removed only by expert workmen with appropriate protection.

Research into providing suitable safe substitutes, notably fibreglass, continues with a substantial degree of success.

Effects of exposure
NORMAL POPULATION STUDIES
Examination of the lungs in routine autopsies has repeatedly demonstrated the presence of asbestos bodies in a high, up to 50%, proportion of urban dwellers: these are of no apparent clinical significance, and the proteinaceous wrapping round the individual fibres appear to represent a successful defensive reaction. It is the uncoated fibre that constitutes the hazard; this is more difficult to detect on microscopy, requiring polarized light, and special extraction techniques for the measurement of quantity.

Effects of light industrial exposure
Light or intermittent exposure over a period of months or years, or heavy exposure over as little as a few days or weeks, may lead to pleural reactions in a substantial proportion of cases. These may present in three ways:

1. PLEURAL PLAQUE FORMATION
These rarely appear in less than 10 years from the initial exposure.

Clinical features. Pleural plaques cause no symptoms or signs, but serve as a firm indicator that asbestos has been inhaled and retained. They are therefore associated with an increased incidence of bronchial carcinoma, which is also seen to a similar degree in individuals exposed to asbestos who have not developed plaques.

Investigations. The *radiographic appearances* are highly characteristic. The early change is due to localized fibrous pleural thickening which does not involve the costophrenic angles: it is best seen in standard radiographs in tangential view in the axillary region, or as bumps on the diaphragms (*Fig.* 2.23).

Twenty or more years after first exposure a high proportion of plaques develop calcification, often presenting a bizarre holly-leaf appearance (*Fig.* 2.24); they are readily seen on the diaphragms, particularly on the lateral view, whilst the pericardium is involved in about one-fifth of cases.

Histologically they consist of avascular collagen tissue almost invariably in the parietal pleura: *biopsy* is unnecessary.

Lung function tests are normal.

Management. The patient should not smoke because of the increased risk of bronchial carcinoma. Care is required to avoid compensation neurosis.

2. DIFFUSE PLEURAL THICKENING: TRANSIENT BENIGN PLEURAL EFFUSION

Clinical features. This lesion may be heralded by transient pleurisy with effusion, often accompanied by a persistent pleural rub during resolution

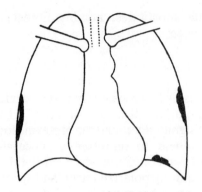

Fig. 2.23 Bilateral axillary and left diaphragmatic fibrous pleural plaques.

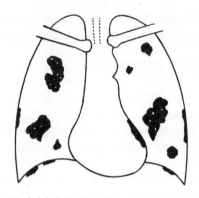

Fig. 2.24 Calcified pleural plaques with pericardial calcification.

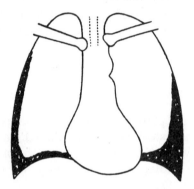

Fig. 2.25 Diffuse pleural thickening.

which may last many weeks: there is no constitutional disturbance and little or no pain. A small proportion show steady progression leading to restrictive impairment of ventilation.

Investigations. Chest radiographs show obliteration of the cardiophrenic angles, with diffuse pleural thickening of varying extent (*Fig.* 2.25): changes on one side may precede the other by several years. Examination of pleural fluid shows increased protein and numerous lymphocytes. Lung function testing in progressive cases will show a restrictive impairment of ventilation. The circulating rheumatoid factor is frequently positive.

Management. Rarely, the lesion may progress steadily and lead to effort dyspnoea: very exceptionally pleurectomy may be indicated. The condition is benign, there being no evidence of later malignancy.

3. MALIGNANT MESOTHELIOMA
This tumour develops on average about 35 years after initial asbestos exposure, which may have been brief and even trivial. In the absence of

asbestos exposure it is a very rare tumour, but it is currently common in shipyard communities and in persons who were involved in gas-mask manufacture during the 1939–45 war. The majority of cases are due to crocidolite, the association having been first recognized in southern Africans who had played on asbestos tips as children. The disease is eligible for compensation.

Clinical features. The onset is with dyspnoea, the majority having a large initial pleural effusion, which is bloodstained in a few. The general condition remains good for a time, but when the chest wall is invaded, deterioration is rapid and pain may then be intractable. Death is usual within about a year of diagnosis, though a few patients may live in relative comfort for three or four years.

Investigations. The *chest radiograph* shows a large pleural effusion in about 90%, the remainder showing gross and irregular pleural thickening (*Fig.* 2.26). Contralateral plaques are a useful pointer, being proof of

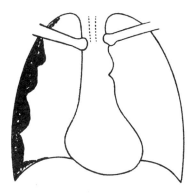

Fig. 2.26 Pleural mesothelioma without effusion.

asbestos exposure. The proof of diagnosis, however, depends on the histology, which is sometimes only obtained at autopsy; the tumour is dimorphic, with glandular elements enmeshed in a malignant fibrous stroma.

Pleural fluid cytology, in expert hands, reveals typical mesothelioma cells, particularly in the early stages, in a high proportion. *Pleural biopsy* is useful, and should be done with a needle which covers the specimen during withdrawal because of the risk of causing seedling tumours along the needle track.

Thoracotomy is at no time justified, as it may accelerate the disease and cause distressing tumour deposits in the wound: it does not prolong life or significantly relieve distress.

Management. This consists of chest aspiration, to be repeated only when the degree of dyspnoea demands it; and adequate analgesics when pain develops. The patient should apply for compensation once the diagnosis is proved; the death must always be reported to the coroner as a case of industrial disease.

Effects of heavy exposure
PULMONARY ASBESTOSIS

Prolonged exposure to a high level of asbestos dust may lead after only a few years to fine lung fibrosis: this is seen most frequently in pipe laggers, and was common in asbestos textile workers until effective measures for dust suppression were instituted. The disease may be progressive and disabling, and the incidence of carcinoma is high. Histologically, there is extensive fibrosis with destruction of the normal alveolar structure; asbestos bodies are usually numerous, and the asbestos fibre content is always greatly increased.

Clinical features. The predominant *symptom* is gradually progressive effort dyspnoea, which may lead to respiratory crippling and premature death from cor pulmonale, if carcinoma of bronchus does not develop in the meantime; alternatively it may never progress or cause disability. The risk of carcinoma is estimated in cigarette smokers to be some ninety times the expected risk in non-smoking subjects who do not have asbestosis; this suggests a synergistic effect, the asbestosis increasing the known risk of cigarette smoking by a factor of three or more. Carcinoma in the presence of asbestosis is eligible for compensation: it is, however, very rare in men with asbestosis who have never smoked. Surveys of shipyard workers show an overall increase in bronchial carcinoma, independently of clinical asbestosis, but which evidently relates to dust exposure also.

The *physical signs* of asbestosis are abundant fine inspiratory basal crepitations, together with finger clubbing, and cyanosis as the disease progresses. Warts on the skin of the wrists are occasionally seen.

Investigations. Chest radiographs show a fine ground-glass hazy loss of translucency over the lung bases due to pleural thickening, with fine nodular and linear shadowing due to lung fibrosis; the cardiac border is ill-defined. The appearance may be indistinguishable from fibrosing alveolitis, particularly if the pleural changes are minimal.

Lung function tests show a progressive impairment of gas transfer; this is helpful in distinguishing between pulmonary and pleural disease, which may coexist and be difficult to distinguish radiologically. There is also restrictive impairment of ventilation; any associated obstructive changes are invariably due to smoking.

The *circulating rheumatoid factor* is positive in as many as 50% of cases with advanced disease, with rheumatoid arthropathy in a small proportion.

This suggests the presence of an immune change in the host which predisposes towards a damaging fibrotic reaction to inhaled fibre, but no more specific serological changes have been identified.

As expected, estimation of fibre content of lung tissue by maceration shows a vast increase.

Management. There is no effective drug treatment. The patient should not smoke. There is no firm evidence that a change of occupation affects the progression of the disease, and such a change, whilst advisable on general considerations, is not always feasible. The patient should receive industrial compensation when disability develops.

Organic dusts

Occupational Asthma

Introduction

Asthma is a common disorder which affects about 5% of the general population. It may therefore be difficult to decide in any individual case whether the asthma is or is not related to exposure to precipitating factors at work. The answer to this question depends on a careful industrial and environmental history, and a knowledge of the types of agent which could be responsible for the asthma. A number of organic dusts have been identified as culpable, and the resulting asthma accepted as a prescribed disease for compensation purposes.

Clinical features

Occupational asthma occurs as a result of exposure to a sensitizing agent at work. It invariably develops only after a period of symptom-free exposure which may last from a matter of days only to many years before the onset of asthmatic symptoms.

The symptoms improve when the patient is away from work, but recur as soon as he returns to it, even if the dust exposure is less than before. Once sensitization has occurred it is permanent; symptoms may diminish only gradually after cessation of exposure, whilst the patient may react permanently thereafter to non-specific factors such as cold air or cigarette smoke or exercise.

Organic agents responsible for occupational asthma include:

1. *Isocyanates,* which are used in the manufacture of polyurethane, plastics, and flexible foams; they may also lead to permanent impairment of function. Sensitization is frequent, affecting perhaps 10–20% of workers exposed.

2. *Proteolytic enzymes,* used in the manufacture of detergents.

3. *Colophony* (pine resin) used in the production of fluxes for soldering.

4. *Laboratory animals*—probably due to sensitizing proteins in the urine.

5. *Flour and grain dusts*—the sensitization is due to associated fungal spores.

6. *Epoxy resin* hardening agents.

Inorganic platinum salts may also cause occupational asthma.

Investigations

Lung function tests will confirm the presence and degree of reversible airway obstruction.

Skin tests are helpful in some instances, e.g. proteolytic enzymes, laboratory animals, but not in others.

Bronchial provocation tests, involving inhalation of a possible antigen, are potentially dangerous: their use should be limited to research departments with experience of the techniques involved.

Management

In the large majority permanent removal from the offending agent is mandatory, as patients tend to remain sensitive to even minute amounts of dust, which usually cannot be adequately controlled by the use of a respirator.

Bronchodilator therapy may be needed, as for any other form of asthma.

Extrinsic allergic alveolitis

Farmer's lung is one of many examples of extrinsic allergic alveolitis resulting from occupational exposure to an organic antigen. It was the first to be described, and is probably the commonest type in the UK. The inhaled dust leads to a type III (Arthus, or serum sickness) reaction in the lung parenchyma.

Clinical features

The *symptoms* are so characteristic as to be diagnostic, and are not infrequently better understood by the farming than by the medical community. They invariably follow the handling of hay which has been stored damp after a wet harvest, to feed livestock in the winter; it has a musty smell associated with the thermophilic organisms which thrive in the high temperatures which develop in the fermenting hay.

Some 4–6 h after exposure, the patient develops malaise, muscle pain, fever, cough and tightness in the chest. The symptoms continue so long as exposure is maintained; because the tissue hypersensitivity is permanent, they recur whenever musty hay is encountered. Permanent and disabling peripheral lung damage may ensue, and is eligible for compensation.

The *physical signs* in the acute stage are widespread fine crepitations, with, in severe cases, evidence of right ventricular strain due to obstruction of the pulmonary vascular bed, with associated central cyanosis and grossly overdistended external jugular veins.

Investigations

Chest radiography in the acute stage shows widespread but not always symmetrical nodular opacities, which may be discrete or soft and ill-defined; in mild cases the radiograph may be normal.

In the less common chronic stage there may be linear and microcystic changes ('honeycomb' appearance) with confluent dense shadowing due to granuloma formation.

Specific *serum precipitins* against the causative organisms, *Thermoactinomyces* or *Micropolyspora faeni,* are readily demonstrated and serve to confirm the diagnosis when the clinical and radiological features are correct, but it should be noted that precipitins may be present in exposed individuals who are quite symptom-free.

Lung function tests show a striking reduction in gas transfer, which, if done at intervals, may be used to monitor progress, and estimate the degree of any permanent residual damage.

Management

Potassium iodide was the traditional remedy for broken winded horses, which are also susceptible to this disease, as well as for man. This has been supplanted by steroids, which are highly effective given in an initial dose of at least 30 mg of prednisolone daily in the acute stage; oxygen therapy may be required in severe cases. The prednisolone should be gradually reduced according to the response, preferably measured by serial gas transfer estimations, and only discontinued when optimal improvement has occurred. The symptoms would subside spontaneously in time, after removal of the patient from the allergen, but steroid therapy is justified by the threat of permanent damage as much as by the frequently severe nature of the acute illness.

Subsequently the most effective way to avoid recurrence is of course to leave farming, but this is neither easy nor always necessary for the small hill farmer who probably has no alternative means of livelihood. He is often able to manage by getting temporary help after a wet harvest, and by the use of a helmet type respirator with electrically driven exhaust ventilation. Keeping the respirator clean, which should be done by somebody else, is very important as enough antigenic dust may otherwise be carried on the device to perpetuate the disease.

Other occupational causes of extrinsic allergic alveolitis

Occupational causes of allergic extrinsic alveolitis other than farming are numerous, and the list is constantly being added to. The possibility of an extrinsic allergen must therefore be considered in all patients with features

Table 2.5 Occupational causes of extrinsic allergic alveolitis

Disease	Occupation	Organism or causal agent
Wheat weevil disease	Handling stored grain	Sitophilus grananus
Bagassosis	Handling mouldy sugar cane waste	Thermoactinomyces sacchari
Mushroom worker's lung	Handling culture media for cultivating mushrooms	M. faeni
Air conditioner lung	e.g. office work with infected ventilation system	M. faeni
Farmer's lung	Handling musty hay	M. faeni; thermoactinomyces
Furrier's lung	Fur hat making	Animal hair protein
Poultry worker's lung	Hens	Feather or faecal protein
Humidifier fever	Factory or office work	? Amoebae in water used in humidifiers in air conditioning plants

suggesting a type III lung reaction, namely with influenza-like symptoms delayed for some hours after exposure, and often accompanied by radiographic nodular shadowing.

A few examples, with the causal organisms, are given in Table 2.5.

Byssinosis

This disorder affects cotton workers (byssus = linen), particularly those involved in using carding machinery, which combs out the fine fibre, a particularly dusty process. It may also affect jute and hemp workers.

Clinical features

The symptoms consist of cough, fever and tightness in the chest. They usually develop only after many years in the industry, and are worst on returning to work after the weekend away from dust, whence the synonym 'Monday morning fever'. The symptoms improve during the working week in spite of continued exposure.

The signs are those of bronchitis, and, later, of emphysema, disease which may well coexist particularly in cigarette smokers.

Investigations

Chest radiography shows no abnormality, and serological investigation is unhelpful in the absence of any precise knowledge as to the causal agent, presumably a fraction of the cotton fibre. Lung function testing shows mainl obstructive disease, but suggests that both type I and type III reactions may be operative. The diagnosis is therefore largely dependent on the clinical history, the unusual pattern of which is well recognized by the workers themselves.

Management

Effective management depends on suppression of cotton dust, or on the patient leaving the industry. Byssinosis is a prescribed disease, eligible for compensation, and is disabling in the long term.

Gases and fumes
Inhalation of irritant gases

Inhalation of irritant gases in substantial amounts may occur in a number of industries as a result of accident: the gases include chlorine, ammonia, sulphur dioxide and nitrogen dioxide.

The clinical features in the acute situation are similar, and include immediate intense sneezing, cough and lacrimation, followed by acute pulmonary oedema with intense dyspnoea and cyanosis. Most current evidence suggests that the likelihood of long-term effects, once the acute stage has subsided, is much smaller than used to be thought, though more observations are required in this connection.

Similarly, the possible effects of long-term low-dosage gas and fume toxicity are incompletely understood, and await further investigation.

Management

After acute exposure, the patient must be removed to clean air, and have any contaminated clothing removed; oxygen therapy is mandatory, with supportive measures for shock. Both chemotherapy to anticipate secondary bacterial pneumonia, and steroids to reduce the inflammatory oedema, are rational measures.

Any long-term symptoms may require lung function tests for evaluation, with a view to reassurance and the avoidance where possible of compensation neurosis.

Metal fumes

Diffuse interstitial fibrosis of the lung may follow the inhalation of fumes of a number of metals, including aluminium and mercury; cadmium may produce a more acute reaction.

Welder's lung

The classic type of welder's lung is the fine reticulation due to siderosis which follows the inhalation of Fe_2O_3 during steel welding. This causes no symptoms or measurable functional impairment, but there is some doubt as to whether or not it is associated with an increase in carcinoma.

Other metals may cause lung fibrosis in welders, and the coating of the metal and of the electrodes also play their part. *Metal fume fever* is a transient febrile illness caused by inhaling the oxidation products of copper or zinc; it may be followed by bacterial pneumonia.

The term 'welder's lung' thus covers a range of hazards which require further study.

2.8 MISCELLANEOUS CONDITIONS

Mycetoma (also called Fungus ball)

Introduction

Conditions within a pre-existing air-containing space in a lung provide the ideal situation for growth of the widespread fungus, *Aspergillus fumigatus*. Usually in a healed patent tuberculous cavity following chemotherapy, or sometimes in a bronchiectatic area, the fungus can propagate to produce a substantial avascular ball several centimetres in diameter. It consists entirely of mycelium, which behaves as a non-invasive saprophyte.

Clinical features

This inert lesion grows very slowly and causes no symptoms for many years, except that in atopic subjects fungus may spill into the bronchial tree leading to the usual features of bronchopulmonary aspergillosis (*see* p. 103). Eventually in a high proportion of cases a major blood vessel in the cavity wall is eroded, leading to massive and sometimes catastrophic and immediately fatal haemoptysis.

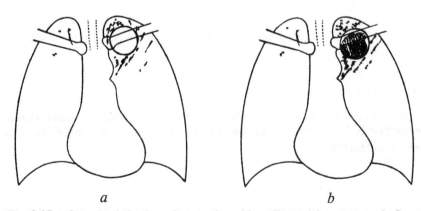

                    a   *b*

Fig. 2.27*a*, Open healed tuberculous cavity with antibacterial treatment. *b*, Same cavity with mycetoma; note air crescent (five years later).

Investigations

Precipitating antibodies are almost always present in the serum, but evidence of skin hypersensitivity is lacking; the fungus is only intermittently present, if at all, in the sputum.

The radiographic appearances are diagnostic (*Fig.* 2.27) as a crescent of air surrounds the fungus ball within the cavity, an appearance seen in no other condition. It is well demonstrated on tomography.

Management

Because of the possibility of fatal bleeding, surgical removal must be considered when lung function is adequate. Antifungal agents are useless as the lesion has no blood supply.

Mucoviscidosis

Introduction

This genetically determined disorder occurs in the offspring of two carriers of a recessive gene, and is believed to affect about 1 in 3000 individuals. All externally secreting glands are involved, and deliver an excess of sodium, which may be measured in the sweat. Death from progressive lung disease commonly occurs in childhood or in the teens; failure of mucociliary clearance is important as well as excessive secretion of viscid mucus, which lead to recurring infections due to retained secretion, with progressive fibrosis and bronchiectasis.

Clinical features

The important organs involved are the pancreas, in which the ducts are dilated and the exocrine tissue is atrophied and replaced by fibrous tissue, leading to pancreatic failure with malabsorption, steatorrhoea and wasting; and the lungs, which are the subject of repeated infections. The abundant sputum is regularly infected with a variety of pathogenic organisms; the fingers are commonly clubbed.

The symptoms start in infancy and commonly lead to death in childhood or adolescence, though with meticulous management survival into adult life is becoming less unusual.

Investigations

A sweat test showing sodium excretion to be more than 70 mEq/l confirms the diagnosis, but the test is less reliable in older patients. Faecal fats should also be measured.

Chest radiographs show patchy fibrotic and cystic change, with softer shadows when acute infection is present.

Sputum culture should be done regularly as a guide to antibiotic therapy. *Staph. pyogenes* and pseudomonas are common pathogens, whilst *Aspergillus fumigatus* infestation is not infrequent.

Management

Pancreatic insufficiency is met by provision of a readily absorbed diet, together with pancreatin taken before each meal; maintenance of adequate nutrition is imperative to sustain resistance, as far as possible, to chest infections.

The lung disease demands regular and conscientious physiotherapy (postural drainage and breathing exercises), which involves detailed instruction of the parents who have to carry out treatment several times a day at home.

Drug treatment includes adequate bronchodilator therapy, with prompt antibiotics according to sputum sensitivity tests. Antibiotic-resistant organisms are a major problem and may call for the administration in hospital of toxic antibiotics of the aminoglycoside group (gentamicin, tobramycin). The place of continuous long-term prophylactic antibiotics is not established, nor is that of mucolytic therapy (acetylcysteine by aerosol), which appears to be helpful in some patients but not others.

Trauma and the thorax

The lungs may be involved in a variety of ways after trauma, some of them involving an immediate threat to life if not promptly recognized and treated.

Fractured rib

Clinical features

Rib fracture commonly follows injury but may be due to coughing in bronchitic subjects, especially in the elderly or when osteoporosis is present, when it usually occurs at the posterior angle. It causes local pain and tenderness. The possibility of metastatic tumour, often from a primary in breast, bronchus or prostate, or of myeloma deposits, should also be kept in mind.

After injury, sharp bone ends may penetrate the lung causing traumatic pneumothorax; a torn intercostal artery may lead to haemothorax.

Investigations

A chest radiograph usually shows the fracture with some displacement, with local callus formation as healing proceeds. Osteolytic destructive lesions must always be looked for.

Management

In simple fracture the pain should be relieved by appropriate analgesic drugs—usually DF 118 (dihydrocodeine tartrate) 30–60 mg 6-hourly by mouth, or pentazocine hydrochloride, 50–100 mg every 4 h, is adequate.

The chest should not be strapped as this restricts bronchial clearance and leads to infection due to retained secretions. Coughing and deep breathing must be encouraged at regular intervals in spite of pain or discomfort.

The pain of fractures due to malignant disease responds to local deep X-ray therapy: hormone treatment has a place in cancers originating in breast or prostate.

Flail chest

When multiple fractures of several ribs occur, the chest wall loses stability, moving in with inspiration and out with expiration (paradoxical movement). This greatly impairs ventilation and may lead to death from acute respiratory failure unless promptly dealt with. Management is by immediate intermittent positive-pressure respiration following endotracheal intubation; as this needs to be continued until the chest wall has been stabilized, tracheostomy is usually necessary.

Haemothorax

Profuse haemorrhage into the pleural cavity with shock and exsanguination is an indication for blood transfusion and emergency thoracotomy. Lesser degrees of bleeding may be dealt with by aspiration, which may be facilitated after active bleeding has ceased by intrapleural streptokinase (100000 units) with streptodornase (25000 units), which liquefies the clotted blood; if this is unsuccessful surgical decortication may be needed later to restore lung function.

Traumatic pneumothorax

A penetrating chest wound allows air to be sucked into the pleura with each inspiration, leading rapidly to asphyxiation unless controlled. If the visceral pleura is breached the pleura must be intubated and drained, pending possible emergency thoracotomy. A persistent pneumothorax is sometimes due to a ruptured bronchus, which may be recognized bronchoscopically.

Shock lung

This term is used to describe multiple areas of oedema and consolidation developing in the lungs, usually a day or more after the initial trauma; the patient is gravely ill with tachypnoea and cyanosis which does not respond to oxygen therapy. The aetiology is multiple: it is particularly common after crush injuries, and may relate to local bruising and haemorrhage, thromboembolism, tissue anoxia, and sometimes oxygen toxicity following therapy. Management depends on maintaining tissue oxygenation by IPPR, with regular monitoring of P_{O_2} levels, together with supportive antibiotic and steroid therapy; the mortality is high.

Fat embolism

Embolism of fat particles from the bone marrow is not uncommon in the first few days after major fractures; it may cause no symptoms, or severe respiratory embarrassment due to obstruction of the pulmonary vascular bed, when widespread miliary or fluffy shadows are seen on radiography; purpura, especially over the shoulders, is a common feature. Treatment is directed to maintaining oxygenation.

Lipid pneumonia

Aspiration of fat into the lungs may cause diffuse nodular shadowing, or a dense localized shadow mimicking bronchial carcinoma. The commonest example is liquid paraffin used in nasal drops or to lubricate bougies used in the management of oesophageal structure. The relevant history is not always volunteered by the patient, and should be sought in any case of unusual shadowing on the chest radiograph; symptoms are few, and the lesions may clear spontaneously after the cause has been removed. The diagnosis may be confirmed by finding fat droplets in the sputum.

Pneumothorax

Introduction

Due to the intrinsic elastic recoil of lung tissue, a negative pressure is maintained in health in the pleural space; when a communication between the space and the atmosphere develops, air will enter and the lung will retract. Such a communication most commonly follows:

1. Rupture of a small bleb in the visceral pleura, the lungs being otherwise healthy;

2. Rupture of sizeable bulla in the presence of advanced chronic obstructive airway disease;

3. Traumatic injury to the lung or bronchus, or a perforating injury to the chest wall;

4. Less commonly, rupture of a tuberculous lesion, or staphylococcal pneumatocele, into the pleura: or as a complication of bronchial carcinoma.

Spontaneous pneumothorax

Clinical features

Spontaneous pneumothorax due to rupture of a superficial bleb is commoner in males and tends to occur early in adult life; siblings may be affected. The characteristic symptom is lateral chest pain of sudden onset, which may be followed by effort dyspnoea depending on the degree of lung retraction. The condition recurs in about a quarter of the cases.

Rarely, a valve mechanism may operate at the site of the rupture, allowing more air to be sucked into the pleural space on each inspiration, but allowing none to escape on expiration; this leads to tension pneumothorax, with complete collapse of the lung and displacement of the mediastinum towards the opposite side, and constitutes a medical emergency.

In the presence of established obstructive airway disease and limited respiratory reserve, even a shallow pneumothorax can precipitate a crisis of respiratory failure; this is particularly likely when multiple bullae are present, or in the presence of advanced fibrosing alveolitis.

The physical signs are usually diagnostic, namely absent breath sounds with normal, or sometimes increased, resonance on percussion; a small left-sided pneumothorax may also produce a clicking sound synchronous with the heart beat. Tension pneumothorax is characterized by severely distressed respiration, with displacement of the trachea and cardiac apex to the other side; a ringing sound may be heard by tapping a coin placed on the chest wall.

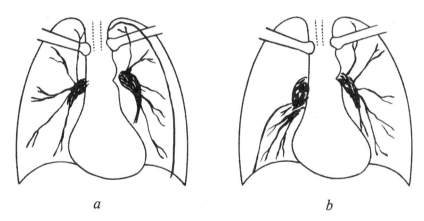

a   *b*

Fig. 2.28*a,* Uncomplicated shallow pneumothorax. *b,* Larger pneumothorax with collapsed right upper lobe.

Investigations

A chest radiograph will show a thin line corresponding to the edge of the lung, with absence of any markings peripheral to it, with or without collapse of a lobe or segment (*Fig.* 2.28). In tension pneumothorax, the whole lung is airless and the mediastinum displaced (*Fig.* 2.29). A shallow pneumothorax is more clearly seen on a film taken in deep expiration.

The blood gases should be estimated to monitor progress if respiratory failure is present due to underlying lung disease.

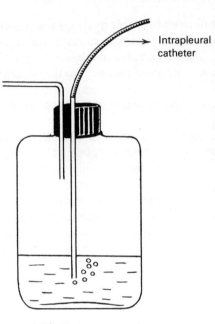

Intrapleural
catheter

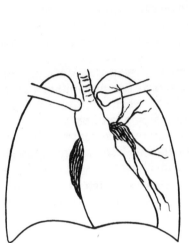

Fig. 2.29 Tension pneumothorax; collapsed right lung; mediastinum displaced
to left.

Fig. 2.30 Underwater seal.

Management

The mild case, with a distance of 2–3 cm between the lung edge and the chest
wall, usually resolves spontaneously in about 3 weeks. No treatment is
required, and there is no evidence that bed rest hastens re-expansion. When
dyspnoea is present, as is usual with greater degrees of collapse, an
intercostal rubber catheter is inserted through a cannula, and held in place by
a skin stitch or plaster after the cannula is withdrawn: this is best done
through the 3rd intercostal space in the midclavicular line, or, alternatively,
in the 5th space in the midaxillary line, a position which is rather less
convenient for the patient. The catheter is connected to an underwater seal
(*Fig.* 2.30), or more conveniently to a ball valve strapped to the skin which
allows the patient to remain mobile. The underwater seal has the advantage
that escaping air can be seen bubbling through the water during cough or
expiration, as can the swing of the water level in the lower end of the glass
tube with each respiration, confirming that the drain is patent.

When a substantial bulla has ruptured in a patient with established bullous
emphysema or other diffuse lung disease, underwater drainage may need to
be supplemented by a suction pump in series with, and distal to, the water
seal bottle. If this fails to achieve re-expansion, thoracotomy is called for so
that the bulla can be excised or oversewn; some patients in this category are
not fit for major surgery because of impaired function, and in this group the
pneumothorax may be a terminal complication.

Management of recurrent pneumothorax

If a spontaneous pneumothorax recurs once, it is likely to do so again. After a second incident, pleurodesis should be considered; in the past this used to be attempted by injecting sclerosing fluid (dilute silver nitrate solution) or talc into the pleura, to promote an inflammatory reaction and later pleural adhesion. There is, however, no firm evidence that this painful procedure affords any useful protection against further attacks. The procedure of choice to prevent recurrence is thoracotomy with extensive parietal pleurectomy.

Epidemic myalgia

First described on the island of Börnholm, this disorder is due to infection with Coxsackie B virus. It presents with fever and sore throat, rapidly followed by prostration and severe pleuritic pain. Cough and sputum are absent, and the lungs are not involved. Resolution follows spontaneously in a few days, but a second spike of fever about 5 days after the onset is not unusual. The diagnosis is confirmed by rising serum antibody levels.

Reactions to ingested agents

Paraquat

Ingestion of even small amounts of this weedkiller gives rise after a few days to acute renal failure, which is accompanied by relentlessly progressive diffuse lung fibrosis, which continues after the poison has disappeared from the serum. Death occurs about 3 weeks after ingestion; the nature of the reaction is obscure.

Many cases occur as a result of self-poisoning, the remainder accidentally, often in children, after drinking from an unlabelled bottle.

Management

Death is due to a combination of renal failure and anoxia. A number of recoveries have occurred, so that intensive respiratory and renal care, including steroid therapy, should be instituted after immediate gastric lavage; large doses of Fuller's earth by mouth are believed to adsorb the poison and reduce absorption, but there is no specific antidote.

Drugs

Diffuse lung reactions may be due to a hypersensitivity response to a number of drugs: the accurate recording of any current or previous drug therapy must never be neglected in any case of diffuse lung disease, despite the difficulty sometimes experienced in obtaining accurate information. The reactions, which vary in type with different drugs, are not all fully understood. The following are some of the commoner examples: new ones are regularly being reported.

1. *Pulmonary eosinophilia* (*see* p. 103) may be due to a number of drugs including sulphonamides and imipramine.

2. A drug reaction resembling *systemic lupus erythematosus* may involve the lungs and pleura; drugs incriminated include procainamide, hydralazine, and methyldopa.

3. *Diffuse interstitial fibrosis* may be due to nitrofurantoin, and some immunosuppressive drugs, notably busulphan and bleomycin: the latter may cause extensive and acute changes which later lead to fibrosis.

4. *Pleural and mediastinal fibrosis* may be due to methysergide, along with retroperitoneal fibrosis.

Management

Success depends on recognizing the possibility of a drug reaction: many are completely reversed after withdrawal of the drug, but, depending on the duration of exposure, there may be permanent residual fibrosis. It is reasonable to exhibit steroids in the acute stage.

FOR FURTHER READING

General

Brewis R. A. L. (1980) *Lecture Notes on Respiratory Disease,* 2nd ed. Oxford, Blackwell.
Crofton J. and Douglas H. (1981) *Respiratory Diseases,* 3rd ed. Oxford, Blackwell.
Cumming G. and Semple S. J. (1980) *Disorders of the Respiratory System,* 2nd ed. Oxford, Blackwell.
James D. G. and Studdy P. R. (1981) *A Colour Atlas of Respiratory Diseases.* London, Wolfe Medical Publications.
Scadding J. G. and Cumming G. (1981) *Scientific Foundations of Respiratory Medicine.* London, Heinemann.

Chapter 2.2

Cameron I. R. and Phillips I. (1980) Pneumonia. In: *Recent Advances in Respiratory Medicine II.* (ed. Flenley D. C.) p. 14. Edinburgh, Churchill Livingstone.
Fox W. (1980) *Short Course Chemotherapy for Tuberculosis.* p. 183. Edinburgh, Churchill Livingstone.

Chapter 2.3

Brewis R. A. L. (1978) Respiratory failure. *Br. Med. J.* **1,** 898–900.
Henley D. C. and Warren P. M. (1980) Chronic bronchitis and emphysema. In: *Recent Advances in Respiratory Medicine.* Edinburgh, Churchill Livingstone, p. 205.

Hugh Jones P. and Whinster W. (1978) Aetiology and management of disabling emphysema. *Am. Rev. Resp. Dis.* **117**, 343.
Sykes M. K., McNichol M. W. and Campbell R. J. M. (1976) *Respiratory Failure.* Oxford, Blackwell.
Third Report from the Royal College of Physicians (1977) *Smoking or Health.* London, Pitman.

Chapter 2.4

Ciba Foundation Guest Symposium (1971) *Identification of Asthma.* Edinburgh, Churchill Livingstone.
Israel H. L. (1980) Granulomatous lung disease. In: *Recent Advances in Respiratory Medicine II.* (ed. Flenley D. C.). Edinburgh, Churchill Livingstone, p. 19.
Turner-Warwick M. (1972) Cryptogenic fibrosing alveolitis. *Br. J. Hosp. Med.* **7**, 697.
Turner-Warwick M. (1976) Diffuse interstitial disease of the lungs. In: *Recent Advances in Respiratory Medicine I.* (ed. Streeton J. B.) Edinburgh, Churchill Livingstone, p. 187.

Chapter 2.5

Miller G. A. H. (1970) Massive pulmonary embolism—medical management. *Br. Med. J.* **1**, 777.
Oakley C. M. (1970) Diagnosis of pulmonary embolism. *Br. Med. J.* **1**, 773.
Parreth M. (1970) Massive pulmonary embolism—surgical management. *Br. Med. J.* **1**, 778.

Chapter 2.6

Stradling P. (1981) *Diagnostic Bronchoscopy,* 4th ed. Edinburgh, Churchill Livingstone.
Third Report from the Royal College of Physicians (1977) *Smoking or Health.* London, Pitman.

Chapter 2.7

Parkes W. R. (1982) *Occupational Lung Disorders,* 2nd ed. London, Butterworths.

Chapter 2.8

D'Arcy P. F. and Griffin J. P. (ed.) (1984) *A Manual of Adverse Drug Interactions,* 3rd ed. Bristol, Wright.
Davies D. M. (ed.) (1981) *Textbook of Adverse Drug Reactions,* 2nd ed. London, Oxford University Press.

3 Common Gastroenterological Problems

R. H. Salter

3.1 INTRODUCTION

Many gastroenterological disorders are transient and subside spontaneously, even without recourse to the prevalent habit of self-medication. However, continuing symptoms are a frequent reason for patients seeking medical advice and account for a substantial percentage of a family doctor's workload. Similarly, gastrointestinal disorders are a common reason for referral to hospital outpatient clinics and emergency admission.

Accurate incidence and prevalence rates for gastrointestinal disorders are not available and the selection of conditions for inclusion in this section has been based on an analysis of the common reason for referral to a District Hospital Gastroenterology Clinic and for emergency admission to a General Medical Unit.

However, it is generally acknowledged that disorders of gastrointestinal function rather than organic disease account for the majority of patients referred to Gastroenterology Clinics and of this group, the irritable bowel syndrome predominates. Equally, acute upper gastrointestinal haemorrhage is probably the commonest gastrointestinal disorder resulting in emergency medical admission.

Clinical assessment

History

Listening to the patient's description of his complaints is time-consuming and is probably the main reason why this part of the assessment tends to be neglected. Nevertheless, more information is usually obtained when a greater proportion of the time available for the clinical assessment is spent on the history rather than the physical examination.

Some patients find it easy to give a concise, coherent account of their complaints with little prompting but others find it much more difficult and a question and answer approach is more appropriate. However, it is essential to be sure that the patient and the doctor are speaking the same language. Words such as 'nausea', 'vomiting', 'regurgitation', 'constipation', 'diarrhoea', etc. frequently need amplification for terms such as these carry many different interpretations.

The *family history* may frequently give useful information. Many gastrointestinal diseases have an increased familial incidence, e.g. gastric

158

cancer, duodenal ulcer, ulcerative colitis and gallstones. Similarly the knowledge that a relative of the patient has recently suffered or died from gastrointestinal malignancy may account for a patient's apparent excessive concern regarding the cause of his own symptoms.

The *social history* is particularly relevant. Stress factors such as marital disharmony, unemployment, school or occupational unhappiness, financial or accommodation problems, etc. may often be a direct cause of gastrointestinal symptoms or, alternatively, act as an aggravating factor even when there is an underlying organic explanation. Details of smoking and drinking habits should also be requested. Alcohol abuse is increasingly common and frequently accounts for early morning nausea and vomiting and the exacerbation of peptic ulcer symptoms.

Details of any *drugs* which the patient is taking must be established for it is no credit to the medical profession that gastrointestinal symptoms are frequently iatrogenic. Dyspepsia is commonly caused by analgesics (salicylates in particular) and this problem is also a frequent complication of many of the non-steroidal anti-inflammatory agents. The same preparations which cause dyspepsia may also precipitate frank ulceration and bleeding from the gastric mucosa. Digoxin is a potent cause of anorexia, nausea and vomiting and is a frequently overlooked explanation for these complaints. Drugs which may cause constipation include codeine, anticholinergics, anti-Parkinsonian preparations (excluding levodopa and amantadine), phenothiazine tranquillizers and tricyclic antidepressants, iron preparations, calcium and aluminium-containing antacids, barbiturates, benzodiazepines, monoamine oxidase inhibitors and diuretics. Many antibiotics cause soreness of the mouth, nausea, vomiting and diarrhoea. Drug jaundice is a significant problem and some cases of acute pancreatitis are iatrogenic. The list is endless. The message is to take a detailed drug history and consider whether each of the preparations in question might be contributing to any of the patient's problems, whether gastroenterological or not.

It might appear that taking such a detailed history is a lengthy undertaking. However, it is salutary to remember that patient mismanagement is much more often a result of inadequate history taking and physical examination than ignorance of the latest biochemical or immunological minutiae. Also time is often saved in the long run by avoiding unnecessary investigations and return visits.

Physical examination

Physical examination is often relatively unrewarding in diseases of the gastrointestinal tract. However, despite the low yield of diagnostic information a general examination is essential in addition to detailed attention to the abdomen. Even when the patient's symptoms suggest alimentary disease, the cause of the patient's illness may often be outside the gastrointestinal tract; for example, liver enlargement may be due to metastases from a bronchogenic carcinoma or consequent on cardiac failure.

Rectal examination is imperative and its omission continues to account for delay in the diagnosis of rectal carcinoma in particular.

Even when no abnormality is found, which is frequently the case, the patient often derives considerable relief from the fact that he has been thoroughly examined and senses that his complaints have been taken seriously. Similarly, a rough assessment of the patient's discomfort threshold can be obtained from his reaction during procedures such as inflating the sphygmomanometer cuff, abdominal palpation and rectal examination.

Multiple pathology

Gastrointestinal disorders frequently coexist and not all may have symptomatic relevance at any particular time. For example, hiatus hernia, duodenal ulcer, gallstones and diverticular disease of the colon may occur singly or in virtually any combination. Similarly, multiple pathology may occur in the same organ; for example, the coexistence of colonic cancer and diverticular disease. This problem re-emphasizes the importance of a thorough clinical assessment. If this is inadequate, the initial clinical impression may be misleading and an inappropriate investigation requested. This may nevertheless reveal an abnormality which may be irrelevant to the clinical problem but to which unjustified importance is attached. Indeed the possibility that an abnormal finding may be a red herring always needs to be considered even when clinical assessment has been extremely thorough.

Psychiatric aspects

The importance of a thorough social history has already been emphasized for environmental stress factors frequently have a major role both as the cause of gastrointestinal symptoms and as an aggravating influence lowering the discomfort threshold even when there is an underlying organic condition. Also the possibility of an underlying anxiety state or depressive illness should always be borne in mind. Depression frequently presents as an apparent alimentary disorder with anorexia, weight loss, upper abdominal pain and constipation. However, the underlying problem can usually be recognized when specific enquiry is made of the sleep pattern, diurnal mood variation, lack of confidence and interest and inability to cope, uncontrollable tendency to weep, etc.

The fear of underlying malignant disease is particularly common in patients with gastrointestinal symptoms. Sometimes this results from contact with relatives or friends who have suffered from carcinoma and this anxiety is rarely volunteered spontaneously. In consequence it is necessary to ask the patient specifically whether this has been a particular concern. Firm reassurance can then be given when appropriate (which is fortunately in the majority of instances) with often visible relief.

Even when no organic disease is found as a result of careful clinical assessment and the completion of appropriate investigations, it is important not to give the impression that the doctor considers the complaints imaginary. To the patient the symptoms are no less real and he still deserves a sympathetic hearing and an explanation of their origin in terms that he is able to understand.

3.2 GASTRO-OESOPHAGEAL REFLUX AND HIATUS HERNIA

Gastro-oesophageal reflux

Gastro-oesophageal reflux is one of the commonest causes of dyspepsia and is often associated with the radiological demonstration of a sliding hiatus hernia. However, reflux can occur in the absence of a hernia and equally by no means all patients in whom a hernia can be demonstrated show a tendency to reflux so there is no clear-cut causal association. Consequently, the demonstration of a sliding hiatus hernia by no means implies that the patient's symptoms are due to reflux and the possibility of coincidental gastrointestinal disease should always be considered.

The tendency to gastro-oesophageal reflux seems much more closely related to the competence of the *lower oesophageal sphincter,* rather than its position in relation to the diaphragmatic hiatus.

The two important *symptoms* of gastro-oesophageal reflux are:

1. *Heartburn,* defined as a burning sensation which starts in the xiphisternal region and radiates up behind the sternum and occasionally into the throat.

2. *Regurgitation* of bitter gastric contents into the mouth.

These symptoms are usually worse after food ingestion and are related to posture, being particularly troublesome on stooping or during recumbency. Retrosternal pain may also be experienced when swallowing hot fluids, this being a useful clinical pointer to the presence of oesophagitis.

Recurrent gastro-oesophageal reflux may result in *oesophagitis,* the complications of which are:

1. *Bleeding,* manifest by the development of chronic iron-deficiency anaemia or, less commonly, acute upper gastrointestinal haemorrhage.

2. *Stricture formation,* indicated by the development of progressive dysphagia (intermittent dysphagia may be due to oesophageal spasm.)

The pulmonary complications of gastro-oesophageal reflux include inhalational pneumonitis and bronchial asthma.

Diagnosis

RADIOLOGY

A barium meal (which should be performed using a double-contrast technique) is usually the first investigation performed in patients complaining of reflux symptoms. Frequently this will demonstrate a sliding hiatus hernia with a tendency to reflux during the examination but the failure to demonstrate either does not exclude the possibility that the patient's symptoms are a result of reflux. In addition, the barium meal examination should also show if there is any significant degree of oesophageal stricture, may reveal evidence of oesophagitis when this is gross, and will also demonstrate any associated gastroduodenal pathology.

ENDOSCOPY

Oesophagoscopy, usually performed with a fibreoptic instrument, allows visualization of the oesophageal lumen when the degree of reflux can be noted and whether or not the regurgitated fluid is bile-stained. Gross oesophagitis can be recognized macroscopically but the correlation between the degree of oesophagitis as judged histologically and the endoscopic appearance of the oesophageal mucosa is not close so that biopsies should be taken in situations of doubt. Specimens should also be taken for histological or cytological examination whenever there is any associated oesophageal stricture.

OTHER INVESTIGATIONS

The most reliable way to demonstrate the reflux of acid gastric juice into the lower oesophagus is continuous recording of the pH of the oesophageal contents but this procedure is not widely available nor very frequently indicated. Perfusion of the lower oesophagus using dilute hydrochloric acid is a simple and reliable way of reproducing pain due to gastro-oesophageal reflux when there is doubt as to the origin of the patient's symptoms.

Differential diagnosis

The frequent occurrence of a sliding hiatus hernia without symptoms and the very loose association between this anatomical variant and symptomatic reflux implies that great care is necessary in deciding its clinical significance when this is reported radiologically. The distinction between *chest pain* of cardiac origin and that resulting from gastro-oesophageal reflux may be extremely difficult, particularly when the two conditions coexist. A detailed history is the mainstay of diagnosis and pain of reflux origin may be reproduced by acid perfusion. Likewise, stress-testing may be useful to establish the suspicion of pain due to ischaemic heart disease when a resting ECG is normal. *Dyspeptic symptoms* may be due to coexisting gastro-intestinal pathology such as gastric or duodenal ulceration and gallstones. Diverticular disease of the colon may be an alternative explanation for the patient's complaints. *Iron-deficiency anaemia*—a sliding hiatus hernia can certainly be the cause of occult blood loss from the gastrointestinal tract even when the patient denies symptoms of reflux and there is little oesophago-scopic evidence of oesophagitis. Nevertheless, as this is such a common finding, the fact that an hiatus hernia has been demonstrated does not automatically imply that it is the source of blood loss and other possibilities, particularly carcinoma of the proximal colon, should also be considered (*Fig.* 3.1).

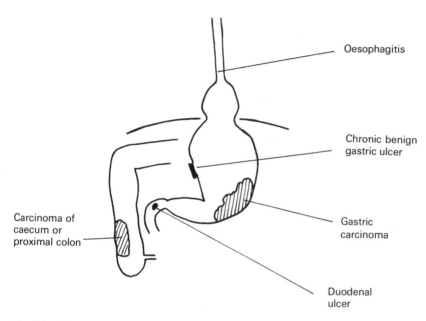

Fig. 3.1. Common causes of occult gastrointestinal bleeding.

Management

Most patients with symptomatic gastro-oesophageal reflux can be managed conservatively. Reassurance and a simple explanation of the origin of the patient's symptoms is important.

General measures include postural advice, raising the head of the bed, weight reduction, the avoidance of tight abdominal supports and giving up cigarette smoking.

Drug treatment

Antacids remain the mainstay of drug treatment and should be given as frequently as symptoms indicate and in adequate dosage. Liquid or tablet preparations appear equally effective although the latter is often more convenient for the patient. More sophisticated preparations which carry theoretical advantages and which some patients find more effective in practice include:

Antacid combined with dimethicone.
Antacid–alginic acid compounds.

Pyrogastrone. This preparation consists of an antacid with alginate and carbenoxolone which is effective not only in relieving the symptoms of gastro-oesophageal reflux but also heals the oesophagitis. The dose is one tablet to be chewed three times a day after meals and two tablets at bedtime for at least 6 weeks.

Metoclopramide 10 mg t.d.s., appears to increase the lower oesophageal sphincter pressure and thus reduce gastro-oesophageal reflux.

H₂-receptor antagonists. Cimetidine 200 mg t.d.s. and 400 mg at bedtime, or alternatively, 400 mg b.d. and ranitidine 150 mg b.d. inhibit gastric acid secretion and are helpful to a varying degree in patients with symptomatic gastro-oesophageal reflux.

Anticholinergic drugs reduce lower oesophageal sphincter pressure and their use should be *avoided* when dyspeptic symptoms are due wholly, or even partially, to gastro-oesophageal reflux.

Surgery

Operative intervention is usually indicated for one of two reasons:

1. The failure of medical treatment to control reflux symptoms.

2. Because of the development of complications, for example stricture or recurrent gastrointestinal bleeding.

When possible the hernia is reduced and the hiatus repaired by an abdominal or transthoracic approach. The former allows the exclusion of coincidental abdominal disorders although employment of the transthoracic route may achieve a better technical result. A fibrous oesophageal stricture usually responds to dilatation which can be repeated as necessary.

Surgery for troublesome reflux symptoms associated with an uncomplicated sliding hiatus hernia should be approached with caution and advised only when:

1. The patient has not responded to a course of intensive medical treatment.

2. The symptoms are genuinely those of gastro-oesophageal reflux.

3. Coexisting intra-abdominal or intrathoracic disorders contributing to the clinical picture have been excluded as far as possible.

Para-oesophageal hiatus hernia (Fig. 3.2)

The considerably less common para-oesophageal or rolling hiatus hernia describes the condition when the gastro-oesophageal junction remains in the normal position below the diaphragm but part of the stomach passes up through the oesophageal hiatus. This may be quite gross and yet is often asymptomatic. The disorder is not usually associated with gastro-oesophageal reflux and symptoms may either be due to the presence of the hernia itself (e.g. breathlessness) or due to complications such as bleeding, ulceration, gastric volvulus, obstruction, strangulation, perforation, etc. Medical management has little to offer and surgical repair is usually advised

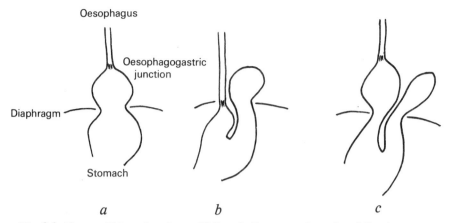

Fig. 3.2. Types of hiatus hernia. *a*, Sliding; *b*, Para-oesophageal; *c*, Mixed.

when the hernia is troublesome, assuming the general condition of the patient permits.

3.3 DYSPHAGIA

Dysphagia, or difficulty in swallowing, is always a symptom to be taken seriously for it usually has an organic basis and malignant disease in particular always needs to be considered when this symptom occurs for the first time in a patient of middle-age or over. The causes of dysphagia are numerous but in adult clinical practice the causes encountered most frequently are (*Fig.* 3.3):

1. Peptic oesophageal stricture.
2. Carcinoma of the oesophagus or upper stomach.
3. Oesophageal spasm, associated with either oesophagitis resulting from gastro-oesophageal reflux or as part of the peristaltic abnormality occurring in old age (presbyoesophagus). Achalasia of the cardia is rare.
4. Extrinsic pressure, e.g. from a bronchogenic carcinoma, aortic dilatation or an enlarged left atrium.
5. Drugs such as emepronium bromide (Cetiprin) doxycycline (Vibramycin) and slow-release potassium preparations may also cause dysphagia, particularly in patients with underlying oesophageal hold-up.

Clinical features

The major complaint is the sensation of food sticking anywhere between the throat and xiphisternum although the site indicated by the patient is not a reliable guide to the anatomical level of obstruction.

Intermittent dysphagia is more suggestive of spasm rather than a fixed obstruction and a previous history of heartburn and acid regurgitation suggests a peptic stricture. Peristaltic disorders often make the swallowing of

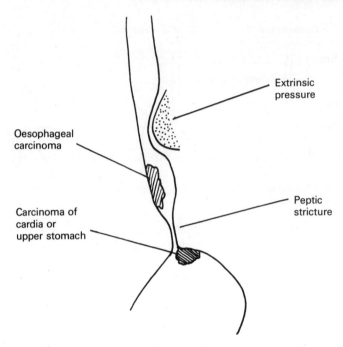

Fig. 3.3. Common causes of dysphagia.

liquids and solids equally difficult whereas a persistent stricture, whether malignant or benign, causes difficulty at least initially with solids only and especially meat and potatoes.

The swallowing difficulty may be associated with retrosternal pain which can be so severe that the patient faints and may not subside until the food bolus either passes the obstruction or is regurgitated. Anorexia and weight loss are often present when the dysphagia is due to malignant disease.

Physical examination is often unhelpful but may reveal weight loss or evidence of underlying bronchogenic malignancy or cardiovascular disease.

Investigations

RADIOLOGY

A chest film should reveal the existence of bronchogenic carcinoma, aortic aneurysm or cardiomegaly and a barium swallow and meal can usually be relied upon to demonstrate the site of obstruction although even with a double-contrast technique it is not possible to differentiate a benign from a malignant structure with confidence.

OESOPHAGOSCOPY

Oesophagoscopy complements radiology in this situation and should always be performed when a patient complains of dysphagia even if the barium swallow and meal is normal. The use of a fibreoptic instrument is preferable which allows the lumen to be inspected together with the cardia and upper stomach. Specimens can be taken by brushing for cytological or histological examination respectively.

Management

The management of patients with dysphagia depends on the underlying cause. Carcinoma of the oesophagus may be treated surgically although squamous lesions also respond to megavoltage deep X-ray therapy. Adenocarcinomas which occur predominantly in the upper stomach and cardia are not radiosensitive and if these cannot be removed surgically then useful palliation may be achieved by the insertion of a Celestin tube which can now be placed using a fibreoptic instrument. Extrinsic pressure from bronchogenic carcinoma may also respond at least temporarily to deep X-ray therapy or cytotoxic drugs. Dysphagia due to a peptic stricture may be helped by oesophageal dilatation as necessary, combined with the use of intensive medical anti-reflux measures (*see* Chapter 3.1). Oesophageal spasm, associated with severe oesophagitis, also usually responds to the use of a preparation such as pyrogastrone. The medical treatment of peristaltic disorders is less satisfactory and firm reassurance is an important aspect of management in this situation.

3.4   CHRONIC GASTRIC ULCER

The management of gastric ulceration, the cause of which is still not clear, is dictated by the difficulty in confidently distinguishing benign from malignant gastric lesions. The possibility of malignancy is particularly high if an ulcer is situated in the gastric antrum or on the greater curve of the stomach and although ulcers on the lesser curve are usually benign this can never be an automatic assumption. The maximal incidence is in middle-age and over, and there is an increased familial incidence. Gastric ulceration also occurs more frequently in patients with chronic bronchitis and other debilitating diseases. Gastric and duodenal ulceration may coexist in a small percentage of patients. Non-steroidal anti-inflammatory drugs are a potent cause.

Clinical features

A gastric ulcer may be completely *silent* clinically, its presence only becoming apparent when complications such as haemorrhage or perforation occur.

More commonly, *dyspeptic symptoms* occur such as epigastric or left hypochondrial pain often related to food ingestion and relieved by antacids. The pain may be periodic and radiate into the back. Vomiting may occur and weight loss can result both as a consequence of fear of eating lest pain is induced or actual loss of appetite.

Physical examination is rarely helpful. Epigastric tenderness is frequently found but of no diagnostic value.

Diagnosis

It is important to realize that the symptoms referred to above are by no means pathognomonic of gastric ulceration and the diagnosis, if suspected, must be confirmed by further investigations.

BARIUM MEAL

The barium meal remains the method of choice for the investigation of a patient suspected of having a gastric ulcer, provided a double-contrast technique is used. It follows that a barium meal report should not simply be taken at its face value for its reliability can only be assessed in the knowledge of the proficiency and interest of the radiologist and the technique used.

GASTROSCOPY

Gastroscopy using a fibreoptic instrument is complementary to radiology, its main use being to assess further a gastric lesion demonstrated by barium meal examination. It is also indicated despite a negative barium meal if the patient's symptoms are persistent, there is a positive family history of peptic ulceration or evidence of gastrointestinal bleeding as indicated by anaemia or the presence of occult blood in the faeces.

Modern fibreoptic instruments allow virtually the whole of the stomach to be inspected so that not only can the presence of the gastric ulcer be confirmed but specimens can be taken from the ulcer edge and base for cytological or histological examination so that malignancy can be excluded with a reasonable degree of confidence. The proximal duodenum can also be inspected during the examination in view of the occasional coexistence of duodenal ulceration.

Complications

These may be the first indication that an ulcer is present or occur on a background of chronic dyspepsia.

GASTROINTESTINAL BLEEDING

This may manifest either by the development of iron-deficiency anaemia or acute upper gastrointestinal haemorrhage (*see* p. 177).

PERFORATION

This classically presents with the sudden onset of severe upper abdominal pain which rapidly becomes generalized and associated with signs of peritonitis. A plain X-ray of the abdomen usually reveals free gas under the diaphragm. Emergency surgery is indicated.

PENETRATION

A gastric ulcer may penetrate through the stomach wall into the surrounding structures, especially the pancreas. Clinically this development is suggested by the pain radiating into the back and becoming more severe and continuous.

HOUR-GLASS STOMACH

Gross scarring as a result of chronic gastric ulceration on the lesser curve may constrict the body of the stomach into an upper and lower loculus. This is suggested clinically by the development of nausea, a sensation of fullness after meals and vomiting.

MALIGNANT CHANGE

A chronic benign gastric ulcer rarely undergoes malignant change and the major problem is to distinguish between a benign lesion and an ulcerating carcinoma from the outset.

Management (Fig. 3.4)

As has been previously emphasized management is influenced by the fear that a gastric ulcer might be a malignant lesion. Surgery may be advisable when the diagnosis is first made on the grounds of ulcer site, chronicity, associated complications, etc. with the operation most commonly employed being partial gastrectomy with a gastroduodenal anastomosis (Billroth I resection). An alternative procedure is vagotomy and drainage combined with ulcer biopsy. However, with the reassurance from radiology and endoscopic biopsy that a gastric ulcer is benign, it is reasonable to try and heal an *uncomplicated gastric ulcer* with *medical treatment.*

Drugs which appear to increase the rate of ulcer healing include cimetidine 200 mg t.d.s. and 400 mg at bedtime or, alternatively, 400 mg b.d.; ranitidine 150 mg b.d.; carbenoxolone 100 mg t.d.s., after meals for one week than 50 mg t.d.s. after meals for a further 4–6 weeks; deglycyrrhizinized liquorice, 2 or 3 tablets chewed 3–6 times daily between meals and potassium dicitrato bismuthate 5 ml diluted with 15 ml of water q.d.s. half an hour before the three main meals and 2 hours after the last meal. Side-effects associated with the use of cimetidine are unusual but carbenoxolone may induce hypokalaemia, sodium retention and oedema, and should be used with care particularly in the elderly and those patients with associated heart disease or renal functional impairment. Deglycyrrhinizinized liquorice is free from these side-effects but its efficacy is doubtful.

Bed-rest and the cessation of cigarette smoking both accelerate ulcer-healing, antacids are helpful for symptomatic relief but the hallowed 'ulcer diet' is not of proven value. However, the temporary omission of dietary items which specifically aggravate the patient's complaints is commonsense.

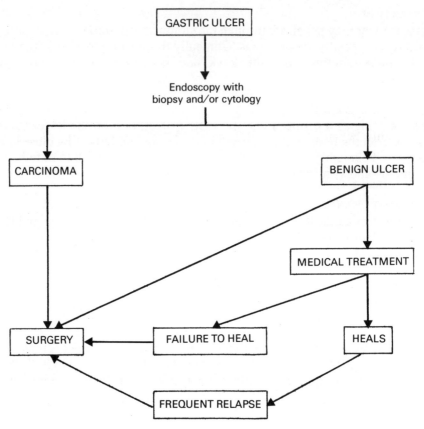

Fig. 3.4. Management of gastric ulceration.

After 6–8 weeks of medical treatment, the patient is reassessed, bearing in mind that the relief of symptoms unfortunately does not necessarily mean that the ulcer has healed. This can only be confirmed by either repeating the endoscopic examination or a double-contrast barium meal.

RELAPSE
Unfortunately, even if medical treatment is successful in achieving ulcer healing, there is a high chance of relapse varying from 30 to 40%. Maintenance treatment with one of the H_2-receptor antagonists in low dosage may delay recurrence.

Surgery
Surgery should at least be considered when medical treatment fails to achieve ulcer healing, when there is any suggestion that the lesion may be malignant, when ulcer complications develop, when gastric ulceration

occurs in association with a chronic duodenal ulcer or rapidly recurs after courses of medical treatment.

3.5 GASTRIC CARCINOMA

Carcinoma of the stomach remains one of the most depressing of the commonly encountered gastrointestinal problems. Results of treatment are poor, mainly because in most instances by the time the growth begins to cause symptoms it has already reached an advanced stage. The results of surgery are considerably better when the malignant process is confined to the gastric mucosa (mucosal cancer) but although diagnosis at this stage is technically possible with the aid of modern radiology and endoscopy, this is rarely achieved in practice as the disease is usually asymptomatic until advanced.

The cause of gastric carcinoma remains unknown although dietary factors may be important and there is considerable interest in the possibility of potential carcinogens such as nitrosamines in the gastric juice. There is a definite association with blood group A, a marked variation in incidence in various parts of the world and occasionally a strong family history is obtained.

Premalignant conditions include pernicious anaemia, atrophic gastritis, adenomatous gastric polyps and previous gastric surgery. The incidence is maximal between the ages of 50 and 70 years, although the younger age groups are by no means completely exempt.

Clinical presentation

As previously mentioned, symptoms are a late feature of gastric malignancy making early diagnosis extremely difficult. Consequently a high degree of clinical suspicion is required and the possibility of carcinoma of the stomach should always be kept in mind when patients with any of the premalignant situations already discussed are encountered. The usual modes of clinical presentation are:

1. The development of anorexia, weight loss, upper abdominal pain and a feeling of fullness after only a small quantity of food in a person of middle-age or over who has not previously complained of dyspepsia. However, a long history of dyspepsia does not necessarily exclude the possibility of gastric malignancy and a change in bowel habit (either constipation or diarrhoea) may be an associated feature.

2. Obstructive symptoms. A high gastric carcinoma involving the cardia or lower oesophagus is particularly likely to cause dysphagia and malignant lesions in the pyloro-antral region are prone to induce vomiting and gastric retention.

3. Gastrointestinal bleeding. This usually occurs occultly and presents as a chronic iron-deficiency anaemia, but occasionally the bleeding may be

acute and result in emergency admission with haematemesis and/or melaena. The development of an iron-deficiency anaemia in a person of middle-age or over should be assumed to be a consequence of gastrointestinal blood loss until there is a more convincing alternative explanation and gastric malignancy must always be considered as a possible underlying cause.

4. Features of secondary spread. An unfortunately all-too-common presentation of gastric carcinoma, this suspicion is raised when a patient presents with the development of enlarged lymph nodes in the left supraclavicular fossa, hepatomegaly, ascites from peritoneal seeding and pulmonary metastases.

It is important to realize that the H_2-receptor antagonists may not only relieve the symptoms of gastric malignancy but also apparently heal a carcinomatous ulcer thus leading to diagnostic delay and diminishing the chances of successful surgical excision.

Physical signs

In the early stages of gastric carcinoma, physical signs are conspicuous by their absence and this possibility should never be dismissed because the patient appears in good health. When the growth is more advanced, any of the following signs may be detected: anaemia, evidence of weight loss, epigastric tenderness, an upper abdominal mass, a succussion splash or signs of secondary involvement (*see above*).

Investigations

A blood count may reveal a hypochromic anaemia and raised ESR but this is not a reliable screening test and when there is a strong clinical suspicion of gastric malignancy the fact that the Hb and ESR are normal should never result in more specific investigations being deferred. The faeces may be positive for occult blood but again a negative result does not obviate the need for further investigation.

RADIOLOGY

A barium meal is the most appropriate initial investigation and as already discussed its reliability is considerably increased if this is performed by an experienced radiologist using a double-contrast technique.

GASTROSCOPY

When there is definite radiological evidence of gastric malignancy, there is little need for further investigation but if the barium meal is doubtful or a negative result conflicts with a high index of clinical suspicion, fibreoptic gastroscopy is mandatory. This examination needs to be particularly thorough and biopsies or cytological material can be taken from any suspicious areas. However, it should be noted that extensive carcinomas are often those from which it proves most difficult to obtain positive histological confirmation.

Management

The treatment of carcinoma of the stomach is surgical but often, even when surgery appears feasible initially, many such operations prove to be only palliative rather than offering permanent cure. So often the disease may have already reached such an advanced stage when the patient is first seen that even palliative surgery may have nothing to offer. In this situation every attempt is made to maintain the patient's quality of life at as high a level as possible by the judicious use of measures such as blood transfusion, analgesics, anti-emetics and tranquillizing preparations.

Radiotherapy is of little value in this situation and the use of cytotoxic drugs in disseminated gastric cancer has not found widespread acceptance.

Dysphagia associated with a high gastric carcinoma or malignancy at the cardia may be relieved at least temporarily by oesophageal intubation using a fibreoptic technique.

3.6   DUODENAL ULCER

Duodenal ulceration is a common cause of recurring dyspeptic symptoms. Although the presence of a duodenal ulcer is usually associated with gastric hypersecretion of acid and pepsin, the fundamental cause of this condition remains unknown. There is a familial predisposition, males are affected more commonly than females and there is a wide age incidence. Duodenal ulceration is rarely associated with hyperparathyroidism or is a consequence of hypergastrinaemia.

Clinical features

As with gastric ulceration, an ulcer in the duodenum may be entirely symptomless and attention only drawn to its presence by the development of a complication such as acute gastrointestinal bleeding or perforation. Usually, however, the patient presents with recurring dyspeptic symptoms, i.e. epigastric or right hypochondrial pain which is commonly relieved by food or antacids. Back pain may be experienced when the ulcer is posterior in situation and penetrating the pancreas. Vomiting is not usually a major problem unless either pyloric stenosis has occurred or the ulcer is situated close to or actually in the pyloric canal.

Unfortunately the presence of a duodenal ulcer cannot be confidently predicted from symptom analysis alone and these complaints are equally likely to be a consequence of gastric ulceration, gastritis, or even biliary tract pathology. However, features which are particularly associated with duodenal ulceration are:

1. A definite periodicity with long symptom-free intervals, at least in the early stages.

2. Nocturnal pain, the patient often being awakened with epigastric pain during the early hours of the morning, relief usually being quickly obtained by taking antacids, milk or a small snack.

The appetite usually remains good and the weight is either static or may actually increase if the patient consumes large quantities of milk in an effort to relieve his discomfort. A disturbance of bowel rhythm is unusual but the association of a duodenal ulcer with diarrhoea should always raise the possibility of a gastrin-secreting tumour although a much more likely explanation is the use of a magnesium-containing antacid or coincidental bowel irritability.

Unfortunately the correlation between a duodenal ulcer and the patient's dyspeptic symptoms is not entirely clear; endoscopic studies have shown that even when an ulcer heals the symptoms may continue unchanged. The problem is even more difficult when the presence of an ulcer, demonstrated either radiologically or endoscopically, is associated with atypical symptoms such as diffuse lower abdominal pain without any clear relation to either food ingestion or antacid therapy. While such symptoms do occasionally seem to be a consequence of a duodenal lesion, the possibility of a coexisting intra-abdominal condition needs to be considered, or even that the symptoms might be due to a functional gastrointestinal disturbance.

Physical examination

Physical examination is essentially negative. Often the only finding is non-specific epigastric tenderness. Signs of anaemia and the presence of occult blood in the faeces suggest the ulcer has bled and a succussion splash several hours after taking food or drink may indicate gastric outlet obstruction. Physical examination is nevertheless important both for patient reassurance and also for detection or exclusion of associated disorders.

Investigations

A *barium meal* is usually the first investigation requested which should preferably be performed using a double-contrast technique. This minimizes the chances of error and, in particular, aids the distinction between scarring and acute ulceration which is virtually impossible to make using the conventional method. The barium meal will also allow an estimate as to the degree of gastric retention, demonstrate associated upper gastrointestinal pathology and may also be the first warning of gastric hypersecretion raising the possibility that a gastrin-secreting tumour might be responsible.

ENDOSCOPY

Fibreoptic endoscopy is complementary to radiology and should be performed routinely during endoscopic examination of the upper gastro-intestinal tract. This technique allows the presence of a duodenal ulcer to be established with a high degree of accuracy and is indicated when the radiological diagnosis remains in doubt or even if the barium meal is negative but the patient's symptoms are strongly suggestive, there is a family history of duodenal ulcer, or occult blood is present in the faeces.

GASTRIC SECRETION STUDIES

Assessment of the basal and maximal acid output after pentagastrin stimulation may be helpful for duodenal ulceration is frequently associated with gastric hypersecretion. This procedure is much less used than formerly, however, for the use of gastric secretion studies to determine which surgical procedure to use is not widely accepted and the Zollinger–Ellison syndrome is more easily excluded by serum gastrin assay which is now widely available.

Complications

1. Acute upper gastrointestinal bleeding (*see* 177).
2. Perforation. A perforated duodenal ulcer classically presents with sudden onset of severe abdominal pain which rapidly becomes generalized and associated with signs of peritonitis. A plain film of the abdomen usually reveals free gas under the diaphragm. Emergency surgery is indicated.
3. Penetration. A posterior duodenal ulcer may penetrate into other surrounding structures, especially the pancreas. Clinically this complication is suggested by the pain becoming more severe and continuous and boring through into the back.
4. Pyloric stenosis. The development of gastric outlet obstruction is suggested by the development of nausea, fullness after meals and vomiting, often occurring against a background of chronic dyspepsia. The vomitus may be copious, is often brownish in colour (often misinterpreted as a haematemesis) and contains recognizable food residue from a meal eaten 24 h or more previously. Associated features include loss of weight, weakness, thirst and constipation. The main *physical signs* are: weight loss, dehydration, visible gastric peristalsis and a succussion splash.

The diagnosis is established by barium meal and endoscopy, the differential diagnosis including pyloric canal ulceration, adult hypertrophic pyloric stenosis, prepyloric gastric ulcer and prepyloric carcinoma. Management includes correction of fluid, electrolyte and acid–base disturbance with gastric aspiration and usually surgery to follow whenever the patient's condition permits.

Management

The majority of patients suffering from duodenal ulceration can be effectively treated conservatively. Reassurance is important, it being stressed to the patient that his condition is not malignant and with no chance of the ulcer becoming so in the future. General advice includes attention to life-style with advice to relax and shelve responsibilities where possible.

Cessation of cigarette smoking and restriction of alcohol is recommended although most environmental stress factors are obviously outwith medical control. Dietary restrictions should be temporary and normal eating habits encouraged during remission. Advice to eat frequent and small meals is more important than the dietary constituents, although many duodenal ulcer sufferers often find their symptoms are aggravated by eating fried, starchy and spicy foods.

Mental and physical relaxation aids relief of ulcer symptoms and a period of bed rest may be necessary during severe ulcer exacerbations.

DRUG THERAPY

A wide variety of drugs have been used in the treatment of duodenal ulceration.

Symptom relief. Antacids remain the mainstay of symptomatic treatment and should be used as frequently as necessary when symptoms are troublesome. There is little to choose between individual preparations and the final decision should take into account cost, patient choice and convenience.

Anticholinergic drugs have little place in the modern treatment of duodenal ulceration and although anxiolytic agents may be helpful if a patient shows pronounced features of anxiety, these are not indicated routinely.

Ulcer healing preparations. The H_2-receptor antagonists both relieve symptoms and heal duodenal ulcers in a high percentage of patients. Either cimetidine 200 mg t.d.s., and 400 mg at bedtime or, alternatively, 400 mg b.d., or ranitidine 150 mg b.d. is appropriate. Carbenoxolone incorporated in a capsule of denatured gelatine which is designed to rupture at the pylorus and discharge its contents into the first part of the duodenum (Duogastrone) has also been shown to heal duodenal ulcers, the dose being a capsule taken with liquid q.d.s., 15–30 min before meals, for 6–12 weeks. Important side-effects of this treatment are electrolyte disturbances including hypokalaemia and sodium retention.

Other preparations which may be helpful to induce ulcer healing include potassium dicitrato bismuthate 5 ml diluted with 15 ml of water q.d.s. (half-an-hour before the three main meals and 2 hours after the last meal), and deglycyrrhizinized liquorice 2–3 tablets chewed 3–6 times daily between meals. New drugs are continually being introduced for this purpose.

Relapse prevention. The natural history of duodenal ulceration is to undergo spontaneous remission and relapse. The long-term use of the H_2-receptor antagonists in low dosage may control this tendency.

SURGERY

Surgical intervention may be indicated either to deal with complications or, even though the ulcer is uncomplicated, the patient's symptoms continue to be troublesome despite intensive medical treatment. Gastric resection (Polya gastrectomy) has largely been replaced by vagotomy (truncal or selective) combined with a drainage procedure (pyloroplasty or gastro-jejunostomy). Highly selective vagotomy (proximal gastric vagotomy; parietal cell vagotomy) obviates the need for a drainage procedure so there is less chance of side-effects such as diarrhoea, dumping or bilious vomiting. However, the incidence of recurrent ulceration is higher than after a more conventional surgical procedure.

Surgical intervention should be approached with caution in the following situations:

1. A young patient with a short history of dyspeptic complaints.

2. When there is associated neurotic or psychotic illness without a competent psychiatric assessment.

3. When there are predominant environmental stress factors such as marital disruption, legal proceedings, financial embarrassment, family bereavements or illness. In this situation there is a possibility that the ulcer symptoms might improve as the stressful situation subsides.

4. When the patient himself is not keen on surgical intervention.

5. When there has been little attempt to co-operate with suggested medical treatment.

6. When the patient admits to little in the way of ulcer symptoms despite the radiological or endoscopic demonstration of a large ulcer with or without evidence of gastric hypersecretion.

7. When the patient's symptoms are not convincingly those of a duodenal ulcer despite the fact that this has been demonstrated either radiologically or endoscopically.

8. When the risk of surgery is unacceptably high, for example in a frail, elderly patient or when there is evidence of associated severe cardio-respiratory disease. In this situation, long-term therapy with H_2-receptor antagonists is usually more appropriate.

3.7 ACUTE UPPER GASTROINTESTINAL BLEEDING

Acute upper gastrointestinal bleeding is an acute medical emergency which is potentially life-threatening. Sudden haemorrhage from the upper gastrointestinal tract usually results in haematemesis (the vomiting of blood which may be either fresh or, as the result of digestion, appears similar to coffee-grounds) and/or melaena (the passing of tarry black stools per rectum, the appearance of the blood having been altered in transit through the small bowel).

'Coffee ground' vomiting need not necessarily be due to the presence of altered blood for recently consumed beer, cocoa, meat extract, etc., may result in a similar appearance. In cases of doubt, testing the vomitus for the presence of occult blood usually settles the matter. Gastric outlet obstruction may also result in the patient vomiting brownish material which is often mistaken for true haematemesis.

Similarly, the passage of black stools may be associated with oral iron therapy or with taking a bismuth-containing antacid preparation rather than due to the presence of altered blood.

Fresh blood passed per rectum may be a result of bleeding from the upper gastrointestinal tract but this complaint is more likely to be due to a colonic or anorectal lesion.

Occasionally a patient is seen having fainted following an acute gastrointestinal bleed but before either an haematemesis or melaena has occurred. A thorough history and physical examination usually clarifies the diagnosis and a rectal examination may be confirmatory by revealing tarry faeces.

All patients who have suffered an acute gastrointestinal haemorrhage should be admitted to hospital, for even if the initial bleed appears trivial it is impossible to predict that a further catastrophic haemorrhage requiring intensive resuscitation will not recur in the near future.

Causes

The commonest causes of acute upper gastrointestinal bleeding are (*Fig.* 3.5):

1. Chronic gastric or duodenal ulcer.
2. Acute gastric erosions. These may be related to the ingestion of aspirin or other salicylate-containing preparations, corticosteroids or the use of non-steroidal anti-inflammatory agents. Alcohol abuse may also be a precipitating factor but often no cause is apparent.
3. Reflux oesophagitis.
4. Oesophageal varices.

Acute gastrointestinal haemorrhage may occasionally be the presenting feature of carcinoma of the stomach and bleeding may also arise from mucosal tears in the lower oesophagus which result from repeated vomiting (Mallory–Weiss syndrome). Other causes include benign oesophageal and gastric tumours, anticoagulant drugs, and any of the haemorrhagic disorders such as thrombocytopenia and familial haemorrhagic telangiectasia. Haematemesis may also be due to blood swallowed from bleeding lesions in the mouth or upper air passages, and occasionally even after full investigation no cause is apparent.

Clinical features

As previously stated, an acute upper gastrointestinal bleed usually presents with a haematemesis and/or melaena, often associated with a feeling of

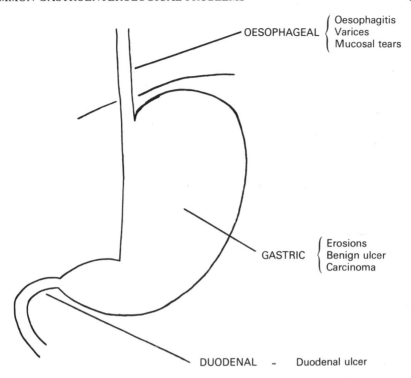

Fig. 3.5. Common causes of acute upper gastrointestinal bleeding.

faintness or actual loss of consciousness, sweating, palpitations, thirst and restlessness.

The main problems are to decide:
1. The cause of the bleeding.
2. The amount of blood lost.

1. CAUSE OF BLEEDING

Even though it is not possible to confidently identify the source of bleeding clinically, it is at least possible to exclude with reasonable confidence many of the possibilities. A long history of dyspepsia relating to meals suggests a chronic duodenal or gastric ulcer. Acute gastric erosions are suggested by the absence of previous dyspeptic symptoms and the recent ingestion of a salicylate, corticosteroid or non-steroidal anti-inflammatory preparation or alcohol abuse.

Reflux oesophagitis is suggested by heartburn occurring on bending or lying down at night, occasionally associated with the regurgitation of gastric contents into the mouth. However, bleeding may also occur from an ulcer in the intrathoracic portion of the stomach in a paraoesophageal hiatus hernia and as the mechanisms which prevent gastro-oesophageal reflux are not disturbed, heartburn is not a prominent feature.

Oesophageal varices should be suspected if the spleen is palpable for splenomegaly is the most reliable sign of portal hypertension. Other signs of chronic liver disease, such as jaundice, liver palms, spider naevi and ascites may also be apparent. It should be noted, however, that there is an increased incidence of peptic ulceration in patients with hepatic cirrhosis so that varices may not necessarily be the source of blood loss.

Gastric carcinoma is suggested by a recent history of anorexia, fullness or discomfort after meals and weight loss. Physical examination occasionally reveals evidence of the tumour itself or hepatomegaly from the presence of metastases.

Careful history taking and physical examination should exclude the more uncommon causes such as anticoagulant drugs, the Mallory–Weiss syndrome, thrombocytopenia, familial haemorrhagic telangiectasia, etc.

2. ASSESSMENT OF BLOOD LOSS

This presents some difficulty for the patient's or relative's description of the amount of blood loss is usually unreliable and there is tremendous variation in the response of different patients to the same degree of haemorrhage. The point at issue is to determine whether or not transfusion is indicated and by comparing the clinical features of haemorrhage with measurement of blood volume it has been found that this is usually required if:

 a. The pulse rate is 110 per min or above.

 b. The systolic blood pressure is 110 mmHg or below.

However, a young, fit patient may lose at least 50% of his blood volume with minimal or no change in the blood pressure and pulse rate. In the case of elderly patients who withstand severe haemorrhage comparatively poorly it is often wise to transfuse if significant blood loss is suspected before a major fall in the blood pressure occurs.

A misleading impression of severe blood loss may be given by a vasovagal reaction superimposed on the background of haemorrhage, the patient initially appearing deathly pale and severely hypotensive, only to improve spontaneously over the next 15–30 min.

As a rule a frank haematemesis indicates a large bleed and melaena alone a smaller bleed. Patients with an initial large bleed are more likely to bleed again than those with an initial small bleed and there is more chance of recurrent haemorrhage occurring after a haematemesis than after melaena only.

Investigations

These can be considered under three headings:

1. CAUSE OF BLEEDING

Theoretically at least the subsequent management of patients with acute gastrointestinal bleeding should be easier if the cause of the haemorrhage is established as early as possible although convincing benefit to the patient by such an approach is hard to demonstrate. Fibreoptic endoscopy is undoubtedly the most accurate technique although double-contrast radiology of the upper gastrointestinal tract can also demonstrate the site of bleeding reasonably accurately. Selective arteriography may occasionally be necessary if endoscopy has not localized the bleeding source but its use is excluded by the recent administration of barium as a contrast medium. Also this technique depends on there being continuing blood loss at the time arteriography is performed. A full haematological assessment is also indicated if a blood dyscrasia or bleeding diathesis is suspected.

2. ASSESSMENT OF BLOOD LOSS

Although a baseline haemoglobin and packed cell volume should be obtained, the results are of no value for this purpose as it may take several hours or days for haemodilution to be completed. Nevertheless, an initial Hb of 10 g or below is a further indication for immediate transfusion. Blood volume measurement using an isotopic technique is rarely available or indicated in the emergency situation but central venous pressure monitoring is readily available and is a useful indicator of oligaemia. This procedure is particularly helpful in minimizing the risk of precipitating cardiac overload by rapid blood transfusion. Likewise, a sudden drop in the central venous pressure may also be the first indicator that re-bleeding has occurred.

3. GENERAL INVESTIGATIONS

Patients presenting with acute upper gastrointestinal bleeding are often elderly with coexisting cardiopulmonary and renal disease which frequently affect management decisions. Urinalysis should be routine and chest radiography and electrocardiography are helpful. The blood urea is frequently elevated after gastrointestinal haemorrhage as a consequence of reduced renal blood flow, absorption of nitrogenous products or digested blood from the gastrointestinal tract and dehydration. In fact, assuming that the renal function prior to admission is normal a blood urea concentration over 8·5 mmol/l appears to indicate considerable blood loss.

Management

Many patients stop bleeding soon after admission and no specific measures are required other than a period of careful observation and investigation in an attempt to establish the cause of the haemorrhage. Bleeding from oesophageal varices is often difficult to control and as gastrointestinal haemorrhage in chronic liver disease carries the additional risk of precipitating hepatic failure, the management of this problem will be discussed in a separate section (*see below*). Patients with evidence of severe or recurrent blood loss are best managed in an intensive care situation with close medicosurgical co-operation.

1. CROSS-MATCHING

A blood sample should be taken at the time of admission for haemoglobin estimation and blood grouping and 2 litres of blood should be cross-matched. If this is transfused, more blood should be cross-matched so that a constant reserve of 1–2 litres is always readily available.

2. OBSERVATION

The pulse and blood pressure should be recorded half-hourly in addition to noting the general appearance of the patient. The nursing staff should be aware that indications of continuing or recurrent haemorrhage, other than the vomiting of blood or passage of a fresh melaena stool are:

    a. A fall in blood pressure.

    b. A rise in pulse rate.

    c. Complaint by the patient of suddenly feeling faint and thirsty, associated with signs such as pallor, restlessness and sweating.

Failure of the nurses to appreciate these points may result in considerable delay before the medical staff are informed that further bleeding has occurred.

3. SEDATION

Sedation is not indicated routinely but if this is judged necessary diazepam 10 mg i.m. is a suitable preparation for this purpose and can be repeated as necessary. The use of opiates for this purpose should be avoided.

4. BLOOD TRANSFUSION

As already stated, the widely accepted indications for immediate transfusion are:

    a. Pulse rate of 110 per min or over.

    b. Systolic blood pressure of 110 mmHg or below.

    c. An initial haemoglobin of 10 g/100 ml or less.

Blood is transfused until the pulse and blood pressure return to normal and until the patient looks pink with warm hands and a full volume pulse. If there is any doubt as to the adequacy of blood transfusion, monitoring the central venous pressure can be helpful.

Occasionally the haemorrhage may be so severe that it is impossible to wait for blood to be cross-matched even by an abbreviated technique and under these circumstances the use of plasma or a plasma substitute needs to be considered. Very rarely, the transfusion of unmatched group O Rh negative blood may be necessary.

When the rate of blood transfusion is rapid, 10 ml of 10% calcium gluconate should be given intravenously for every litre of blood transfused. The elevation of the serum potassium by the rapid transfusion of large volumes of stored blood is rarely a problem and can, in any case, be minimized by the use of as much fresh blood as possible.

5. H₂-RECEPTOR ANTAGONISTS

The role of preparations such as cimetidine and ranitidine remains to be defined. There seems little evidence that they are effective in preventing re-bleeding in patients with established chronic gastric or duodenal ulceration but may be of value when the haemorrhage occurs from gastric erosions or reflux oesophagitis.

Investigations to establish the cause of haemorrhage are instituted as soon as practically possible. Nasogastric aspiration is not indicated routinely but is useful in selected patients, in particular to give early warning of further haemorrhage. A light diet can be quickly introduced and it is important to maintain an adequate state of hydration.

With such measures, many patients stop bleeding soon after admission. However, apart from blood replacement, continuing blood loss demands measures to stop further gastrointestinal bleeding. Endoscopic laser photocoagulation is neither generally available nor convincingly effective for this purpose but selective arteriography used in conjunction with therapeutic embolism or intra-arterial infusion of vasopressin should certainly be considered in selected patients, particularly those who are unfit for surgical intervention. In practice, however, the only widely available method of stopping continuing or recurrent gastrointestinal haemorrhage is operative intervention. Conventional indications include bleeding from a chronic gastric ulcer, a longstanding duodenal ulcer with previous episodes of bleeding or other complications, any suspicion of gastric malignancy and continuing or recurrent haemorrhage 48 h after hospital admission. Relative contraindications are coexisting severe cardiac, respiratory or renal disease but the factors both for and against surgery must be carefully considered in each individual case. Surgical mortality undoubtedly increases with advancing age when the chance of coexisting disease is also at its highest.

Emergency management of bleeding oesophageal varices

It should be re-emphasized that in patients with oesophageal varices as a complication of hepatic cirrhosis, gastrointestinal bleeding may not necessarily be variceal in origin, alternative possibilities being reflux oesophagitis, chronic gastric or duodenal ulceration and gastric erosions. However, gastrointestinal haemorrhage from any site in a patient with cirrhosis is potentially serious in that the possibility of hepatic coma being precipitated is always present.

The first essential as described above is adequate blood transfusion to maintain the circulatory blood volume. In addition, the following precautions must be taken to prevent the development of hepatic coma:
1. The avoidance of sedative drugs.
2. Oral neomycin—6 g daily in divided dosage.
3. Evacuation of the colon by enema.
4. All dietary protein must be stopped and nutrition maintained with

glucose to provide 1600 calories per day. This is preferably given orally but may be administered by a nasogastric tube or as a 20–40% solution infused into a caval drip.

If the bleeding fails to stop spontaneously 20 units of vasopressin in 100 ml 5% dextrose should be infused intravenously over 10–15 min. Alternatively, this can be administered through a catheter in the superior mesenteric artery.

If the bleeding fails to stop after vasopressin infusion or quickly recurs, then variceal compression using the Sengstaken–Blakemore triple-lumen double balloon tube should be attempted. Before use the balloons should be checked for any leaks by inflating them under water. The tube is then lubricated and passed through the mouth into the stomach. The lower balloon is inflated with 200 ml of air and its position in the stomach checked by a plain radiograph of the abdomen. The oesophageal balloon is then distended with air to a pressure of 300 mmHg, gentle traction is exerted on the tube which is then fixed to the cheek by adhesive tape. In consequence, the lower balloon compresses the submucosal veins in the upper part of the stomach and the oesophageal varices are compressed by the upper balloon. The stomach contents may be aspirated via the third lumen and repeated pharyngeal suction is also required to remove saliva and other secretions.

Disadvantages of this technique are: it is unpleasant for the patient, there is a risk of asphyxia from upward displacement of the tube and ulceration of the lower oesophagus may occur.

Unfortunately there is a high risk of recurrent bleeding both after vasopressin infusion or variceal compression when injection scleropathy should be considered, the varices being injected through a fibreoptic endoscope. Shunt procedures to decompress the portal venous system are potentially hazardous in an emergency situation and when liver function is impaired. Likewise, surgical ligation of oesophageal varices or oesophageal transection confers temporary benefit only. None of these methods is ideal and the outlook for cirrhotic patients with recurrent upper gastrointestinal haemorrhage remains poor.

3.8   CHRONIC GASTROINTESTINAL HAEMORRHAGE

The commonest consequence of chronic blood loss from the gastrointestinal tract is iron-deficiency anaemia. This may be of recent onset or recurrent over many years and is occasionally interspersed with episodes of melaena. Chronic gastrointestinal bleeding may also be detected by chance if the faeces are screened for the presence of occult blood.

Clinical features

1. ANAEMIA

The symptoms and signs are those of anaemia from any cause, i.e. tiredness, lack of energy, breathlessness, faintness, dizziness, palpitations and leg

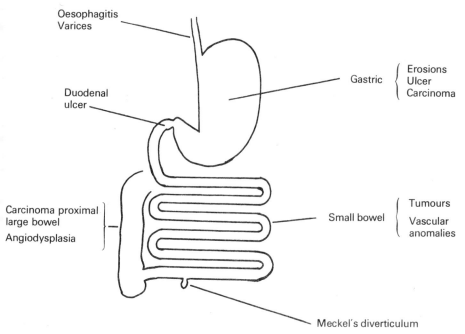

Fig. 3.6. Causes of chronic gastrointestinal bleeding.

swelling. Physical signs include pallor of the conjunctivae and mucous membranes, tachycardia, a haemic murmur, peripheral oedema and, if the anaemia is severe, heart failure. The tongue may be sore and the nails flat and brittle or spoon-shaped if the iron deficiency is of long-standing.

2. FEATURES OF THE UNDERLYING CAUSE

Some of the many causes of chronic blood loss from the gastrointestinal tract are shown in *Fig.* 3.6. The patient may complain of symptoms of the underlying lesion but it is important to note that reflux oesophagitis, chronic gastric ulceration, duodenal ulceration, gastric malignancy and carcinoma of the colon may be asymptomatic. Carcinoma of the caecum or right half of the colon is notoriously silent and is particularly likely to be missed if the upper gastrointestinal tract is investigated first by either radiology or endoscopy and too much significance attached to minor abnormalities, such as an hiatus hernia or gastric erosions.

Diagnosis

This depends on:
   1. Confirming that the anaemia is due to chronic blood loss from the gastrointestinal tract.
   2. Localizing the source of blood loss.

1. CONFIRMATION OF GASTROINTESTINAL BLEEDING

There are many causes of iron-deficiency anaemia including lack of dietary iron, malabsorption, recurrent nose bleeding, menstrual blood loss, etc. but whenever there is no other convincing explanation the possibility of chronic bleeding from the gastrointestinal tract must be considered. The anaemia is associated with hypochromic and microcytic red cells and if necessary iron deficiency can be confirmed by estimation of the serum iron or iron-binding capacity, serum ferritin or staining a bone marrow smear for the presence of iron. Haematological indicators that chronic haemorrhage is the cause include polychromasia and a persistent reticulocytosis in the absence of haemolysis or haematinic therapy. Serial faecal specimens should be tested for the presence of occult blood, but it should be noted that even if this is negative it does not exclude the possibility of chronic gastrointestinal bleeding for this may be intermittent. If there is still any doubt whether or not the anaemia is due to chronic gastrointestinal bleeding the red cells can be tagged with a suitable radioisotope and an assessment made of the radioactivity in a subsequent faecal collection.

2. LOCALIZING THE SOURCE OF BLOOD LOSS

Even if clinical assessment does not allow an accurate diagnosis as to the source of chronic gastrointestinal bleeding it often allows a reasonably confident prediction as to whether the cause is in the upper or lower gastrointestinal tract. Haemorrhoids may be apparent at proctoscopy but care should be exercised in attributing chronic bleeding to this cause for so often there may be coincidental pathology elsewhere in the gastrointestinal tract.

a. Barium studies. Disorders of the upper and lower gastrointestinal tract are by far the commonest cause of chronic blood loss and both barium meal and enema provide a high diagnostic yield in this situation. So often it is necessary to perform both these investigations (which need to be done using a double-contrast method), for both a sliding hiatus hernia and diverticular disease of the colon are such common radiological findings that care needs to be exercised in attaching too much clinical significance to their demonstration.

b. Fibreoptic endoscopy. Fibreoptic endoscopy of the upper gastrointestinal tract is essentially complementary to radiology, being particularly indicated when there is any diagnostic doubt resulting from a barium meal examination, and on occasions even when the radiologist is confident that the barium meal is negative, but no other obvious source of blood loss is apparent. For example, even quite severe oesophagitis may not be apparent radiologically and occasionally gastroduodenal lesions may be missed. Both sigmoidoscopy and colonoscopy may also be useful in this situation although a good quality double-contrast barium enema is a fairly reliable guide that there is no significant colonic pathology present.

c. *Small intestinal radiology.* When endoscopy and barium studies have revealed no source of bleeding in the upper and lower gastrointestinal tract, a lesion of the small intestine, for example tumour, ulcer, arteriovenous malformation, Meckel's diverticulum, should be considered. Radiology of the small intestine is indicated in this situation, the examination being performed using an intubation technique which is not only quicker but much more accurate than the conventional barium follow-through examination.

d. *Scintiscanning.* A preparation such as isotopically labelled sulphur colloid is injected intravenously, this being rapidly cleared from the circulation by the liver, resulting in a fast decrease in background activity. Concomitantly at the bleeding site there is a local area of increasing activity which can be identified with the gamma camera. The method is simple and non-invasive but it is nevertheless sometimes very difficult to localize the source of bleeding accurately. A Meckel's diverticulum lined with gastric-type mucosa may also be demonstrated by this method.

e. *Selective arteriography.* When the preceding investigations have failed to identify the site of bleeding, selective arteriography is of great value, particularly in demonstrating small gut disorders, such as tumours or vascular malformations, and also the microvascular abnormality referred to as angiodysplasia, which occurs most frequently in the right side of the colon. The procedure is relatively safe and well-tolerated in experienced hands.

f. *Laparotomy.* It must be admitted that even after the most intensive investigations it is sometimes still not possible to localize the source of gastrointestinal bleeding. Provided the patient is well and can adequately compensate for the bleeding with an iron supplement, it may be reasonable to follow an expectant course. However, if the patient suffers from recurring anaemia despite iron supplements and if blood transfusion is frequently necessary then a laparotomy may be justifiable. If still no obvious cause is apparent, the diagnostic yield of laparotomy may be increased by systematically inspecting the lumen of the gastrointestinal tract using a fibrescope at the time of surgery.

Management

The two essentials of management are:
1. Correction of the iron-deficiency anaemia. If mild, an oral iron supplement may be sufficient. More severe anaemia may require a total dose iron infusion but if the patient is severely anaemic intermittent transfusion of packed cells may be necessary.

2. Identifying and treating the cause of bleeding on its merits with surgical intervention as indicated.

3.9 DYSPEPSIA AFTER PEPTIC ULCER SURGERY

The recurrence of dyspepsia after peptic ulcer surgery is a disappointment to both patient and doctor. The keystone to effective management in this situation is *accurate diagnosis*. Two main questions required to be answered:

1. Is the patient's dyspepsia a consequence of recurrent peptic ulceration?

2. If not, are the patient's complaints due to organic pathology other than peptic ulcer or a consequence of a functional disturbance of the gastro-intestinal tract?

Apart from recurrent ulceration, alternative causes of dyspepsia in this situation include:

1. Gastro-oesophageal reflux
2. Bile gastritis and vomiting
3. Gallstones
4. Gastric carcinoma.

Diagnosis depends on a careful assessment of the clinical features and the use of appropriate investigations (*Fig.* 3.7). When these various possibilities have been excluded there remains a hard core of patients in whom no organic cause can be discovered for the persistence or recurrence of dyspeptic symptoms. This is particularly likely when no convincing evidence of peptic ulceration was found at the time of initial surgery.

Clinical features

Dyspepsia recurring after ulcer surgery is no exception to the rule that it is frequently not possible to diagnose the cause of the patient's complaints from clinical features alone. However, careful symptom analysis in particular often provides information that considerably narrows the diagnostic field.

1. RECURRENT PEPTIC ULCERATION

The site of recurrent peptic ulceration depends largely on the preoperative diagnosis and the previous surgical procedure performed. After vagotomy and pyloroplasty a recurrent ulcer is usually found in the pyloroduodenal region. Recurrent ulceration following either vagotomy and gastroenter-ostomy or a Polya gastrectomy usually occurs at or close to the stoma on the efferent side of the anastomosis. An ulcer may occur in the gastric remnant after a Billroth-I gastrectomy for chronic benign gastric ulceration. The incidence of recurrent ulceration also varies with the operative procedure, this being lowest after gastrectomy or vagotomy combined with antrectomy

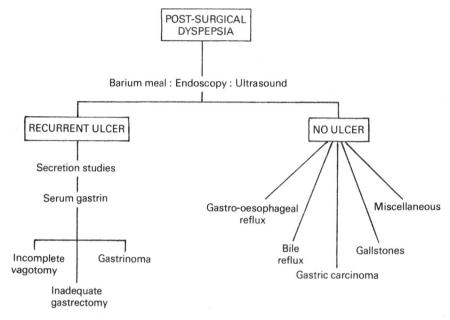

Fig. 3.7. Assessment of dyspepsia after peptic ulcer surgery.

and highest after the various vagotomy variants with or without a drainage procedure.

The possibility of recurrent ulceration is suggested by the return of dyspeptic symptoms similar to those experienced by the patient pre-operatively (*see* Chapters 3.4 and 3.6). Gastrointestinal bleeding, whether overt or occult, associated with the return of dyspeptic symptoms is a particularly strong pointer to recurrent peptic ulceration being the underlying explanation. Physical examination is usually negative or the findings non-specific.

2. GASTRO-OESOPHAGEAL REFLUX

The main features of gastro-oesophageal reflux, whether or not these are associated with the radiological demonstration of an hiatus hernia, are *heartburn* and *regurgitation* (*see* Chapter 3.2). Following ulcer surgery the refluxed gastric contents may still be acid or, alternatively, the pH may be alkaline due to the presence of pancreatic secretions and bile. The latter is particularly noxious to the oesophageal epithelium and may result in severe oesophagitis with its attendant complications—bleeding and stricture formation.

3. BILE REFLUX AND VOMITING

Apart from highly selective vagotomy where no anastomosis is created and no gastric drainage procedure required, all surgical procedures employed in the management of gastric and duodenal ulceration allow the reflux of bile and pancreatic juice back into the stomach. When severe, this may be associated with symptoms such as upper abdominal discomfort or fullness after meals, nausea and the vomiting of green or yellow fluid (bile) rather than food. The latter usually promptly relieves the patient's discomfort and may be self-induced to obtain pain relief. Often the symptoms are worse in the early morning, the patient feeling considerably better when, soon after rising he vomits a large quantity of bile-stained fluid.

Again physical examination is usually negative or reveals only non-specific upper abdominal tenderness.

4. GALLSTONES
The clinical features of gallstones are discussed in Chapter 3.11. The evidence suggesting there is an increased incidence of gallstones after vagotomy or gastric resection is not conclusive but nevertheless this condition is sufficiently common in its own right to require consideration as a possible explanation for the development of dyspepsia after ulcer surgery.

5. GASTRIC CARCINOMA
This is suggested by the complaints of anorexia, weight loss, a feeling of upper abdominal discomfort or fullness with inability to finish a meal, and vomiting. There appears to be an increased incidence of gastric malignancy after previous operations, such as gastrectomy and gastroenterostomy. Physical examination may be negative or, alternatively, there may be evidence of weight loss or anaemia. Occasionally an upper abdominal mass may be palpable (*see* Chapter 3.5).

6. FUNCTIONAL DYSPEPSIA
This is essentially a diagnosis of exclusion (*see* Chapter 3.10). It is particularly likely when the patient complains of recurrent symptoms within a few weeks or months of surgery similar to those experienced preoperatively and when a check of the operation note reveals that no convincing evidence of peptic ulceration or other intra-abdominal pathology was discovered at the time of laparotomy. The patient's complaints are often vague with diffuse upper abdominal pain unaffected by either food ingestion or the use of antacids. Physical examination is essentially negative and a detailed history is particularly important in this situation to search for background stress factors or features of hypochondriasis, anxiety or depression.

Investigations
The main stages in the assessment of patients with recurrent dyspepsia after peptic ulceration are shown in *Fig.* 3.7. The two most useful investigations as in the diagnosis of dyspepsia prior to surgery are:

1. BARIUM MEAL

When performed by the conventional technique the barium meal is notoriously unreliable in the post-operative situation. The use of a double-contrast technique by an experienced radiologist undoubtedly improves the diagnostic accuracy of radiology but whenever possible this procedure should be complemented by endoscopy.

2. FIBREOPTIC ENDOSCOPY

Endoscopy is particularly helpful in this situation although it is technically more difficult than when performed preoperatively. Endoscopy is undoubtedly the most accurate diagnostic technique postoperatively but the two methods are essentially complementary.

Hopefully as a result of these two investigations it should be possible to establish with a fair degree of uncertainty whether or not the patient's complaints are due to recurrent peptic ulceration. If the presence of a recurrent ulcer has been established, the next step is to ascertain the cause, if possible. The most likely explanations are an incomplete vagotomy or an inadequate gastric resection. Rarely, recurrent peptic ulceration is a consequence of a gastrin-secreting pancreatic tumour (Zollinger–Ellison syndrome). Gastric secretion studies aid this distinction although the results are often difficult to interpret in the postoperative situation. The assessment of basal acid secretion and the maximal gastric output after pentagastrin stimulation may provide evidence of gastric hypersecretion and the Zollinger–Ellison syndrome may be suspected if there is little difference between the basal and stimulated levels. This possibility can be further checked by assaying the serum gastrin concentration.

The standard method of checking whether or not a vagotomy has been completed is the 'Hollander' or insulin test where, after a basal collection of gastric juice has been made, hypoglycaemia is induced by the intravenous injection of insulin. This acts as a stimulant to gastric acid secretion, the vagi providing the sole efferent parasympathetic pathway. Complete section of the vagi is indicated by the ineffectiveness of the induced hypoglycaemia as a gastric acid stimulant.

When barium meal and endoscopy do not reveal any evidence of recurrent peptic ulceration this combination of investigations may nevertheless provide useful information to support any of the following as the explanation of the patient's complaints:

1. Gastro-oesophageal reflux
2. Bile reflux and vomiting
3. Gastric carcinoma

If neither recurrent ulceration nor any of the above possibilities appear to be the explanation for the patient's symptoms, the possibility of gallstones should be checked by radiology (cholecystography, cholangiography) and/ or ultrasonic scanning. Functional dyspepsia is suggested by the recurrence of symptoms within a few weeks or months of surgery, when the organic conditions discussed above have been excluded and when no convincing evidence of peptic ulceration was apparent at the time of surgery.

Occasionally the possibility of pancreatic disease may need to be considered and also diseases of the small and large intestine may require exclusion as the explanation of symptoms in selected patients.

Management

It has been repeatedly emphasized that an essential prerequisite for the effective management of recurrent dyspepsia after peptic ulcer surgery is an accurate diagnosis.

Recurrent peptic ulceration may initially be treated medically with H_2-receptor antagonists such as cimetidine 200 mg t.d.s., with 400 mg at night or ranitidine 150 mg b.d., but as in the preoperative situation the risk of ulcer recurrence when treatment is withdrawn is very high and maintenance treatment may be required indefinitely. The use of such treatment in the management of recurrent peptic ulceration has not been fully assessed and this situation is still frequently regarded as an indication for further surgery, particularly in view of the morbidity amd mortality associated with complications such as bleeding, gastrojejunocolic fistulae and perforation. Gastro-oesophageal reflux can usually be controlled by medical measures (Chapter 3.2) although surgery may be necessary if the patient's symptoms do not respond to such treatment or if complications such as stricture occur. The tendency to bile regurgitation and vomiting may improve spontaneously or be helped by metoclopramide 10 mg t.d.s. When bile vomiting and epigastric pain are persistent, however, and really make life a misery for the patient, further operation should be considered to minimize this tendency.

The demonstration of gallstones is usually an indication for cholecystectomy although if the patient's symptoms are solely those of flatulent dyspepsia there is no guarantee that operation will be followed by symptom relief. Further surgery should also be considerd when the diagnosis proves to be one of gastric carcinoma. Management of dyspeptic symptoms in the absence of organic pathology is particularly difficult, the approach being similar to that outlined in Chapter 3.10. Further surgery in this group of patients should be avoided if at all possible.

3.10   FUNCTIONAL DYSPEPSIA

Dyspepsia is a useful term to describe the complaint of upper abdominal pain and discomfort related to food ingestion, although this definition is often widened to include other symptoms such as nausea, flatulence, vomiting, heartburn and acid regurgitation. The commonest causes for this symptom complex are gastro-oesophageal reflux, gastric and duodenal ulceration, gastric cancer and gallbladder disease. Other gastrointestinal disorders which may cause dyspepsia include pancreatic disease, Crohn's disease and colonic disorders, and dyspepsia may also result from cardiac failure or chronic renal insufficiency. Many drugs induce dyspepsia (for example salicylates, non-steroidal anti-inflammatory drugs) and alcohol abuse is an often denied, although a frequent, explanation for early morning nausea and vomiting.

However, in many patients presenting with dyspepsia no underlying organic explanation can be found and it is assumed that their symptoms are a consequence of a *functional disturbance* of the upper gastrointestinal tract, i.e. the diagnosis is made by the exclusion of possible organic explanations. The pathophysiological basis of these symptoms is not clear although a disordered motility pattern of the upper gastrointestinal tract is probably one factor and pyloric incompetence leading to duodenogastric reflux may also be relevant.

The large number of possible causes of dyspepsia, both intra- and extra-abdominal, can easily lead to over-investigation in this particular clinical situation. Far from providing reassurance, the patient's anxiety is frequently intensified as the investigational process gathers momentum and the need for detailed investigation needs careful assessment in each individual situation.

Clinical features

Detailed analysis of the patient's symptoms is important although there are no characteristic features which reliably indicate the patient's complaints are a consequence of a functional disturbance rather than organic disease. Particular attention should be paid to:

1. Features suggesting psychiatric illness or cancer phobia.
2. Details of any drugs the patient may be taking.
3. Smoking and drinking habits.
4. Social factors including family stresses, employment problems, financial insecurity, marital disruption, etc.

Features suggesting that dyspeptic symptoms may arise from a functional disturbance of the upper gastrointestinal tract rather than organic disease are:

1. A long history of dyspepsia with preservation of general health combined with previous repeatedly negative investigations.
2. Associated features of neurotic or depressive illness or vague symptoms in patients with known hypochondriacal or hysterical tendencies. Unfortunately, however, it is inevitable that a patient will be encountered who cries 'wolf' once too often.
3. Significant background problems, such as marital disruption, employment unhappiness or dissatisfaction, financial embarrassment, etc.
4. Continuous vague upper abdominal pain with little or no relief by

antacids and the complaint of recurrent vomiting without weight loss or dehydration.

5. The patient's own observation that his symptoms are only present or certainly exaggerated when he is exposed to a stressful situation and eased or even absent when this no longer operates.

Conversely, two situations where the diagnosis of functional dyspepsia is fraught with danger are:

1. The onset of troublesome and persistent dyspepsia in a previously fit patient of middle age or over.

2. When the patient is obviously unwell and, in particular, complains of *anorexia* and *weight loss.*

Other clinical situations where particular care needs to be taken before the diagnosis of functional dyspepsia is made are:

1. When there is a strong family history of peptic ulceration, gastric carcinoma or gallstones.

2. When the patient is known to suffer from pernicious anaemia.

3. When dyspepsia recurs after peptic ulcer surgery.

4. Persistent dyspeptic complaints in an otherwise stoical patient or when there is no suggestion of psychiatric illness and when no background stress factors can be identified.

5. When dealing with an inarticulate or unintelligent patient where the history may be positively misleading.

Physical examination

A thorough physical examination is essential both to reassure the patient that his complaints have been taken seriously and, in particular, to exclude some of the major possible extra-abdominal causes of dyspepsia. By definition, physical examination must be essentially negative although diffuse upper abdominal tenderness may be detected and possibly a succussion splash if there is a significant degree of pylorospasm. The features of nervous tension might be conspicuous, such as an inability to relax, tachycardia and exaggerated tendon reflexes or, alternatively, the patient may appear obviously depressed.

Investigations

It has already been stated that functional dyspepsia is a diagnosis of exclusion and cannot confidently be made on clinical grounds alone. The difficulty is to steer a course between intensive over-investigation which may simply aggravate the patient's fear that he is suffering from some sinister disease, and under-investigation with the inevitable risk of missing an organic explanation for the patient's complaints. Routine investigations should include:

1. A full blood count, including the erythrocyte sedimentation rate (ESR).

2. Estimation of the serum urea, electrolytes and liver function tests.
3. Urine examination for protein, sugar bile etc.
4. Chest radiograph.
5. Faecal occult blood.

These are basically screening tests and particularly valuable to exclude causes of dyspepsia, such as cardiac or renal disease. It has been emphasized, however, that even gastric malignancy may be present with a normal haemaglobin and sedimentation rate and almost invariably one or more of the following investigations will be required:

1. BARIUM MEAL

This is by far the most useful radiological investigation and reliance can be placed on a negative report if the procedure has been done by an experienced radiologist using a double-contrast technique. Should neither of these factors apply, a negative barium meal can by no means be taken to exclude organic disease in the upper gastrointestinal tract.

2. FIBREOPTIC ENDOSCOPY

This is also a particularly useful investigation which is safe, well-tolerated and can be done as an outpatient procedure. The yield of clinical abnormalities is small in patients with dyspepsia in whom a double-contrast barium meal has been negative, but nevertheless this procedure should be considered when the symptoms are particularly troublesome, clinically strongly suggestive of peptic ulceration, there is a family history of ulcers or if there has been any evidence of overt or occult gastrointestinal bleeding.

3. BILIARY TRACT INVESTIGATIONS

These include radiography of the biliary tract or ultrasonic gallbladder scan.

When the above investigations are negative it is prudent to review the clinical situation before deciding whether the possibility of underlying physical disease should be further pursued. If the patient has obviously been reassured by what has been done and the fact that nothing sinister has been found, and, in particular, if his symptoms are not unduly troublesome, it is reasonable to maintain a watching brief although a deterioration in the patient's condition should be a signal to review the diagnosis.

Alternatively, if it is still felt likely that there could be an organic explanation for the patient's symptoms, the possibility of a more unusual cause for dyspepsia should be considered, such as Crohn's disease, pancreatic disorders, diverticular disease of the colon, colonic cancer, etc. necessitating further investigations, such as pancreatic function studies, small and large bowel radiology, etc.

Laparotomy may still occasionally be necessary when the patient's symptoms continue to be troublesome and organic disease cannot be confidently excluded despite a series of negative investigations.

Management

The majority of patients with functional dyspepsia are relieved to have had their symptoms taken seriously, to have been thoroughly examined and know that the appropriate investigations have been done with negative results. This allows them to receive the reassurance they are hoping to hear that they are not suffering from malignant disease in particular. It is then important, having stressed that neither clinical examination nor investigations have revealed any organic disease, not to let the patient feel that he has been given the impression that his symptoms are imaginary. It should be stressed that pain, nausea, vomiting, etc. can be just as much a result of an abnormal behaviour of the upper gastrointestinal tract as they can of organic disease and are none the less real in consequence.

Drug treatment is helpful and any of the following may be found beneficial individually or in combination:

1. Antacids. These can be taken as often as necessary. A vast number of preparations is available but there is little evidence that the more recently introduced sophisticated expensive preparations are any more efficacious than the cheaper, well-established products.

2. Metoclopramide, 5–10 mg t.d.s. is a particularly useful preparation for vague dyspepsia associated with nausea and vomiting.

3. Occasionally a minor anxiolytic such as lorazepam 1–4 mg daily in divided doses or chlordiazepoxide 30 mg daily in divided doses or an antidepressant preparation may be helpful if there is clear evidence of either excessive anxiety or a depressive illness respectively.

Long-term adherence to a strict 'gastric' diet should be discouraged although it is reasonable for patients to omit selected dietary items if these are consistently associated with symptom production. Cigarette smoking and excess alcohol consumption should be discouraged and drugs which may be contributing to patient's symptoms should be withdrawn whenever possible. Social problems are less easy to influence but simply getting the patient to realize their possible significance is helpful.

It also needs re-emphasizing that once a diagnosis of functional dyspepsia has been made it does not meant that this should be accepted for all time and the diagnosis should be periodically reviewed, particularly when the patient's symptoms prove to be resistant to therapy or if his condition should be seen to deteriorate in any other way.

3.11 GALLSTONES

Gallstones are common and increase in frequency with age. Although there is a higher incidence in females, this decreases in later years so that in the elderly the sex incidence is almost equal. There is also a geographical variation with a particularly high incidence of gallstones in the USA and Western Europe. Parity, obesity, diabetes mellitus, ileal dysfunction or excision and drugs such as clofibrate and oestrogen-rich contraceptives are also associated with an increased incidence of gallstones.

Clinical features

Gallstones may be symptomless, be responsible for dyspepsia or result in specific complications. The diagnosis will be frequently missed if they are only suspected in fertile, flatulent, fat ladies of forty.

1. SILENT

Gallstones, whether in the gallbladder or common bile duct may be symptomless and discovered by chance as a result of radiography or as a consequence of abdominal surgery for other reasons.

2. DYSPEPSIA

Gallstones may be associated with dyspeptic symptoms such as epigastric and retrosternal pain, flatulence, abdominal distension, nausea and intolerance of fatty food. However, such complaints are non-specific and equally likely alternative explanations, such as gastro-oesophageal reflux, gastric and duodenal ulceration, frequently coexist and must be excluded before gallstones are assumed to be of symptomatic significance.

Even when no other abdominal disorder is discovered, the symptom complex of flatulent dyspepsia appears to be the result of a loosely associated pyloroduodenal motility disturbance resulting in the reflux of duodenal juice into the stomach and occasionally into the oesophagus.

Physical examination is usually unhelpful, frequently being negative or revealing non-specific findings, such as epigastric or right subcostal tenderness.

3. COMPLICATIONS

More specific clinical features of gallstones, associated with biliary infection or gallstone migration include:

a. Biliary colic. This is suggested by the complaint of extremely severe upper abdominal and right subcostal pain which often radiates into the back and to the tip of the right shoulder blade. The patient is usually unable to find a comfortable position and either rolls about the bed or walks around the room. Associated features are sweating, nausea and vomiting. Usually the pain is continuous rather than spasmodic and eventually subsides spontaneously or results in a call for medical aid. Often there is a residual feeling of upper abdominal soreness lasting for several hours after the acute attack. The severity of the episode usually results in the patient being able to recall the details of the attack in considerable detail and he is usually frightened lest he should suffer a repetition.

b. Cholecystitis and cholangitis. Acute cholecystitis usually presents with upper abdominal pain which tends to be localized to the right hypochondrium and may sometimes begin with an episode of biliary colic. Nausea, vomiting and fever are usually associated features. The main findings on physical examination are fever, a tachycardia, occasionally slight jaundice (suggesting the presence of a stone in the common duct) and tenderness with rebound in the right upper abdominal quadrant. Less frequently, an inflammatory mass may be palpable in the right hypochondrium. Major differential diagnoses include pancreatitis, perforated peptic ulcer, appendicitis and myocardial infarction.

Sequels to acute cholecystitis include:

i. Resolution.

ii. Suppuration leading to empyema or gangrene and perforation of the gallbladder with resultant spreading peritonitis.

iii. Chronic cholecystitis (which may be silent or associated with flatulent dyspepsia, recurrent bouts of biliary colic or repeated bouts of acute inflammation).

Cholangitis may occur as the complication of a common duct stone in the presence of infection when the characteristic clinical features are fever, rigors and fluctuating jaundice.

c. Mucocele. Cystic duct obstruction unaccompanied by infection results in distension of the gallbladder with mucus. This abnormality may be palpated in a patient complaining of chronic right subcostal discomfort after a previous episode of biliary colic.

d. Jaundice. The presence of a stone in the common bile duct may be associated with obstructive jaundice (*see* Chapter 3.12) which may resolve spontaneously if the stone is passed into the duodenum or progress in severity if the obstruction is complete and persistent.

e. Pancreatitis. In the UK gallstones are the single most common cause of acute pancreatitis, a disease with a mortality rate of about 10%. This complication is suggested by the development of severe upper abdominal pain radiating into the back associated with nausea, vomiting and prostration.

Less common complications of gallstones are:

1. Intestinal obstruction (gallstone ileus) consequent on the ulceration of gallstones from the gallbladder into the duodenum and subsequent impaction in the intestinal tract—usually the terminal ileum.

2. Carcinoma of the gallbladder.

Investigations

In addition to a full blood count, the conventional biochemical tests of liver function should be checked whether or not the patient is clinically jaundiced. The urine should also be checked for the presence of bile.

RADIOGRAPHY

A plain film of the abdomen will only reveal approximately 10–20% of gallstones and contrast radiology of the biliary tract is essential when there is clinical suspicion of this diagnosis. The standard method is the *oral cholecystogram.* After preliminary films of the gallbladder area, the patient takes the contrast medium in tablet form on the evening prior to the examination. Unless obvious gallstones are demonstrated a fatty meal is then given and further films taken. A good concentration of contrast medium in the gallbladder with no stones visible is a reliable indicator of a normal gallbladder. Similarly, non-visualization is a reliable index of gallbladder pathology if the following causes of spurious non-function can be excluded:

1. Failure of the patient to take the contrast medium.
2. Vomiting or diarrhoea induced by the tablets.
3. Pyloric stenosis, pylorospasm or malabsorption.
4. A serum bilirubin greater than 2 mg/100 ml (35 μmol/l).

The *intravenous cholangiogram,* the contrast agent being injected directly into a peripheral vein, avoids the problems associated with absorption from the alimentary tract, is quicker than the oral technique and carries the additional advantage of demonstrating both the gallbladder and duct system. As with the oral cholecystogram the biliary tract will not be outlined if the patient is clinically jaundiced (serum bilirubin higher than 2–3 mg/100 ml (35–50 μmol/l)).

When the patient's complaints are those of flatulent dyspepsia rather than more specifically suggestive of gallstones, a barium meal (preferably double contrast) is a wise precaution to exclude the presence of coincidental pathology in the upper gastrointestinal tract.

ULTRASONIC SCAN

The increased availability of and experience with ultrasonic scanning has shown that this technique which is non-invasive and independent of the level of the serum bilirubin, is at least as reliable as cholecystography for detecting the presence of stones in the gallbladder.

The radiological techniques of use in the differentiation of jaundice are discussed in the next section.

Management

Symptomatic gallstones are usually an indication for cholecystectomy. When the patient's symptoms are those of flatulent dyspepsia alone, surgical intervention should be approached with caution. As previously emphasized, alternative causes for the patient's complaints, such as gastro-oesophageal reflux, gastric or duodenal ulceration or diverticular disease of the colon should be excluded. Even when there is no evidence of coincidental intra-abdominal pathology, cholecystectomy for flatulent dyspepsia associated with gallstones does not carry a guarantee of symptom relief.

Pethidine, 50–100 mg intramuscularly, is probably the drug of choice to relieve biliary colic and should be repeated as necessary. Acute cholecystitis usually responds to a regime of bed rest, oral fluids and antibiotics, e.g. ampicillin 500 mg q.d.s., but close observation and repeated abdominal examination are essential to detect any sign of extension of the inflammatory process as early as possible. Cholangitis usually responds to a similar regime.

The management of obstructive jaundice is discussed in the next section.

Stones in the common bile duct can be removed by endoscopic sphincterotomy of the ampulla of Vater in specialized centres although this technique is still reserved predominantly for elderly patients whose general condition renders conventional surgery inadvisable.

Medical dissolution of gallstones is a possibility but three major prerequisites are:
1. The stones must be of the cholesterol type.
2. There must be a functioning gallbladder.
3. The liver function must be normal.

Other disadvantages are that stone dissolution is slow and stones tend to reform when treatment is discontinued. Drugs available for this purpose include chenodeoxycholic acid 15 mg/kg body weight/day in divided doses and ursodeoxycholic acid 300 mg b.d. after meals with one administration always after the evening meal. The advantages of the latter preparation are the absence of liver dysfunction and less tendency to cause diarrhoea.

The main value of medical dissolution lies in the management of patients who cannot, or will not, be considered for cholecystectomy but not surprisingly surgery remains the treatment of choice in the vast majority of gallstone sufferers. The management of patients with symptomless gallstones remains controversial but cholecystectomy should at least be considered in this situation to prevent the development of complications in the future.

3.12   JAUNDICE

Jaundice is said to be present when the serum concentration of bilirubin is raised and has a number of causes. From the management point of view the issue of cardinal importance is whether or not the cause of the jaundice requires surgical intervention.

The simplest classification of jaundice depends on whether the excess of serum bilirubin is unconjugated or conjugated to glucuronide:
1. *Unconjugated hyperbilirubinaemia* may be caused by haemolysis and, less frequently, hepatocellular disease. Unconjugated hyperbilirubinaemia also occurs in Gilbert's syndrome in which patients have reduced bilirubin glucuronyl-transferase activity.

2. *Conjugated hyperbilirubinaemia* may result from liver cell disease or from obstruction to bile flow. However, the biochemical features of both these disorders may be identical and are referred to as 'cholestasis' (conjugated hyperbilirubinaemia with elevated serum alkaline phosphatase and gammaglutamyl-transferase). The cause of cholestasis may lie in the liver (intrahepatic cholestasis) or result from extrahepatic biliary obstruction.

Hepatocellular causes of jaundice include acute and chronic hepatitis, the various forms of cirrhosis, secondary malignant disease of the liver and drug reactions. Causes of extrahepatic biliary obstruction include stones in the common bile duct, carcinoma of the head of the pancreas and strictures or malignant disease of the bile duct.

Clinical features

The cardinal clinical features of *cholestasis* (whether intra- or extrahepatic) are jaundice, associated with pruritus, dark urine and pale stools. A past history of upper abdominal pain suggests gallstones but painless jaundice by no means excludes extrahepatic biliary obstruction due to a duct stone.

Fever and rigors suggest cholangitis and jaundice associated with anorexia, weight loss and back pain is suggestive of pancreatic malignancy.

In the history particular attention should be paid to:

1. Possible exposure to hepatitis viruses.

2. Details of *any drugs* which the patient may have been taking for whatever cause. If the patient is at all unsure as to the drugs he may have been taking, this aspect needs to be double-checked with relatives and the family doctor. The list of drugs which may be responsible for jaundice continues to increase and includes preparations which interfere with bilirubin metabolism (e.g. methyldopa, sulphonamides, rifampicin), preparations which have direct hepatotoxicity (e.g., carbon tetrachloride, tetracycline, paracetamol), preparations which result in unpredictable hypersensitivity type reactions (e.g. halothane, methyldopa, oxyphenisatin, antituberculous drugs, monoamine oxidase inhibitors) and drugs which produce cholestatic reactions (e.g. oral contraceptives, phenothiazines, oral hypoglycaemic agents, non-steroidal anti-inflammatory agents and certain testosterone derivatives). This list is by no means comprehensive and the safest policy is to suspect any drug which the patient may be taking as contributing to the jaundice until disproved.

3. Details of alcohol ingestion.

Careful clinical examination is essential. A combination of slight jaundice with anaemia is suggestive of haemolysis. Scratch marks suggest cholestasis. Signs of chronic liver disease include palmar erythema, spider naevi, finger clubbing, leukonychia, gynaecomastia and oedema.

The abdomen should be carefully examined for enlargement of the liver or spleen and whether or not the gallbladder is palpable. The liver may be enlarged, hard and with an irregular edge suggesting underlying malignancy. Portal hypertension is suggested by splenomegaly and ascites, although the latter may be due to intra-abdominal malignant disease.

Investigations

1. BLOOD

Full blood count. A full blood count is essential, a hypochromic anaemia being suggestive of gastrointestinal bleeding. A combination of anaemia with a high reticulocyte count suggests haemolysis as an explanation for the patient's jaundice and further haematological investigations will then be appropriate. The prothrombin time may be prolonged when the jaundice is either due to liver cell disease or extrahepatic biliary obstruction.

Conventional biochemical liver function tests. These are useful (serum bilirubin (conjugated and unconjugated), aspartate transaminase, gammaglutamyl-transferase, alkaline phosphatase, albumin) but are by no means totally reliable in differentiating biliary obstruction from other causes of jaundice.

Immunology. A variety of immunological and serological tests are available which are often helpful in the differential diagnosis of jaundice. Particularly valuable are the various serological markers of hepatitis B infection, HBs Ag, HBc Ag and their respective antibodies. The Paul–Bunnell test is also worth checking if there are any other clinical pointers to infectious mononucleosis. A high titre of smooth muscle antibodies is suggestive of chronic active hepatitis and a significant antimitochondrial antibody titre is strongly suggestive of primary biliary cirrhosis.

2. RADIOLOGY

A plain film of the abdomen may show radio-opaque gallstones but even when these are demonstrated it cannot be automatically assumed that these are responsible for the jaundice. Contrast radiography of the biliary tract (cholecystography or cholangiography) are of no value in the presence of jaundice.

Ultrasonography. Ultrasonic scanning of the liver and biliary tree by an experienced radiologist, using the real time technique is of great value in the differential diagnosis of jaundice. The technique is quick, non-invasive and is particularly useful in the differentiation of extrahepatic biliary obstruction from other causes of jaundice on the basis of whether or not the bile duct system is dilated. Useful information can also be obtained regarding the liver texture and the possibility of metastases and stones in the gallbladder can also be reliably detected although, as with the plain film, even when these are shown it should not be assumed that they are necessarily the cause of jaundice.

Percutaneous transhepatic cholangiography. Using a fine bore Chiba needle, the biliary tree can be outlined accurately and the site and cause of the obstruction identified in the majority of patients with extrahepatic biliary obstruction. The technique is safe, provided appropriate precautions are taken to correct any significant bleeding tendency and the patient needs careful watching after the procedure to detect any significant haemorrhage or bile leak from the puncture site in the liver.

Endoscopic retrograde cholangiopancreatography. With the aid of a fibreoptic endoscope passed into the second part of the duodenum, the ampulla of Vater is cannulated and radio-opaque contrast medium introduced into the pancreatic and common bile ducts. Considerable technical expertise is required and the technique is not without hazard. However, the yield of information is high, pancreatic juice can be obtained for biochemical and cytological analysis and it is also possible to remove stones from the common bile duct by endoscopic papillotomy.

Liver biopsy. Percutaneous liver biopsy is safe and is usually indicated when the presence of extrahepatic biliary obstruction has been excluded. The platelet count and prothrombin time should be checked as preliminaries and any deficiences corrected by either the administration of intramuscular vitamin K or the infusion of fresh plasma or whole blood.

Management (Fig. 3.8)

The effective management of a patient with jaundice depends on making a definite diagnosis and, in particular, as to whether or not extrahepatic biliary obstruction is the underlying cause. It should again be stressed that conventional biochemical liver function tests do not allow this distinction to be made with confidence and further investigation is nearly always required.

When there is a possibility of the jaundice being drug-induced, the suspected preparation should be withdrawn immediately. The management of haemolytic jaundice depends on the underlying haematological cause and Gilbert's syndrome is a benign condition requiring only firm reassurance and a warning that the patient may look yellow from time to time, particularly during any intercurrent illness.

The management of extrahepatic biliary obstruction is essentially surgical although in selected cases it may be possible to remove stones from the common bile duct by endoscopic sphincterotomy (*see* Chapter 3.11).

The management of hepatitis A is symptomatic with almost invariably complete recovery and when the problem is liver metastases the main emphasis is on making the patient's remaining time as comfortable as possible. Jaundice due to alcoholic liver disease demands abstinence and nutritional support. The management of chronic active hepatitis and the various forms of cirrhosis of the liver is outside the scope of this book.

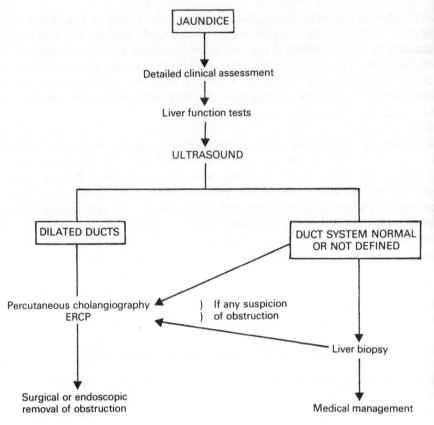

Fig. 3.8. Management of jaundice.

3.13 ULCERATIVE COLITIS

Ulcerative colitis (or idiopathic proctocolitis) is an inflammatory disease of unknown cause confined to the mucosa and submucosa of the large bowel. In a large proportion of patients the disease process is limited to the rectum and may remain so for many years. Once established, ulcerative colitis often pursues a chronic relapsing course with troublesome flare-ups alternating with symptom-free remission of varying duration.

Clinical features

Ulcerative colitis may occur at any age although the majority of first attacks occur in young adults. The clinical features vary from a comparatively trivial upset to an illness presenting as a life-threatening emergency. Characteristic symptoms are:

1. *Diarrhoea,* the faeces being loose, watery and often containing mucus. Nocturnal diarrhoea is also a characteristic feature.

2. *Rectal bleeding*. When the disease process is confined to the rectum bleeding may be the predominant symptom associated with the infrequent passage of a constipated stool.

A *moderately severe* episode of colitis may be associated with nausea, anorexia and abdominal pain and when the illness is *severe,* lassitude, rapid weight loss, general malaise and fever are often associated features.

On direct questioning the patient may admit to similar previous self-limiting episodes and there may be a family history of inflammatory bowel disease.

Physical examination

When the illness is mild, physical examination is commonly negative although there may be evidence of anaemia, a loaded bowel palpable proximal to the affected segment and rectal examination may reveal blood and slime on the examining glove. Findings accompanying a severe episode may include anaemia, weight loss, dehydration, fever, tachycardia, abdominal tenderness and distension. The latter is of particularly ominous significance and may indicate bowel perforation or toxic dilatation of the colon.

Extra-colonic manifestations

Systemic disorders which may occasionally be encountered in conjunction with ulcerative colitis, thought to be due to the deposition of immune complexes of antigens absorbed from the inflamed gut, include:

1. SKIN

Erythema nodosum and less commonly pyoderma gangrenosum which may progress to large areas of ulceration. Drug eruptions may also be encountered with sulphasalazine being the commonest offender.

2. EYES

These may be inflamed as a consequence of either conjunctivitis or uveitis.

3. JOINTS

Ulcerative colitis may be associated with sacroiliitis, ankylosing spondylitis or a polyarthritis involving the large joints.

4. LIVER

Inflammatory disorders of the liver may occur including pericholangitis and chronic active hepatitis. Progression to cirrhosis may develop and fatty change in the liver may also occur.

Complications

The complications of an acute attack include colonic perforation, toxic dilatation and massive haemorrhage. The complications of chronic ulcerative colitis include pseudopolyposis, fibrous stricture of the colon which may give rise to obstructive symptoms and colonic cancer although the risk of malignant change seems to have been over-stressed in the past.

Investigations

It is essential to realize that the clinical features described are not pathognomonic of ulcerative colitis but may be encountered in other large bowel disorders, such as infection, diverticular disease, malignancy, irritable bowel, Crohn's disease and as a consequence of sudden ischaemia. Antibiotic-associated colitis may easily be confused with ulcerative colitis and the distinction from Crohn's disease may be particularly difficult.

It follows that whenever ulcerative colitis is suspected on clinical grounds investigations are indicated to confirm the diagnosis before the patient is labelled a 'colitic'.

BLOOD INVESTIGATIONS

These are more of value to assess the severity of the disease process rather than establishing the cause of the symptoms and should include a full blood count with ESR, serum urea and electrolytes, serum proteins and mucoproteins.

EXAMINATION OF FAECES

The faeces are usually loose and bloodstained with mucus and sometimes pus. Microscopy confirms the presence of pus and red cells. Stool culture and microscopy is also indicated to exclude bacterial infection and infestation.

SIGMOIDOSCOPY

This is probably the single most important investigation when ulcerative colitis is suspected and can usually be performed without special preparation. A rectal mucosal biopsy should be taken at the time of sigmoidoscopy for confirmation of the diagnosis by histological examination. Apart from establishing the diagnosis, sigmoidoscopy may also determine the extent of the inflammation when this is confined to the rectum and normal mucosa can be seen above the diseased area.

COLONOSCOPY

Colonoscopy is of value in selected cases allowing the whole of the large bowel to be visualized and, in particular, biopsies can be taken from any part of the colon. This technique is particularly useful for long-term surveillance in patients with longstanding whole colon disease where the risk of complicating malignancy is greatest. It is also of value in the differentiation between malignant and benign strictures of the large bowel in a patient with colitis.

RADIOLOGY

A plain film of the abdomen is helpful in severe cases and aids the distinction between colonic dilatation and perforation when abdominal distension is present. However, the main role of radiology is to ascertain the extent of the disease process using a double-contrast barium enema (this, however, being contraindicated when the patient is acutely ill).

Differential diagnosis

Acute bacillary dysentery should be easily distinguished from a first attack of ulcerative colitis by stool culture. Ulcerative colitis may be extremely difficult to distinguish from Crohn's disease when the latter is confined to the large bowel although features which suggest Crohn's disease rather than ulcerative colitis include abdominal pain as a prominent symptom, infrequent rectal bleeding, finger clubbing, anal disease, fistulae and the absence of gross rectal involvement. Elevation of the serum mucoproteins also favours Crohn's disease and radiology may aid the differentiation as does histological examination of rectal or colonic biopsies. Antibiotic-associated colitis appears to be the result of pathogenic clostridial organisms (*Clostridium difficile*) becoming established in the colon and secreting an exotoxin which exerts a necrotizing effect on the colonic mucosa. A history of prior antibiotic therapy is suggestive and sigmoidoscopy may reveal diffuse inflammatory change with pseudomembranous plaques. Ischaemic colitis is suggested when a patient of middle-age or over suddenly develops abdominal pain associated with bloody diarrhoea. Amoebic colitis should always be kept in mind and certainly cannot be excluded by the lack of recent travel abroad although a history of a visit to a highly endemic area is suggestive. A fresh stool specimen should be examined for cysts or vegetative forms of amoebae and serological tests should be arranged if there is any doubt.

Management

Three important aspects of general patient management include reassurance, explanation and a sympathetic approach.

Firm reassurance is vital in this situation for most patients' concept of colitis is that of a chronic disabling disease resulting in a life of invalidism and dietary restriction. An optimistic approach is justifiable with encouragement to the patient to live as normal a life as possible. It also helps if the patient can be given a simple explanation to help him understand his illness and he should be warned that this may be a relapsing problem. Otherwise, the patient may become severely disheartened if he has been given the impression that because an attack has been checked the disease has been eradicated. A confident and sympathetic medical approach is also important for many patients are still embarrassed when discussing bowel problems and they need to be given support and encouragement. It is also important that the patient should feel able to seek medical advice immediately when a symptomatic relapse occurs.

SPECIFIC TREATMENT

With the aetiology of ulcerative colitis remaining obscure, the treatment is essentially empirical.

TREATMENT OF AN ACUTE ATTACK

This depends on the severity and extent of the large bowel involved in the disease process. When the symptoms are mild, there is no associated systemic upset and the disease process is confined to the distal large bowel, there is little need for restriction of normal activities.

Very localized proctitis with the upper limit of the disease being visible on sigmoidoscopy can often be relieved by steroid or sulphasalazine suppositories. This particular variant of the disease is commonly associated with gross constipation and a bulk laxative is often helpful.

Even localized disease may occasionally be associated with severe anaemia due to iron deficiency from chronic blood loss and can usually be corrected with oral iron.

A mild attack, associated with *more extensive left-sided disease,* requires treatment with steroid foam or retention enemas. The patient should be carefully instructed how these preparations should be used. Oral sulphasalazine 1 g t.d.s. or q.d.s. is also useful, the preference being for the enteric-coated form which minimizes the risk of gastric intolerance. It should be noted, however, that sulphasalazine may cause male infertility which is reversible when this preparation is withdrawn. Sulphasalazine enemas may be useful for patients who are intolerant of the oral preparation. Associated anaemia requires treatment by iron replacement and failure to respond is an indication to start oral prednisolone.

A moderately severe attack with the bowel open up to 12 times in 24 h and associated with evidence of mild constitutional upset is treated along the same lines, except that systemic steroids (prednisolone 40 mg daily in divided doses) is started immediately and hospital referral advisable. Dehydration and electrolyte imbalance may require intravenous fluids and blood transfusion is indicated if the haemoglobin falls below 10 g/100 ml.

A severe attack of ulcerative colitis is a medical emergency requiring immediate hospital admission and intensive treatment consisting of intravenous fluids and electrolyte replacement, blood transfusion, intravenous hydrocortisone, steroid retention enemas, parenteral antibiotics and occasionally parenteral feeding. The patient should preferably be under close joint medicosurgical observation to carefully monitor progress and also to watch for early signs of complications such as toxic dilatation or colonic perforation. If the patient's condition improves, intravenous steroids are replaced by oral prednisolone and sulphasalazine. The development of major complications or clinical deterioration or a failure of the patient to respond to such an intensive treatment regime after this has been continued for a few days, is an indication for surgery.

DIET

There is no evidence to suggest that a low residue diet is in any way helpful other than for symptomatic benefit and should not be continued when the patient is in remission. In fact a low-residue regime may be harmful by aggravating constipation which is so often a prominent feature of ulcerative colitis when the disease process is limited to the rectum. Dietary factors seem to be of little relevance to the aetiology of ulcerative colitis other than in a small percentage of patients who benefit from the exclusion of milk and milk products.

PREVENTION OF RELAPSE

Recognized factors which trigger a relapse include psychological and emotional stress, gastrointestinal infection and certain drugs such as oral broad-spectrum antibiotics. Concerning drug therapy, sulphasalazine is the only preparation which has been clearly shown to reduce the relapse rate and if it can be tolerated by the patient is worth continuing indefinitely in the lowest dose necessary to maintain the patient in good health. It should be noted that long-term steroid therapy does not reduce the frequency of relapse and the use of steroids for other than short-term courses should be avoided if possible.

INDICATIONS FOR SURGICAL TREATMENT

Reference has already been made to the role of surgery in the management of a severe attack of colitis and is recommended whenever the patient fails to show significant improvement after a short period of intensive medical treatment or in the event of complications such as perforation or toxic dilatation of the colon. Indications for elective surgery include recurrent severe attacks of colitis or when the patient's quality of life is impaired by continuous symptoms which do not respond to medical treatment and which result in chronic invalidism.

Ulcerative colitis is a premalignant condition, the risk of carcinoma being largely confined to patients in whom virtually the whole of the colon is involved in the disease process, the duration of the disease is longer than ten years and the onset during childhood or adolescence. The regular histological scrutiny of biopsy material obtained by sigmoidoscopy or colonoscopy to detect dysplastic change has been advocated as a suitable method for detecting impending or established malignancy but this has not yet been universally accepted. Surgical intervention implies a colectomy with either ileorectal anastomosis or ileostomy and removal of the rectum together with the colon. The advantage of the former is that the need for a stoma is avoided but disadvantages are the disease may remain active in the rectal stump and the risk of a rectal carcinoma remains. The standard of ileostomy care has improved with the training of nurses with a particular responsibility for this problem and through the efforts of the Ileostomy Association. Various forms of continent ileostomy are still under development.

3.14 DIVERTICULAR DISEASE OF THE COLON

Diverticular disease is the commonest pathological process of the large bowel in Western industrialized countries. The incidence is particularly high in the elderly but is now being recognized increasingly frequently in the younger age group.

The most consistent pathological feature of diverticular disease is *thickening of the colonic muscle* with the sigmoid being most commonly affected. The muscle abnormality is associated with excessive segmentation

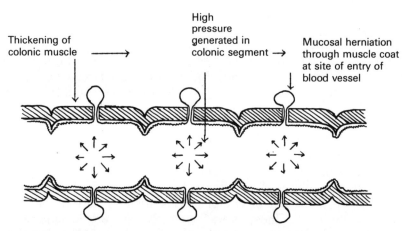

Fig. 3.9. Pathogenesis of diverticular disease of the colon.

which appears to result in the colon acting as a series of small bladders, the outflow being effectively obstructed · at both ends. In consequence the intraluminal pressure is raised with the tendency to produce mucosal blowouts (diverticula) through the muscle coat at its weakest point, this usually being the site of entry of the segmental blood vessels which pierce the muscle at regular intervals (*Fig.* 3.9).

It has been suggested that the major cause of diverticular disease is a deficiency of dietary fibre, this resulting in reduced faecal bulk and a consequent disturbance of colonic motility allowing excessive segmentation to occur and diverticula to develop.

Clinical features

Diverticular disease of the colon may be asymptomatic or associated with *vague dyspeptic complaints* such as nausea, flatulence, abdominal distension and discomfort. The symptom complex of flatulent dyspepsia, however, is just as likely to be a consequence of disorders of the upper gastrointestinal tract such as gastro-oesophageal reflux, peptic ulceration or gallstones which frequently coexist with diverticular disease (*Fig.* 3.10).

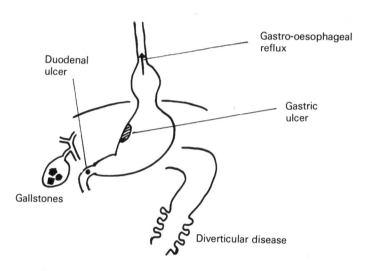

Fig. 3.10. Common causes of flatulent dyspepsia.

Symptoms more recognizably of colonic origin include:

1. *Abdominal pain.* This is often dull and cramping in character and felt diffusely throughout the abdomen or localized in particular to the left iliac fossa. The pain may be associated with the feeling of distension and is often relieved by defaecation or the passage of flatus. It is now recognized that the pain resulting from diverticular disease is commonly a consequence of disturbed colonic motility and by no means implies the development of true diverticulitis'.

2. *Altered bowel habit.* The disturbance may be either a tendency to diarrhoea or constipation or an alternation from one to the other.

3. *Rectal bleeding.* This varies in severity from being mild and infrequent to a sudden severe haemorrhage which might necessitate emergency admission to hospital.

Such symptoms have often been present intermittently for several years and the patient's health is usually preserved with a normal appetite and steady weight.

Physical examination

Often no abnormality is detected although the colon may be palpable and tender in the left iliac fossa. Rectal examination is mandatory to exclude rectal carcinoma and hard faecal pellets are often felt in the rectal lumen.

Acute diverticulitis

This term is reserved for the development of inflammation usually precipitated by a faecolith becoming impacted in a diverticulum. Almost invariably the sigmoid colon is affected and the clinical picture resembles 'left-sided appendicitis'. The clinical features include lower abdominal pain and tenderness, constipation, fever, tachycardia, tenderness and guarding in the left iliac fossa and sometimes a tender mass palpable on deep palpation. The possible complications of acute diverticulitis include local peritonitis or pericolic abscess formation, perforation of the colon with generalized peritonitis, fistula formation and intestinal obstruction.

Investigations

Preliminary investigations should include:

1. FULL BLOOD COUNT

A hypochromic anaemia may result from blood loss associated with diverticular disease and a raised ESR and polymorpholeucocytosis suggest true diverticulitis.

2. URINE EXAMINATION

Recurrent attacks of urinary infection may herald the development of a vesicocolic fistula which presents classically as pneumaturia with or without the passage of faecal matter in the urine. Hence the urine should be examined for the presence of pus cells and organisms.

3. FAECAL OCCULT BLOOD

This can be conveniently checked as a follow-on from rectal examination. A negative result does not imply the absence of large bowel pathology and although a positive result suggests a bleeding lesion in the gastrointestinal tract this carries no discriminant or localizing value.

4. SIGMOIDOSCOPY

Sigmoidoscopy is rarely helpful in making a positive diagnosis of diverticular disease and its main value is to exclude other disorders (particularly malignancy) in the rectum and lower sigmoid. A rigid or fibreoptic instrument can be used.

5. RADIOLOGY

The diagnosis of diverticular disease of the colon is made essentially by a barium enema examination, a plain film of the abdomen only being of value when complications such as perforation or obstruction are suspected. As with the barium meal, considerably more reliance can be placed on a barium enema report when a double-contrast method has been used and when the examination has been performed and the films interpreted by an experienced radiologist. Apart from demonstrating the presence of diverticular disease, a barium enema may also give useful information as to the presence of complications, such as localized perforation or fistula formation.

6. COLONOSCOPY

Examination of the colon using a flexible fibreoptic colonoscope may be helpful in selected cases, particularly in the clarification of equivocal barium enema findings.

Differential diagnosis

Diverticular disease of the colon frequently coexists with other disorders elsewhere in the gastrointestinal tract, e.g. gastro-oesophageal reflux, peptic ulceration, gallstones. It follows that the radiological demonstration of the presence of diverticular disease by no means necessarily implies that this condition is the cause of the patient's complaints. Both a barium meal (preferably double-contrast) and radiology of the biliary tract should be considered if the patient's symptoms are not convincingly of large bowel origin (*Fig.* 3.10).

Diverticular disease may also coexist or be confused with other colonic disorders, e.g. carcinoma of the colon and inflammatory bowel disorders, particularly Crohn's disease. Carcinoma of the colon and diverticular disease may coexist and their distinction may be impossible to make even when the large bowel is inspected and palpated at laparotomy.

Management

Even if not openly admitted, patients with diverticular disease of the colon are frequently worried lest their complaints are a consequence of malignant disease. Accordingly, the patient should be firmly reassured that this is not the case, this usually producing considerable therapeutic benefit in its own right.

Secondly it is often helpful to give the patient a simple explanation of the origin of his complaints which increases the chance of cooperation over matters such as dietary alteration.

The majority of patients with symptomatic uncomplicated diverticular disease respond to medical treatment. The keystone of management is a *high fibre diet,* this being achieved with liberal quantities of fresh fruit and vegetables and a bran supplement daily. This can either be incorporated in cooking, sprinkled on food, etc. but may be more palatable in the form of wholewheat cereals and wholemeal bread. A less preferable alternative to dietary change is the use of bulking agents such as methylcellulose, sterculia, ispaghula husk or compressed fibre.

Antispasmodics such as propantheline bromide 15 mg t.d.s. before meals, or mebeverine 135 mg t.d.s. before meals may be helpful. Severe painful episodes may necessitate analgesia with pethidine 50–100 mg i.m. Morphine is contraindicated as it raises the sigmoid intraluminal pressure and may precipitate perforation in a patient with genuine diverticulitis.

Inflammation is not an invariable concomitant of diverticular disease and antibiotics are not likely to be helpful unless there is convincing evidence of an inflammatory process, for example, fever, polymorpholeucocytosis or an elevated ESR. A combination of ampicillin 500 mg 6-hourly and metronidazole (Flagyl) 400 mg 8-hourly is an appropriate regime.

Complications such as perforation, pericolic abscess and fistulae usually require surgical intervention although massive haemorrhage from the large bowel due to diverticular disease usually subsides spontaneously and emergency resection is rarely required.

Surgery, whether sigmoid myotomy or resection of the diseased colonic segment, should also be considered when the patient fails to respond to medical treatment.

3.15   CARCINOMA OF THE COLON AND RECTUM

Carcinoma of the large bowel is potentially the most curable malignant growth affecting the gastrointestinal tract. Consequently, early diagnosis is of crucial importance so that the tumour can be dealt with while it is still operable.

The risk of carcinoma of the rectum and colon increases with age although the condition is by no means rare in the younger age group. The frequency of tumour occurrence in various parts of the large bowel is illustrated in *Fig. 3.11.*

Conditions which predispose to malignant change include:

1. *Ulcerative colitis.* Patients particularly at risk are those suffering from longstanding whole colon disease and when the onset was during childhood or adult life. Prophylactic colectomy to prevent the development of malignancy is no longer recommended for such patients for the advent of colonoscopy and more sophisticated histopathological interpretation of rectal and colonic biopsies aiding the recognition of pre-carcinomatous change has resulted in a more conservative approach.

2. *Familial polyposis coli.* There may be no family history in up to one-third of patients suffering from this condition where the polyps are not present at birth but often occur in the early teens, at which time they are symptomless. Treatment is colectomy with ileorectal anastomosis, the rectal

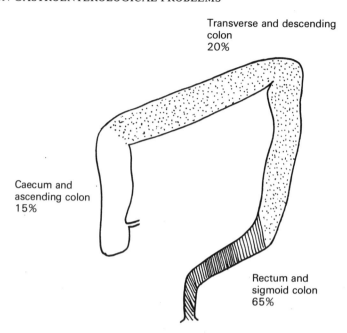

Transverse and descending
colon
20%

Caecum and
ascending colon
15%

Rectum and
sigmoid colon
65%

Fig. 3.11. Frequency of tumour occurrence in various parts of large bowel.

stump subsequently being kept under regular sigmoidoscopic surveillance.

3. *Simple adenomatous polyp.* This type of polyp is always potentially malignant, the risk escalating rapidly as the polyp increases in size. Accordingly, all polyps within reach of the sigmoidoscope should be removed for histological examination and likewise polyps of 1 cm or more in diameter elsewhere in the colon should also be excised. Fibreoptic colonoscopy allows the removal of multiple polyps which can be retrieved for histological examination using a diathermy snare. This technique obviates the necessity for an abdominal operation with its attendant risk.

Cholecystectomy also seems to increase the risk of carcinoma of the colon, particularly right-sided and there is a marked geographical variation in incidence, being common in north-west Europe, North America and Australasia but low in Africa, Asia and most of South America. Some features of the western diet appear to increase the likelihood of carcinoma of the large bowel and the low fibre content is particularly suspect.

Clinical features

The cardinal symptoms of *distal large-bowel cancer* are:
1. Rectal bleeding.
2. Alteration in bowel habit.
3. Abdominal pain.
These may be present singly or in any combination.

1. RECTAL BLEEDING

Every case of rectal bleeding occurring in an adult should be suspected as a consequence of carcinoma of the rectum or distal colon until proved otherwise. The bleeding will often prove to be from a benign anorectal lesion but a high index of suspicion is necessary to achieve the diagnosis of malignancy as early as possible. In particular, the passage of dark red blood, clots or blood mixed with or adherent to the faeces should never be dismissed as a consequence of haemorrhoids.

The bleeding may also be associated with a mucous discharge from the rectum.

2. ALTERATION IN BOWEL HABIT

The same dictum applies as for rectal bleeding, i.e. a change in bowel habit in a person of middle-age or over should be assumed to be a consequence of large-bowel cancer until this is disproved. The disturbance of bowel habit may be either diarrhoea or constipation with the need to use increasing amounts of aperients or an alternation from one to the other. Rectal incontinence may also be encountered.

3. ABDOMINAL PAIN

This is usually described as a diffuse ache in the lower abdomen but may tend to be localized in the left iliac fossa often with an associated feeling of distension. On occasions the pain may be more recognizably colicky and on direct questioning the patient may admit to the discomfort being eased or sometimes aggravated by defaecation or the passage of flatus.

Not infrequently the pain may be upper abdominal in situation aggravated by food ingestion and relieved by antacids, i.e. the symptoms initially suggest a lesion in the upper gastrointestinal tract with the danger that when a barium meal and biliary tract radiology prove negative an erroneous diagnosis of functional dyspepsia is made (*see* Chapter 3.10).

Carcinoma of the proximal large bowel (caecum to transverse colon) is notoriously silent until it reaches a comparatively advanced stage. Presenting features of malignant neoplasms in this situation include:
1. An unexplained iron-deficient anaemia.
2. Anorexia and weight loss.
3. General malaise.
4. Right-sided or upper abdominal pain and/or an abdominal mass.

More distal colonic neoplasms may also be accompanied by anorexia, weight loss and the symptoms of anaemia.

Physical examination

1. GENERAL ASSESSMENT

Frequently the patient appears well but there may be evidence of either anaemia or weight loss. Assessment of the cardiorespiratory state is particularly important in view of the subsequent possibility of surgical intervention.

2. ABDOMINAL EXAMINATION

Any distension should be noted and careful palpation is essential to exclude a mass anywhere along the colonic outline. A 'disappearing abdominal mass' (felt on one occasion but not confirmed at the next examination) does *not* exclude a neoplasm, possible explanations for this phenomenon being a self-reducing intussusception or faeces proximal to a partially obstructing lesion which subsequently clear.

3. RECTAL EXAMINATION

Careful digital examination of the rectum is an essential part of the assessment of any patient with gastrointestinal symptoms but is particularly important when these are rectal bleeding or a change in bowel habit. Failure to perform an adequate rectal examination remains a significant cause of delay in the diagnosis of rectal carcinoma in particular. Even if a tumour is not felt, an empty rectum should raise the suspicion of an obstructing lesion higher in the colon.

4. SIGNS OF SECONDARY SPREAD

Patients should be examined for evidence of dissemination of the disease with the following signs particularly suggestive that this has occurred:

a. Hepatomegaly, an enlarged liver with a hard irregular edge being highly suggestive of liver metastases.

b. Ascites from peritoneal seeding.

c. Supraclavicular node involvement.

d. 'Frozen pelvis' resulting from secondary deposits in the pelvic floor.

Complications

The major complications of carcinoma of the large bowel are intestinal obstruction, fistula formation and perforation with peritonitis.

Investigations

1. BLOOD INVESTIGATIONS

The haemoglobin and ESR may be normal in patients with carcinoma of the large bowel but often a degree of iron-deficiency anaemia is detected and the ESR may be raised. The tumour marker carcino-embryonic antigen (CEA) is of no value for the purpose of either screening or in the diagnosis of carcinoma of the colon but the regular and sequential assay of plasma CEA is the best presently available non-invasive technique for the postoperative surveillance of patients to detect disseminated tumour recurrence.

2. FAECAL OCCULT BLOOD

Testing the faeces for the presence of occult blood is a simple useful technique but it should be noted that a negative result by no means excludes the possibility of a large bowel tumour although a positive result obviously supports the possibility of a bleeding lesion somewhere in the gastro-intestinal tract.

3. SIGMOIDOSCOPY

This should be done at the time the patient is first seen at hospital without any prior preparation. If a tumour is seen a biopsy can be taken for histological examination. Even when there is no direct evidence of a neoplasm this may be strongly suspected when blood and mucus are observed trickling down from above. Failure to obtain adequate visualization, either because of patient intolerance or faecal retention, necessitates the procedure being repeated after bowel clearance and preferably under anaesthesia when the opportunity can also be taken to palpate the abdomen thoroughly with the patient relaxed.

The flexible fibreoptic sigmoidoscope is particularly useful when it is not possible to pass the rigid instrument round the sharp rectosigmoid bend.

4. RADIOLOGY

A plain film of the abdomen is rarely of value unless there are any features of intestinal obstruction or perforation.

The barium enema is the most important radiological investigation in the diagnosis of large bowel malignancy and it is essential that a double-contrast technique is used.

5. COLONOSCOPY

Fibreoptic colonoscopy is useful in selected cases. Although relatively time-consuming and needing thorough preliminary cleansing of the colon, this technique may aid the diagnosis of colonic cancer in patients with persistent rectal bleeding or change in bowel habit when barium enema has been negative and also when the radiological findings are equivocal.

Particular diagnostic problems

In the majority of cases, the diagnosis of carcinoma of the rectum and colon can be established by a combination of careful clinical assessment, sigmoidoscopy and a double-contrast barium enema. However, diagnostic delay is likely to arise when the clinical features do not immediately point to the possibility of large bowel malignancy. For example:

1. THE PROBLEM OF UNEXPLAINED IRON-DEFICIENCY ANAEMIA

This should always be assumed to be a consequence of chronic gastro-intestinal blood loss, whether or not the faecal occult blood test is positive and regardless of whether or not the patient complains of alimentary symptoms (*see* Chapter 3.8).

A barium meal is usually the first radiological investigation requested in this situation and the danger is that an abnormality such as a sliding hiatus hernia may be demonstrated which is assumed to be the source of bleeding but which is, in fact, a 'red herring'. The possibility that a carcinoma of the caecum or right side of the colon may be an alternative source of chronic intestinal blood loss should always be considered in this situation and a barium enema requested even when there are no clinical pointers to large bowel pathology. Similarly the occurrence of melaena stools in the absence of haematemesis and when there is no radiological or endoscopic evidence of an upper gastrointestinal source of blood loss, should again raise the possibility of a caecal or right-sided colonic lesion as the explanation.

2. VAGUE DYSPEPTIC SYMPTOMS

It has already been emphasized that a significant percentage of patients with large bowel malignancy present with dyspeptic symptoms. Understandably the first investigations likely to be requested in this situation are barium meal, endoscopy or biliary tract radiology and if these prove negative the diagnosis of functional dyspepsia may be made. This diagnosis is always dangerous in patients of middle-age or over presenting with dyspepsia for the first time and the possibility of a large bowel malignancy as the explanation in this situation is always worth considering.

3. THE DIFFERENTIAL DIAGNOSIS OF A STRICTURING LESION

On occasions it may be difficult to differentiate a malignant stricture from that caused by other colonic disorders and a consequence of diverticular disease, Crohn's disease or ulcerative colitis in particular. In most cases a careful study of good double-contrast barium enema films by experienced radiologists, consideration of the sigmoidoscopic appearance and biopsy material allows the distinction to be made but there are occasions when even laparotomy may not solve the problem. It should also be remembered that carcinoma of the colon and diverticular disease frequently coexist.

Management

The treatment of carcinoma of the colon and rectum is surgical excision in the hope that a cure can be achieved. The earlier the diagnosis is made the greater the chance that the tumour can be removed.

Even when there is evidence of tumour dissemination and there is no hope of a cure, surgery may nevertheless be advisable as the best method of palliation and, similarly, some instances of recurrent disease may best be dealt with by further operation. When the growth is advanced, cytotoxic drugs and radiotherapy also have their use in the individual patient as do pain-relieving, antiemetic and tranquillizing drugs.

3.16 SIMPLE CONSTIPATION

The wide variation in normal bowel habit makes constipation difficult to define. The term is usually taken to mean irregular infrequent defaecation or the difficult passage of hard faeces or a combination of both. Alternatively, the term may be used to refer to the impression that the stool volume is inadequate or the sensation that the bowel has not been properly evacuated. Frequently constipation is transient and induced by travel or other changes in everyday routine. Persistent constipation, however, is common and frequently leads to self-medication or request for medical advice.

Classification

Constipation may be conveniently classified as:
1. Simple, when there is no apparent primary cause.
2. Secondary, the constipation being a result of any of a wide variety of underlying causes.

Simple constipation

The major factors leading to the development of so-called simple constipation are a diet low in fibre content and ignoring the call to stool. Lack of exercise, unfavourable working conditions or toilet facilities and a low fluid intake may also contribute. Simple constipation is particularly common in geriatric practice when both the poor tone of the intestinal musculature and loss of tone of the anterior abdominal wall muscles are also relevant.

Secondary constipation

Constipation may develop as a consequence of:

1. COLONIC AND ANORECTAL DISORDERS

These include diverticular disease of the colon, carcinoma of the large bowel, distal proctitis and common anal problems such as fissure, haemorrhoids and anorectal strictures.

2. COLONIC MOTILITY DISORDERS

This group includes the irritable bowel syndrome, idiopathic megarectum and megacolon and constipation associated with pregnancy.

3. PSYCHIATRIC DISORDERS

Constipation is common in depressive states and in association with the chronic psychoses and anorexia nervosa.

4. SPINAL LESIONS

Constipation may be associated with both congenital or traumatic spinal disorders.

5. METABOLIC, ENDOCRINE AND TOXIC

Hypothyroidism, diabetes mellitus, dehydration and lead poisoning may all have constipation as a prominent feature.

6. DRUG THERAPY

Drugs that may cause or aggravate constipation include codeine, anti-cholinergics, anti-Parkinsonian preparations (excluding levodopa and amantadine) phenothiazine tranquillizers and tricyclic antidepressants, iron preparations, calcium and aluminium-containing antacids, barbiturates, benzodiazepines, monoamine oxidase inhibitors and diuretics.

Clinical features

Most patients with constipation complain of irregular infrequent defaecation and the passage of hard motions which are passed with difficulty. Frequently patients also complain of less specific symptoms such as general malaise, loss of appetite, tiredness and headache.

Alternative presentations include:

1. ABDOMINAL PAIN

Discomfort in the right iliac fossa or diffusely throughout the abdomen may result from faecal stasis and the patient may obtain partial relief as a consequence of defaecation. Abdominal distension is also a common complaint.

2. SPURIOUS DIARRHOEA

This is suggested by a history of episodes of explosive diarrhoea, the faeces being liquid and interspersed with periods of constipation.

Elderly patients are particularly prone to *faecal impaction* resulting in any of the following: faecal incontinence, urinary retention, restlessness and confusional states, rectal bleeding (although an underlying neoplasm needs to be carefully excluded before haemorrhage is assumed to be a consequence of stercoral ulceration) and intestinal obstruction.

It is important to establish whether or not the constipation is of recent onset or long standing. When the former is the case it is particularly important to exclude a secondary cause and in a patient of middle-age or over with a previously normal bowel rhythm the possibility of underlying bowel malignancy should always be suspected. Enquiry should also be made for symptoms suggestive of depression or neurotic illness and details of current drug therapy.

Physical examination

A thorough general physical examination is essential since constipation may result from so many disorders. The abdomen may be distended, a loaded colon palpable or a discrete mass felt as the result of organic colonic

pathology. Rectal examination is mandatory. An anal fissure or haemorrhoids may be apparent and the extent of faecal impaction can be assessed.
Also the majority of rectal carcinomas can be felt on digital examination.

Investigations

1. BLOOD INVESTIGATIONS

A full blood count, ESR, serum urea and electrolytes should be checked
routinely. A hypochromic anaemia or elevated ESR indicates the need for
further investigation although a normal blood count by no means excludes
underlying organic disease. A raised serum urea may point to dehydration as
a contributory factor and a low serum potassium at least raises the possibility
of purgative addiction. Thyroid function studies are also indicated if
hypothyroidism seems remotely possible.

2. URINE EXAMINATION

Examination of the urine may provide evidence of underlying renal disease or
the discovery of glycosuria may lead to the diagnosis of diabetes mellitus.

3. FAECAL OCCULT BLOOD

Examination of the faeces for the presence of occult blood can be checked as
a follow-on from rectal examination. A negative result does not exclude an
underlying gastrointestinal lesion but a convincing positive points to the need
for further investigation.

4. PROCTOSCOPY AND SIGMOIDOSCOPY

If there is any suspicion of a lesion in the anal canal or at the anorectal
junction, proctoscopy is easily performed without prior preparation. These
remarks also apply for sigmoidoscopy, this procedure being particularly
important if there has been any history of rectal bleeding or if there is any
cause to suspect a lesion in the rectum or lower sigmoid. When, for any
reason, unprepared sigmoidoscopy does not allow adequate examination,
this must be repeated after adequate bowel clearance and, if necessary,
under anaesthesia. Sigmoidoscopy with a flexible fibreoptic sigmoidoscope is
becoming increasingly available and fibreoptic colonoscopy may also be
indicated in selected patients.

5. RADIOLOGY

A plain radiograph of the abdomen is often of value in demonstrating the
extent of faecal accumulation in severe constipation. When there is a need to
exclude an underlying large bowel disorder, a double-contrast barium enema
is essential.

Management

It has been emphasized that in addition to establishing whether or not the
patient is constipated, the possibility of an underlying cause must be

excluded. If the change in bowel habit proves to be secondary to an underlying colonic disorder the primary problem must also be treated wherever possible in addition to achieving bowel clearance (*see* Chapters 3.13, 3.14, 3.15 and 3.17 for discussion of the management of distal proctitis, diverticular disease, carcinoma of the colon and rectum and irritable bowel syndrome respectively).

The management of simple constipation includes:

1. DIET

A diet high in fibre content is probably the most important aspect of therapy. This is achieved with a bran supplement or the use of wholemeal bread, wholewheat cereals and a high dietary content of fruit and vegetables. A high fluid intake is also helpful.

2. LAXATIVES

Laxatives retain an important place in the management of simple constipation, the aim being to wean patients off these preparations when a normal bowel habit is gradually restored. Particularly useful preparations are standardized senna 2–4 tablets at bedtime, bisacodyl 5–10 mg at night, and lactulose 15–30 ml daily. Bulking agents such as methylcellulose, sterculia and ispaghula husk are useful supplements or alternatives to a high fibre diet and bran itself can also be given in tablet form. Stool softeners such as dioctyl sodium sulphosuccinate 37·5–200 mg daily are also occasionally useful.

3. SUPPOSITORIES

Severe constipation verging on faecal impaction usually requires suppositories in addition to the measures outlined above. Bisacodyl suppositories are more effective than the longer established glycerine variety.

4. ENEMAS

Enemas are used mainly for the relief of impaction. Disposable phosphate enemas are usually effective but a preliminary oil retention enema may be necessary to soften impacted faeces.

5. MANUAL REMOVAL

This is occasionally necessary when the rectum is loaded with a hard faecal mass which cannot be evacuated after enema.

The patient should also be encouraged to take an increased daily fluid ration and physical exercise is beneficial. Similarly, patients should be encouraged not to ignore the call to stool—getting up a little earlier in the morning with consequently less rush to get to school or work is the obvious remedy but easier to achieve in theory than in practice! Also it is less easy to deal with poor toilet facilities and unfavourable working and living conditions which are unfortunately still widespread.

3.17   THE IRRITABLE BOWEL SYNDROME

Probably the commonest cause of recurrent abdominal complaints, the irritable bowel syndrome, is defined as the presence of bowel symptoms in the absence of any evidence of organic disease. The fundamental cause is obscure but the clinical features appear to be a consequence of disturbed intestinal motility. Less preferable synonyms for the irritable bowel syndrome include spastic colon, mucous colitis, nervous diarrhoea and colon spasm.

The incidence is much greater in females than males and is commonly found in the younger age group. Bowel symptoms first occurring during middle-age or after are much more likely to be a consequence of organic disease and in this situation the diagnosis of the irritable bowel syndrome should be accepted only with the utmost caution.

The condition may occur in isolation or follow a severe attack of dysentery. There may be an associated psychiatric disturbance, for example emotional stress, anxiety neurosis or a depressive illness and the syndrome may also occur in association with other gastrointestinal disorders such as peptic ulceration, gastro-oesophageal reflux, biliary tract disease or after peptic ulcer surgery.

Clinical features

The major symptoms of the irritable bowel syndrome are:

1. ABDOMINAL PAIN

This is commonly felt in the lower abdomen or left iliac fossa but may be diffuse, predominantly upper abdominal or felt particularly in the right iliac fossa. The pain varies in severity and when situated in the upper abdomen may be aggravated by food ingestion and relieved by antacids. Helpful pointers localizing its origin to the colon include a relationship of the pain to either defaecation or the passage of flatus. The pain is often described as a cramp or dull ache and may be associated with the complaint of abdominal distension. Often the patient seeks to relieve the latter by belching but without benefit.

2. DISTURBANCE OF BOWEL HABIT

Either constipation or diarrhoea may be the predominant complaint or an alternation from one to the other. Diarrhoea may occur in the absence of abdominal pain but in contrast to diarrhoea as a result of organic disease, rarely disturbs the patient at night. Diarrhoea associated with the irritable bowel syndrome is commonly worse in the early morning either just before or after breakfast and the patient may then be virtually free of trouble for the rest of the day. When constipation is the major problem the faeces are hard, ribbon-like or pellety.

3. MUCOUS DISCHARGE

Varying amounts of mucus may be passed per rectum together with, or separate from, hard faeces.

Any of these symptoms will usually have been present intermittently for several years without any obvious deterioration in the patient's general health. There may also be symptoms suggestive of an underlying anxiety state or depressive illness, or there may be a history of stress associated with marital difficulties, employment problems, financial or housing worries.

Symptoms that are conspicuously *absent* include anorexia, weight loss, rectal bleeding and general malaise. Whenever any of these features are present organic disease should be strongly suspected.

Physical examination

This is chiefly important in excluding evidence of serious organic disease. Patients with the irritable bowel syndrome usually appear well generally although may be anxious or depressed. Abdominal examination is usually negative although there may be tenderness over the whole or part of the colonic outline. Rectal examination is negative. It is also worth noting any scars of previous abdominal surgery for in this condition there is a high incidence of removal of normal appendices, minor gynaecological procedures for vague abdominal symptoms with the patient rarely gaining relief for more than a few months before the symptoms recur.

Investigations

The basic principle should be to limit the investigations to the minimum consistent with the exclusion so far as possible of underlying organic disease. Unfortunately the danger is that the minimum commonly becomes the maximum and when the clinical features point strongly to a disturbance of bowel motility the diagnosis of the irritable bowel syndrome should not be accepted with reluctance. In the majority of patients with this problem the investigations can be limited to the following:

1. FAECAL OCCULT BLOOD

When this is negative it obviously does not rule out the possibility of organic disease but the appearance of occult blood in the stool demands an explanation.

2. SIGMOIDOSCOPY

This can be performed with either the rigid or fibreoptic instrument as a follow-on from physical examination. The appearance of the rectal mucosa should be normal but if there is the slightest suspicion of inflammatory bowel disease, a rectal mucosal biopsy can be taken. Air insufflation during sigmoidoscopy may reproduce the abdominal pain of which the patient complains.

3. BLOOD INVESTIGATIONS

The haemoglobin level, white cell count and ESR should be within normal limits as should the serum proteins. The serum thyroxine should be checked if there is any clinical pointer of thyroid dysfunction.

4. BARIUM ENEMA

A double-contrast barium enema is essential to exclude organic colonic pathology. Also there may be radiological pointers to a diagnosis of the irritable bowel syndrome, for example, reduction in the size of the lumen, exaggerated haustral markings and areas of intense bowel spasm.

In a minority of patients further investigations may be necessary to exclude upper gastrointestinal tract pathology, biliary disease, small intestinal abnormalities, etc. but the temptation to over-investigate should be kept firmly under control.

Differential diagnosis

The diagnosis of the irritable bowel syndrome is made chiefly by exclusion of organic disease and disorders of the large bowel in particular, e.g. polyp, carcinoma, diverticular disease, inflammatory bowel disease (Crohn's or ulcerative colitis). A barium meal and radiology of the biliary tract may be indicated when the site of pain is predominantly upper abdominal and small intestinal studies (radiology, faecal fat, xylose excretion, peroral mucosal biopsy) may be indicated in selected patients with persistent diarrhoea when there are other suggestive features of malabsorption. The possibility of food allergy may need consideration and also lactose deficiency. As previously mentioned, however, the temptation to over-investigate patients where the irritable bowel syndrome is suspected needs resisting, the exception being in a patient of middle-age or over presenting with bowel symptoms for the first time when the possibility of an underlying organic explanation is extremely high. In this situation the diagnosis of the irritable bowel syndrome should only be made with the utmost caution.

Management

Undoubtedly the two most important aspects of management are reassurance and explanation.

1. REASSURANCE

The great majority of patients with gastrointestinal symptoms are worried lest they are suffering from cancer even if this fear is not openly expressed. Once the irritable bowel syndrome has been diagnosed on the basis of careful clinical assessment with the minimum of investigations necessary to exclude organic disease, the patient should be strongly reassured that he is not suffering from malignant disease. Colitis is another fear and strong reassurance frequently brings visible relief to the patient who has usually been frightened that either of these alternatives may be present.

2. EXPLANATION

After the relief of hearing that he is not suffering from any serious bowel disorder, the patient will then require an explanation as to the origin of his symptoms. Simply to state that 'there is nothing wrong with you' is not sufficient. Understandably patients find it difficult not to equate pain which may be severe with the presence of serious disease and when they learn that no organic disease has been found they quickly conclude that the doctor considers their complaints to be imaginary. This misapprehension can usually be overcome by making a comparison with severe nocturnal leg cramps, which most people will have experienced and found very painful. They accept, however, that these are not due to serious disease and they can then understand how the intestinal musculature can also be painful without being diseased in the accepted sense. Similarly, painless diarrhoea is more readily accepted as being of no sinister significance when the patient is reminded of the link between nervous tension resulting from commonly experienced stressful situations and the gastrointestinal tract.

It is also essential to warn the patient that symptoms may recur intermittently in the future and not promise a dramatic and miraculous cure.

Drug therapy

Drug therapy is relatively less important than constant reassurance and a simple explanation of the mechanism of symptom production but a variety of preparations may be helpful in selected cases.

1. Bulking agents such as methylcellulose, sterculia, ispaghula husk derivatives or bran preparations are often of value to 'normalize' the bowel rhythm and faecal consistency when the complaint is either one of diarrhoea or constipation.

2. Painless diarrhoea may be helped by anti-diarrhoeal preparations such as codeine phosphate 15–30 mg t.d.s., diphenoxylate hydrochloride 5 mg t.d.s. or loperamide 2 mg t.d.s.

3. Antispasmodics are occasionally effective for the relief of colicky abdominal pain, mebeverine 135 mg t.d.s. before meals probably being the preparation of choice in view of its direct action on the smooth muscle fibre, thus avoiding the unpleasant effects of the anticholinergic preparations such as propantheline. A peppermint oil preparation (Colpermin 1–2 capsules with water t.d.s. before meals) also seems to be useful for this condition.

4. Short courses of anxiolytic agents such as diazepam 2 mg t.d.s., lorazepam 1 mg t.d.s. or chlordiazepoxide 10 mg t.d.s. may be helpful when there is evidence of a pronounced anxiety state and a tricyclic antidepressant is indicated when there are features of an underlying depressive illness.

DIET

There is no evidence that dietary restriction is of any value in the management of this condition and patients with the irritable bowel syndrome should be encouraged to eat as normally as possible apart from particular emphasis on an increase in the fibre content. This can be achieved by the inclusion of fresh fruit and vegetables, the use of wholemeal rather than white bread and the use of wholewheat cereals. Unprocessed miller's bran is a cheap source of additional dietary fibre but many patients find this unpalatable.

Prognosis. The irritable bowel syndrome is a chronic relapsing condition but the majority of patients find it easier to cope with their symptoms when they no longer fear the presence of cancer or other intra-abdominal disease and are reassured that their symptoms are not regarded as imaginary. The fact that the symptoms do occur intermittently should not be an indication for further investigations which can be safely deferred unless the symptom complex changes or there is a deterioration in the patient's general health.

FOR FURTHER READING

Chapter 3.2

Leading Article (1979) Oesophageal reflux and its myths. *Br. Med. J.* **1**, 3–4.
Reed P. I. (1980) Oesophageal reflux. *Practitioner* **224**, 357–363.

Chapter 3.4

Leading Article (1981) Gastric ulcer: benign or malignant? *Br. Med. J.* **282**, 843.

Chapter 3.5

Fielding J. W. L., Ellis D. J., Jones B. G. et al. (1980) Natural history of 'early' gastric cancer: results of a 10-year regional survey. *Br. Med. J.* **281**, 965–967.
Sherlock P. and Zamcheck N. (ed.) (1976) Cancer of the G.I. tract. *Clinics in Gastroenterology.* Vol. 5. No. 3. Saunders, London.

Chapter 3.6

Baron J. H., Langman M. J. S. and Wastell C. (1980) Stomach and duodenum. In: Bouchier I.A.D. (ed.) *Recent Advances in Gastroenterology.* Edinburgh, Churchill Livingstone, pp. 23–86.

Chapter 3.7

Dykes P. W. and Keighley M. R. B. (ed.) (1981) *Gastrointestinal Haemorrhage.* Bristol, Wright.

Thomas G. (1980) The clinical presentations of acute upper gastrointestinal bleeding. *Br. J. Hosp. Med.* **23**, 333–337.
Venables C. W. (1980) Advances in the management of gastrointestinal bleeding. *Br. J. Hosp. Med.* **23**, 338–346.

Chapter 3.8

Dykes P. W. and Keighley M. R. B. (ed.) (1981) *Gastrointestinal Haemorrhage.* Bristol, Wright.

Chapter 3.9

Blum A. L. and Siewert J. R. (ed.) (1979) Postsurgical syndromes. *Clinics in Gastro-enterology.* Vol. 8. No. 2. London, Saunders.
Steinberg D. M., Masselink B. A. and Alexander-Williams J. (1975) Assessment and treatment of recurrent peptic ulceration. *Ann. R. Coll. Surg. Engl.* **56**, 135–140.

Chapter 3.10

Almy T. P. and Fielding J. F. (ed.) (1977) The G.I. tract in stress and psycho-social disorder. *Clinics in Gastroenterology.* Vol. 6. No. 3. London, Saunders.

Chapter 3.11

Bateson M. C. (1982) Dissolving gallstones. *Br. Med. J.* **284**, 1–2.
Kupfer R. M. and Northfield T. C. (1981) Gallstones. *Practitioner* **225**, 449–506.

Chapter 3.12

Bouchier I. A. D. (1981) Diagnosis of jaundice. *Br. Med. J.* **283**, 1282–1284.
Thomson A. D. (1981) Cirrhosis of the liver. *Practitioner* **225**, 449–459.
Zuckerman A. J. (1981) Acute viral hepatitis. *J. R. Coll. Phys.* **15**, 88–94.

Chapter 3.13

Farmer R. G. (ed.) (1980) Inflammatory bowel disease. *Clinics in Gastroenterology.* Vol. 9. No. 2. London, Saunders.
Jewell D. P. (1982) Diagnosis and medical management of ulcerative colitis. *Br. J. Hosp. Med.* **27**, 456–462.

Chapter 3.14

Parks T. G. (1982) The clinical significance of diverticular disease of the colon. *Practitioner* **226**, 643–654.

Chapter 3.15

Roy D. (1982) Common epithelial tumours of the intestine. *Practitioner* **226**, 665–672.
Sherlock P. and Zamcheck N. (ed.) (1976) Cancer of the G.I. tract. *Clinics in Gastroenterology.* Vol. 5. No. 3. London, Saunders.

Chapter 3.16

Leading Article (1980) Investigating constipation. *Br. Med. J.* **1,** 669–670.
Painter N. S. (1980) Constipation. *Practitioner* **224,** 387–391.

Chapter 3.17

Almy T. P. and Fielding J. F. (ed.) (1977) The G.I. tract in stress and psycho-social disorder. *Clinics in Gastroenterology.* Vol. 6. No. 3. London, Saunders.
Ritchie J. (1982) The irritable bowel syndrome. *Practitioner* **226,** 633–641.

4 *Common Neurological Problems*

D. Bates

4.1 INTRODUCTION

Neurological symptoms invariably result in a large proportion of the referrals of patients to hospitals. The common symptoms of pain, abnormalities of movement, sensation and balance, together with those involving the special senses of vision, hearing and smell, comprise the majority of such problems. Among the most difficult are those involving disturbances of consciousness and the epilepsies, and those problems of communication seen in the aphasias and dementias. A patient tends to present with a series of symptoms and a reasonable approach to the common neurological disorders is a symptomatic one.

4.2 PAIN

Pain is probably the single most common symptom which makes a patient consult his doctor, and headache is in many regards the most worrying and certainly amongst the most frequent of such symptoms. With any symptom of pain the most important features to ascertain are those of the site, severity, character and periodicity of the pain, together with those phenomena which act to precipitate or relieve the symptom.

Headache

Headache is a frequently poorly localized symptom and never originates in the brain itself but rather from pressure on, or inflammation of, the meninges or sensory intracranial nerves, the bones of the cranial cavity or the muscles and vessels of the cranium.

Raised intracranial pressure
Undoubtedly the most important of all headaches is that due to raised intracranial pressure whether due to a cerebral tumour, abscess, haematoma, brain swelling or hydrocephalus. Characteristically the pain is occipital in nature due to pressure on the meninges of the posterior fossa and tentorial or foraminal herniation. It is most severe in the early morning, often wakening the patient from sleep and lessening as the erect posture is assumed during the day. This, like most organic pain, does respond to analgesics, is severe enough to make the patient present early in the disease and may be increased

by manoeuvres which increase the intracranial pressure, such as coughing, sneezing, straining and bending. Other associated features include vomiting, often without nausea, dizziness due to brainstem pressure and visual blurring due to the development of a VIth nerve palsy, eventually resulting in diplopia. Rarely, episodes of blindness on bending (obscuration) may occur.

The most important, but not invariable, clinical finding in raised intracranial pressure is papilloedema characteristically without visual disturbance. There may also be VIth nerve palsies causing failure of abduction of the eye and neck stiffness due to pressure in the region of the foramen magnum. Patients will usually have brisk reflexes, often including the jaw jerk, and may show focal signs related to the site of the pressure. The absence of focal signs suggests hydrocephalus or diffuse brain swelling as in benign intracranial hypertension.

Focal symptoms or signs may be positive due to irritative lesions such as seizures (either motor or sensory), complex partial seizures and visual disturbances, or negative such as paralysis, numbness, visual loss, deafness, dizziness or ataxia and diplopia. As the condition progresses there will usually be depression of the conscious level due to brainstem pressure.

The investigation of patients with raised intracranial pressure is now ideally by CT scan which has largely replaced the earlier investigations of skull X-ray, technetium scan and EEG, though the latter may still be indicated to identify a focal problem. In some circumstances angiography is indicated to further identify the nature of the lesion shown on CT scan and nuclear magnetic resonance scanning, when more widely available, may also have a part to play. If the CT scan is normal in the patient suspected of raised intracranial pressure then a lumbar puncture is obligatory to check the pressure of the CSF and to exclude a chronic meningitis of infective or neoplastic origin.

Subarachnoid haemorrhage

Probably the most dramatic of all headaches is that due to a subarachnoid haemorrhage from either a berry aneurysm or arteriovenous malformation. The headache is of dramatic onset and may be likened to a blow to the head. It may cause loss of consciousness and is a cause of sudden death but when the patient is able to give a description of the pain, the onset and severity, with particular reference to neck pain, usually makes the diagnosis evident.

Examination will typically reveal neck stiffness and usually a positive Kernig's sign (pain on straight leg raising) both indicative of meningism. There may be evidence of subhyaloid haemorrhage on fundoscopy and focal signs, if present, may give a clue as to the site of the bleed. Thus a IIIrd nerve palsy with subarachnoid haemorrhage suggests a posterior communicating artery aneurysm, a hemiparesis, an aneurysm at the middle cerebral artery trifurcation, and a paraparesis, a lesion of the anterior communicating artery.

The investigations indicated are a CT scan which will usually show the presence of subarachnoid blood and may indicate the site of the bleed; a lumbar puncture to reveal bloodstained fluid with the presence of xanthochromia; and an angiogram to identify the site and nature of the vascular lesion. The importance of angiography and consequent neuro-surgery is inversely proportional to the conscious level of the patient. Thus those who are alert and well are regarded as neurosurgical emergencies whereas those with deficits, altered consciousness and coma are believed to have significant spasm, and angiography can be reasonably deferred.

Meningitis

The headache of meningitis is classically of subacute onset and associated with general malaise and fever. There may be an associated alteration in conscious level indicating an associated encephalitis, and focal symptoms can occur due to localized collections of pus, venous sinus thrombosis or local encephalitis. Photophobia is a common symptom and again the pain is most prominent in the occipital and cervical regions.

The patient will usually be febrile, frequently toxic with a tachycardia and may have evidence of systemic infection. Neurologically there will be neck stiffness and a positive Kernig's sign. Focal signs may also be detected and raise the possibility of an abscess or empyema.

If there is the suspicion of a focal brain swelling or a collection of pus, the investigation of choice is a CT scan but most patients with meningitis can be safely subjected to lumbar puncture which is the diagnostic test and should reveal a polymorpholeucocytosis with elevated protein and low sugar in the pyogenic infection or a lymphocytic leucocytosis with minimal protein elevation and a normal sugar in viral meningitis. It is important to remember that lymphocytic pleocytosis may occur in tuberculous meningitis and other rarer meningitic disease such as those due to fungi. In patients without focal signs but with altered consciousness and generalized hyper-reflexia a CT scan may still be indicated to exclude the complication of hydrocephalus.

Temporal arteritis

In patients over the age of 50 with a severe, frequently well localized headache usually described as tenderness of the scalp, the possibility of temporal arteritis must be considered. The commonest sites for such headaches are in one or both temporal regions though occasional headache occurs in the occipital region with this syndrome. The patient usually presents early in the illness, frequently appears generally ill and can usually describe discomfort on simple manoeuvres such as chewing and brushing the hair. The temporal or occipital arteries may be exquisitely tender and are frequently palpated as non-pulsatile cords.

The diagnosis is supported by the finding of a high ESR and may be confirmed by biopsy of the affected vessels. The treatment of choice is steroids and the importance of early diagnosis and rapid treatment lies in the fact that this extracranial arteritis may result in the complications of blindness or focal cerebral deficit.

Migraine

Undoubtedly one of the most common headaches is that described by the patient or diagnosed by the physician as migraine. Classic migraine commonly occurring early in life frequently with the history of childhood biliousness or with a family history of migraine headache is not difficult to diagnose. The prodrome of malaise, visual disturbance with fortification spectra, followed by the unilateral headache, nausea, photophobia and vomiting lasting characteristically for less than 48 h makes the diagnosis relatively easy.

There are, however, other migrainous headaches variously described as common migraine or headache of vascular aetiology which may occur at any age in life and which are periodic, frequently unilateral and may be associated with photophobia or nausea.

The more important variants of migraine are those related to evident precipitants such as coffee or chocolate and those occurring either during pregnancy or when taking the contraceptive pill. The occurrence of migraine in a young lady taking the contraceptive pill is a relative contraindication to such treatment.

It must always be recognized that migraine may be complicated, in that it involves focal neurological disturbances ranging from field defects, blindness in an eye, ophthalmopareses or loss of motor or sensory function in a limb and occasionally dysphasia. These episodes probably reflect the vasospastic phase of the migraine episode and can be regarded as a specific contraindication to the use of ergotamine therapy. Such complicated migraine may in fact be symptomatic of an underlying arteriovenous malformation, aneurysm or meningioma. The occurrence of frequent episodes of complicated migraine always involving the same series of symptoms should always raise this possibility and may indicate the need for further investigation with a CT scan or angiogram.

The diagnosis of migraine is one which is essentially made historically, the therapy may be symptomatic with the use of analgesics and anti-nauseants and occasionally with ergotamine agents.

If interval therapy is required then the use of anti-serotonin agents is indicated, simple tricyclics sometimes help and methysergide, probably the most specific therapy, should be reserved in view of its known complication of retroperitoneal fibrosis.

Tension

The most common of all headaches causing referral to neurological clinics is the tension headache. It is characteristically diffuse, ill-defined and often difficult for the patient to describe. The symptoms frequently used are those of a band-like headache persisting day after day and unrelieved by simple analgesics. The history is characteristically long, the patient has frequently undergone numerous investigations and seen many other physicians and the problem is refractory to therapy. There are no signs of raised pressure nor evidence of focal neurological problem and the periodicity of migraine, the specificity of temporal arteritis and the associated symptoms of other headaches are absent. Such headaches are frequently difficult to treat but the use of anxiolytics or antidepressants is most likely to give benefit.

Post-traumatic

A rare but severe form of headache is that seen after significant head injury. Usually only after concussive head injuries the patient may develop a persisting and relentless headache occasionally related to the site of the injury but more frequently diffuse. Some authors believe that this headache is of non-organic nature but others recognize that the problem, though occasionally complicated by the process of litigation, is a genuine one and may persist for 3–5 years following the injury.

Medical causes

There are several varied medical causes of headache which should always be excluded historically and on examination of the patient presenting with this symptom. Perhaps the most common and most serious is that of hypertension though uraemia, hypocortisolaemia and other general medical problems need to be taken into account.

Facial pain

Pain in the face is most frequently related to dental problems or acute sinusitis but several of the more severe and chronic facial pains do have a neurological cause.

Trigeminal neuralgia

A lancinating pain arising most typically from the maxillary or mandibular division of the trigeminal nerve and occurring spontaneously or in response to stimuli such as cold, touch, talking and chewing suggests the diagnosis of trigeminal neuralgia. The pain is short-lived and shoots from its trigger point up or down the face. It is usually unilateral and may be so severe as to stop the patient bathing, talking and even feeding. The abruptness of the pain may make the patient wince and hence its alternative name of tic douloureux.

The syndrome is rare in the ophthalmic division of the trigeminal nerve and when occurring in a patient under the age of 50 years should raise thoughts of other pathologies, non-neurological, the rare trigeminal neuroma or multiple sclerosis. It is never bilateral. The cause of the pain is unknown and is assumed either to be due to a scar in the nerve itself or possibly to a small blood vessel which is lying against the nerve in its intracranial path.

Therapy initially consists of medical treatment most usefully with carbamazepine though surgical treatment is gaining in popularity and includes the creation of a lesion in the Gasserian ganglion either with cryoprobe or with radio frequency, or by performing a formal posterior craniotomy and attempting to release the pressure caused by the vessel lying against the nerve. The technique of nerve section or of alcohol injection is now largely of historical interest.

Painful ophthalmoplegia

Pain in and around the eye associated with an abnormality of eye movement is a not uncommon symptom which demands investigation. Possible causes include orbital or retro-orbital tumours, one of the most frequent of which is a nasopharyngeal carcinoma. The possibility of an aneurysm on the posterior communicating artery should not be forgotten and these structural pathologies make a CT scan obligatory and occasionally an angiogram indicated. If no structural cause is identified the possibilities of ophthal-moplegic migraine, unilateral Grave's disease or the Tolosa–Hunt syndrome due to an orbital apicitis have to be considered. The ill-defined syndrome of orbital pseudotumour may also cause pain in the eye together with restriction of eye movement.

Episodic eye pain

In young adult males the occurrence of episodes of severe orbital pain lasting for hours and classically occurring at night raises the possibility of periodic migrainous neuralgia. This is also called cluster headache and tends to occur daily for weeks followed by months or years of remission. The eye is usually inflamed, there is epiphora and nasal stuffiness on the same side and these phenomena are believed due to vasodilatation. The syndrome may be helped by the use of an anti-serotonin agent though occasionally ergotamine injections and even oxygen therapy are needed.

Other episodic pain with less typical features is also believed to be of vascular origin and termed cephalgia. It, too, may be helped by the use of anti-serotonin agents and occasionally by beta-blockade.

Atypical facial pain

Chronic pain which is poorly localized, remorseless and unresponsive to analgesic therapy is seen frequently in elderly and usually edentulate patients. Whilst the possibility of malocclusion must always be considered, the likelihood is that this form of continual pain has no overt organic cause and is as likely to respond to tricyclic medication as to any form of analgesia.

Herpes zoster

Shingles of the first division of the trigeminal nerve may cause severe unidentifiable pain for 1–2 days before the diagnostic rash appears. Similar problems may occur with shingles in the high cervical segments or when the facial nerve and brain stem are involved in the Ramsay Hunt syndrome.

Facial pain of non-neurological origin

The typical lancinating or aching nature of dental pain is usually very accurately localized to the site of tooth pathology and its relationship to eating hot or cold foods tends to confirm the diagnosis. Adequate radiological and dental investigations are indicated but if there is doubt as to the cause of the symptom it is incorrect, though common, to begin therapy with dental extraction or refilling.

Perhaps the most over-diagnosed condition causing facial pain is sinusitis. Infection in either the maxillary or frontal sinus can cause severe local pain which tends to be acute and well localized. There is pain to percussion over the infected sinus and there may even be reddening of the skin. It should be remembered that acute sinusitis tends to occur in association with an upper respiratory tract infection and may be identified by radiology. It is the exception for sinusitis to be the cause of chronic facial pain though in some instances the presence of a mucocele within a sinus or a neoplasm in a sinus might cause this symptom.

Pain in the back

Most patients with backache in the cervical, dorsal or lumbar spinal region have localized musculoskeletal pain due to the presence of spondylosis, arthritis and consequent muscle spasm. Most neurogenic causes for back pain cause some radiation of pain into the arm or leg due to radicular involvement by the pathology. There are, however, some causes of spinal pain which, by their nature, also affect the neuraxis.

Neck pain

Cervical spondylosis is the commonest cause of such pain though an increase may occur with an acutely prolapsed cervical disc which will tend to cause radicular pain into an arm. The other possibilities of intrathecal and extramedullary or even intramedullary tumours need to be excluded. Other structural abnormalities like syringomyelia may cause pain but the associated signs and symptoms should make this diagnosis evident. Sometimes a transverse myelitis or an acute exacerbation of multiple sclerosis may begin with severe localized cervical pain.

If there is any suspicion of structural abnormality then radiology of the cervical spine is obligatory and myelography should be seriously considered.

Pain in the thoracic spine

Such pain is much less common than in the cervical or lumbosacral regions. It frequently has non-neurological causes and should always raise suspicion of thoracic or abdominal tumours. However, extradural lesions such as bone secondaries, dorsal discs and extradural haematomas do occur as do intradural lesions such as a neurofibroma or meningioma. The latter is most typically seen in middle-aged females. Intramedullary tumours, though less commonly causing pain, may also present in this way. The characteristic of neurological lesions in the cervical and dorsal spine which cause pain is that they result in radicular pain extending to the arm from the cervical region or in a girdle fashion in the dorsal region. They are frequently associated with an evolving para- or tetraparesis in which case both radiology and myelography are obligatory.

Pain in the lumbosacral spine
Pain in the low back is a common cause of prolonged disability and most patients do not have a significant neurological lesion. Indeed, the presence of pain in the low back without radiation into the legs, though sometimes seen in gliomas of the conus, is usually due to musculoskeletal problems.

The symptoms which indicate potentially neurogenic pain are radiation into the legs in either sciatic or femoral nerve distribution, disturbances of bladder or bowel function, evidence of motor and sensory loss in the lower limbs and saddle area and an increase in pain occasioned by manoeuvres which raise the intraspinal pressure.

Lesions damaging the conus at the dorsolumbar junction cause a mixture of upper and lower motor neurone signs in the legs with brisk reflexes, absent reflexes, spastic muscles and wasted and flaccid muscles. Lesions in the cauda equina simply affect the lower motor neurones causing weakness, wasting and loss of reflexes. The commonest causes are prolapsed intervertebral discs, tumours in the lumbar spine and the newly recognized syndrome of claudication of the cauda equina due to a narrow lumbar canal, ischaemia to the lumbar theca or the after-effects of surgical operations. The possibility of an intraspinal lesion causing low back pain indicates the need for radiology and possibly myelography.

Pain in the arm

The symptoms of pain in the arm may be local or referred. Local causes such as bone and joint disease, ischaemic and rheumatological problems should be excluded and the referred pain of myocardial ischaemia and diaphragmatic irritation must be remembered.

Radicular pain
Pain arising due to damage to the cervical roots in the cervical spine tends to be constant and sharp and relates to neck movement or factors which raise the intraspinal pressure. It is well localized and more common in the upper roots of the arm, notably the fifth, sixth and seventh cervical segments. Possible causes include a cervical disc, a cervical spine tumour, secondary

deposit or a syrinx. Rarer causes include extradural or intramedullary haematomas which tend to arise after injury and again pain in radicular distribution in the upper limbs may herald by some days the onset of the typical rash of shingles.

Plexus

Pain arising from lesions in the brachial plexus may be postinfective as in a brachial plexitis or in neuralgic amyotrophy when it commonly affects the upper part (C5/6) of the plexus, or due to structural damage such as the rare syndrome of cervical rib or Pancoast's tumour arising in the apex of the lung when the lower plexus (C8/T1) is more often involved.

Nerve pain

The most important causes of pain arising in the peripheral nerve in the upper limb are the entrapment neuropathies. The median nerve is commonly compressed in the carpal tunnel at the wrist and results in dysaesthesiae in the thumb, index and middle fingers, particularly common during the night. There is weakness of median nerve innervated muscles and the treatment is decompression of the nerve in the tunnel. The ulnar nerve is most frequently damaged at the elbow in the olecranon groove and causes pain and numbness in the little and ring finger. Ulnar nerve transposition may be performed for this though its effectiveness is dubious. The radial nerve may be trapped in the radial groove of the humerus, is usually painless but may cause pain radiating into the back of the hand. The anterior interosseous nerve may be trapped at the interosseous membrane or the head of the pronator and typically causes pain on pronation and supination of the forearm with weakness of the long flexors of the hand.

Though these neuropathies commonly arise due to local pressure, it should be remembered that they may also be caused by conditions such as the arteritides or diabetes resulting in nerve infarcts, and the concurrence of a generalized neuropathy such as seen in diabetes or alcoholism may make these particular nerves more liable to trauma.

Other neurogenic pain

It should always be remembered that spasticity in the upper limb may cause cramps and pain arising from any cause of upper motor neurone disturbance in the limb. In addition, some examples of muscle disease, particularly the metabolic myopathies and polymyositis, are associated with pain in the arm. Post-traumatic pain in the arm may arise due to disturbance of nerve function particularly when involving the autonomic nerves and this intractable pain causes great problems in management.

Pain in the leg

It is again important to exclude those causes of local pain including bone and joint disease and ischaemia which commonly result in pain on movement of the limb and may occur at rest. It should be recognized that exercise pain is not confined to syndromes of vascular disease in the legs.

Radicular pain

The most typical cause of radicular pain in the lower limb is that due to a prolapsed intervertebral disc. The most common discs to prolapse are those between the L4/5 and L5/S1 vertebrae resulting in the syndrome of sciatica. The pain characteristically radiates down the posterior aspect of the leg into the ankle or foot. The pain is made worse by factors which increase intraspinal pressure or those which stretch the nerve roots involved. More rarely the roots of the femoral nerve are involved in a prolapsed intervertebral disc but this syndrome is more commonly seen with other lesions affecting the higher lumbar roots including diabetes mellitus and intraspinal tumours.

Plexus pain

The most common cause of pain in the lumbosacral plexus is the presence of infiltration or tumours in the pelvis. A rectal and/or pelvic examination is obligatory in such causes of lower limb pain and other investigations including ultrasound, body scanning and intravenous pyelography may be indicated.

Peripheral nerve pain

Peripheral nerve pain in the lower limb is less common than in the upper limb but similar causes of mononeuropathies should be considered: the entrapment of the lateral cutaneous nerve of the thigh at the inguinal ligament causes the syndrome of meralgia paraesthetica with paraesthesiae over the thigh, damage to the lateral popliteal nerve at the head of the fibula can cause pain in the outer aspect of the leg and the tarsal tunnel syndrome may cause pain in the foot. Digital pain in the foot may be caused by the presence of a neuroma on one of the digital nerves (Morton's metatarsalgia) and generalized peripheral neuropathies can cause dysaesthetic pain in both lower limbs commonly seen in diabetes mellitus.

Other neurological pain

The condition of intermittent claudication of the cauda equina has already been mentioned and this may present with pain in the lower limb which is often increased by standing and walking and may only be relieved by flexing the lumbar spine. In addition, cramp in the lower limb is a common cause of pain in patients with spasticity from any cause. The metabolic and inflammatory myopathies may also present with pain in the lower limb and recently the possibility of ischaemia affecting peripheral nerves in the case of generalized arterial disease has also been raised as a cause of pain in the lower limbs.

Pain in an arm and leg

The occurrence of pain in a hemi-distribution affecting both the arm and leg is uncommon but occurs occasionally in patients who have suffered thalamic infarcts where the contralateral side may be rendered anaesthetic and dysaesthetic. This particular pain is frequently intractable to therapy and can at times make patients suicidal. The types of medical treatment which sometimes are effective include the use of carbamazepine or phenytoin, tricyclic medications and the physical application of a stimulator to a particularly painful area.

Another rare, though important, cause of pain in one side of the body occurs with lesions affecting the spinothalamic tract in multiple sclerosis where it is frequently seen in an association with spasms and may be expected to respond to treatment with carbamazepine.

4.3 DISORDERS OF MOVEMENT

Disturbances of the motor system provide another group of symptoms which commonly result in neurological referral. The most obvious of these symptoms is paresis or weakness which may result from lesions in the upper motor neurone, the lower motor neurone, the neuromuscular junction or the muscle itself. A further problem of altered tone and posture, including the development of involuntary movements, is seen in patients with disturbances of the basal ganglia and lesions affecting the cerebellum and its connections result in disturbances of equilibrium which may also compromise movement (*Fig.* 4.1)

Weakness

Although the complaint of weakness is not always organic and can be very non-specific and varied, it is among the most important and potentially the most revealing of all the patient's complaints. The initial distinction which the clinician has to make is between weakness due to damage affecting the upper motor neurone and that affecting the lower motor neurone, neuromuscular junction and muscle (*Table* 4.1).

The upper motor neurone

Damage to the upper motor neurone characteristically results in the symptoms of spasticity of the muscle without evident wasting, brisk reflexes and loss of power. The power loss characteristically follows a particular pattern, being most marked in the extensor muscles of the upper limb and therefore resulting in the flexed posture of that limb, and the flexor muscles of the lower limb resulting in an extensor posture of that limb. Tone is increased in a clasp-knife fashion and the reflexes in the affected limb are

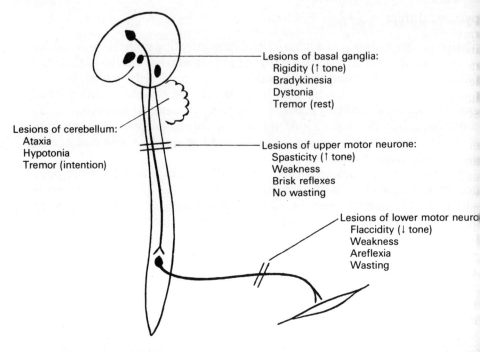

Fig. 4.1. Disturbances of movement.

Table 4.1 Patterns of weakness

Lower motor neurone	Peripheral symmetrical weakness	Peripheral neuropathy
	Weakness in distribution of single nerve	Mononeuropathy
	Weakness in distribution of single root	Radiculopathy
Upper motor neurone	Pyramidal weakness — paraplegia	Spinal cord
	— hemiplegia	Hemisphere or high cord
	— tetraplegia	High cord or bilateral cerebrum
	Apraxia	Cerebral cortex
	Proximal weakness	Muscle disease

brisk. An exception to this general rule may be seen with truly cortical lesions in which the weakness may appear peripherally in the limb but the clue remains the finding of extremely brisk reflexes and usually an extensor plantar response.

Once the nature of an upper motor neurone lesion is established the site is determined by the limb involved and whether or not there is sparing of the face. A monoplegia causing weakness of the limb implies damage to the pyramidal tract supplying that limb in the internal capsule, spinal cord or rarely at the level of the cortex. The most common causes of such problems include cerebrovascular accidents, stroke and multiple sclerosis and the necessary investigations undertaken are decided by the putative site of the lesion. Thus if a spinal cord problem is suspected then myelography or lumbar puncture may be indicated, if a cerebral lesion is suspected then a CT scan and angiography may be the investigations of choice.

The more common symptom of hemiplegia involving weakness of an arm and leg implies a lesion either high in the cervical cord or in the brain itself and is most commonly seen in stroke and cerebral tumour. An important clue as to the level of the lesion is given by the involvement or sparing of the face which, because of the bilateral innervation of the upper part of the facial nerve nucleus will usually be included as weakness of the lower face ipsilateral to the hemiplegia indicating a contralateral hemispheric lesion. Involvement of the whole of the face implying a lower motor neurone problem, usually on the contralateral side to the hemiplegia, suggests that the lesion is in the brainstem and sparing of the face suggests the lesion is in the cervical spine. In this way the physician is able to direct his further investigations towards either the cerebrum, the brainstem or the spinal cord and undertake the relevant tests.

A paraparesis, that is involvement of both lower limbs, is most frequently seen with lesions in the spine and it is important to note that spastic weakness of both lower limbs implies a lesion in the cervical or dorsal spine since lesions arising in the lumbar spine will necessarily cause lower motor neurone problems. The relevant investigation is likely to be that of myelography though the possibility of the rare parasagittal lesion causing such damage in the interhemispheric fissues to the leg portions of both the left and right homunculus should also be considered.

Tetraparesis or involvement of all four limbs is most commonly seen in high cervical lesions such as multiple sclerosis or tumours though it may also occur in bilateral strokes and in system degenerations such as motor neurone disease. The involvement of the upper motor neurones bilaterally in the cerebral hemispheres will also result in the syndrome of pseudobulbar palsy causing a spastic paralysis of muscles innervated by the Xth and XIIth nerves and resulting in a spastic dysarthria and dysphagia. This condition also implies bilateral disease and is seen in multiple strokes, multiple sclerosis and system degeneration.

The lower motor neurone

The cardinal features of damage to the lower motor neurone include weakness and wasting of muscles together with loss of reflexes and occasionally the finding of fasciculation in the affected muscle. Once these features are established most importance is placed on the pattern of weakness. Thus a lesion involving the muscles supplied by a single peripheral nerve identifies the presence of a mononeuropathy due to local nerve entrapment, trauma or to a nerve infarct as in the arteritides or diabetes. A diffuse peripheral lower motor neurone weakness is seen in the generalized peripheral neuropathies which may be toxic, metabolic, inherited or postinfective as in the Guillain–Barré syndrome.

Weakness of muscles innervated by a single nerve root suggest a radicular lesion and if more than one root is involved the possibility of plexus involvement should be considered. Usually lesions affecting the roots or plexus are painful and investigations to be undertaken may include nerve conduction studies and EMG, scanning techniques and radiology.

When a diffuse weakness of the lower motor neurone type is detected particularly in the presence of muscle fasciculation in more than one limb and classically if the reflexes are paradoxically brisk the diagnosis of motor neurone disease is almost certain.

Lower motor neurone lesions affecting the cranial nerves may present in different ways. Involvement of the lower motor neurone of the facial nerve is seen most commonly in Bell's palsy and is usually unilateral. The lower motor neurone nature of the lesion is shown by the involvement of both the lower facial muscles and frontalis which muscle is bilaterally innervated at the level of the nucleus and therefore spared in upper motor neurone lesions. Lower motor neurone involvement of the bulbar muscles result in a true bulbar palsy with a flaccid dysarthria and dysphagia.

The neuromuscular junction

The cardinal feature of disease of the neuromuscular junction is the phenomenon of fatigue. Thus patients who may show no evidence of weakness early in the day develop increasing weakness with use of muscles and show an improvement with rest and a deterioration with exercise. The most common cause of this problem is myasthenia gravis and the diagnosis is confirmed by the use of electrophysiological techniques, ideally single fibre EMG, and also by the assessment of the presence of acetylcholine receptor antibodies in the blood.

Muscle disease

The myopathies and muscular dystrophies most commonly manifest with muscle weakness which is particularly evident in the proximal muscles. Pain may also be a feature of muscle disease, particularly in the relatively common condition of polymyositis and less commonly with certain of the metabolic myopathies. Most muscle disease causes, apart from weakness and loss of reflexes, wasting of the involved muscles. Some muscle diseases however, are associated with apparent hypertrophy of muscles as seen in Duchenne dystrophy.

The suspicion of a myopathy or dystrophy is confirmed by EMG studies assessment of creatinine kinase and myoglobin in blood and ultimately by muscle biopsy.

Rigidity

The symptom of stiffness is frequently used by patients with an upper motor neurone lesion to describe the spasticity present in a limb. However, true stiffness or rigidity is a cardinal feature of disturbance of basal ganglia function. Patients may initially develop pain in the affected limb or limbs and will then become aware of a difficulty in movement predominantly due to an alteration in tone. Unlike the spastic limb, this alteration in tone is rigid and may be associated with the finding on examination of cog-wheeling. Other factors are likely to include a relatively expressionless face, a dorsal kyphosis causing a stooped posture and the loss of associated arm movement on walking. The finding of these features indicates the likelihood of Parkinson's disease and they are frequently associated with a rest tremor which is abolished by movement. The diagnosis remains essentially clinical and distinction should be made between idiopathic Parkinson's disease, that secondary to toxic agents such as carbon monoxide poisoning or manganese, the rare post-encephalitic Parkinson's disease and the more common finding of extrapyramidal disturbance in patients with diffuse vascular disease.

Some patients with evident disturbance of basal ganglia function will show associated features of an autonomic neuropathy as in the Shy–Drager syndrome or of gross eye movement disturbance and possible dementia as in the syndrome of progressive supranuclear palsy.

The therapy consists of dopaminergic agents, most commonly the combination of L-dopa and dopa decarboxylase inhibitor, but also with anticholinergic agents, and with direct dopaminergic agents such as bromocriptine.

Involuntary movements

Most involuntary movements reflect a degree of disturbance of the basal ganglia system, either primary or in response to drug therapy.

Chorea

Relatively fast and so-called semi-purposive movements of the limbs are seen in chorea, most commonly as part of the degenerative condition, Huntington's chorea, which is inherited as an autosomal dominant, though rarely in association with rheumatic fever as Sydenham's chorea or in pregnancy and during the use of the contraceptive pill as chorea gravidarum.

It is not uncommon to see choreic-like movement occurring in patients treated with phenothiazines and in patients with Parkinson's disease who are overdosed with dopaminergic agents.

Athetosis

The more writhing and slower involuntary movements of athetosis are most commonly seen as a complication of cerebral palsy though they may also occur in adults after anoxic insult.

Hemiballismus

The syndrome of unilateral chorea, typically seen in elderly patients after presumed vascular lesions in the subthalamic nucleus, is termed hemiballismus.

Tremor

Tremor is one of the clinical symptoms which can be relatively easily assessed into three kinds, each of which gives some indication of the underlying pathology.

Resting tremor

The possibility of a resting tremor in Parkinson's disease has already been identified and the occurrence of a fine and compound tremor frequently described as pill-rolling is strongly suggestive of Parkinson's disease. Characteristically this particular symptom is made better by movement and may even cease when the patient's attention is drawn to it.

Intention tremor

An intention tremor is most apparent at the end of movement and is best shown on the finger–nose test. It is strongly suggestive of disease affecting the cerebellum and its connections and in its most severe form indicates a lesion in the connections between the dentate and red nuclei. It may cause the patient only minimal inconvenience at its most mild but can be totally disabling, preventing feeding, bathing and movement when most severe. It is frequently seen in multiple sclerosis and also in toxic and degenerative conditions affecting the cerebellum.

Action tremor

The most common of all tremors present on action and throughout movement is the action tremor. It may be physiological as in states of anxiety or when seen as benign familial or senile tremor, or pathological in which case the cause may be metabolic as in thyrotoxicosis, renal and hepatic failure and hypercapnia or toxic as in the effects of alcohol and certain drugs.

Tremor can be a disabling symptom and though the resting tremor may frequently be helped by the exhibition of dopaminergic agents and an action tremor by the correction of the underlying metabolic or toxic abnormality or the use of beta blockade the intention tremor is usually refractory to therapy.

4.4 DISORDERS OF SENSATION

Sensory disturbances provide a common presenting symptom but sensory signs are often very difficult to demonstrate and, with few exceptions, are entirely subjective. In considering abnormal sensory symptoms it is important to recognize the distinctive pathways of the different sensory modalities and therefore to recognize which particular modalities should be tested. In general the symptoms of anaesthesia, pain, dysaesthesiae, paraesthesiae and loss of thermal sensation are seen in disturbances of the small fibres in the peripheral nerves which synapse shortly after their entry to the spinal cord and then cross to ascend in the contralateral spinothalamic tract to the thalamus. Here they again synapse before ascending to the cortex. These modalities are tested with touch, pinprick and the use of warm and cold objects. Symptoms of the loss of proprioception or loss of vibration sensation and those of tightness or band-like sensations occur with lesions in the large sensory fibres of the peripheral nerve which ascend ipsilaterally in the posterior column of the spinal cord, synapse in the gracile and cuneate nuclei of the medulla and then cross to make their second synapse in the contralateral thalamus before ascending to the cortex. They are tested by the application of a tuning fork to the limb and by assessing joint position sense.

Clinically the type of symptom suffered by the patient and its distribution are the factors which help identify the nature and site of the neurological lesions causing those symptoms (*Table* 4.2).

Table 4.2 Patterns of sensory loss

Glove and stocking anaesthesia	Peripheral neuropathy
Single nerve numbness	Mononeuropathy
Single root numbness	Radiculopathy
Posterior column loss	Large fibre neuropathy
	Dorsal column spinal cord
Spinothalamic loss	Small fibre neuropathy
	Central cord disease
Anaesthesia contralateral to proprioceptive loss	Hemisection of spinal cord
Hemianaesthesia	Cerebral hemisphere lesion
Agnosia	Cortical disease

Peripheral sensory symptoms

Sensory symptoms beginning in the feet and gradually spreading proximally to the knees, at which stage the hands also become involved, is characteristic of a peripheral neuropathy. The symptoms may be predominantly of numbness as seen in many of the inherited neuropathies but in the toxic and paraneoplastic neuropathies there may also be a distressing dysaesthetic sensation. If the large peripheral nerve fibres are also involved then there may be loss of proprioception in the feet and hands resulting in the symptoms of unsteadiness, a tendency to fall and clumsiness.

Such symptoms of peripheral neuropathy are usually associated with depression of reflexes and frequently with a peripheral lower motor neurone weakness also. The investigations indicated include nerve conduction studies and EMG, relevant haematological investigations and possibly even nerve biopsy. One syndrome which deserves special mention is the predominantly proprioceptive loss in the hands and feet together with areflexia but with extensor plantars as seen in subacute combined degeneration of the spinal cord due to vitamin B_{12} deficiency (*Fig.* 4.2).

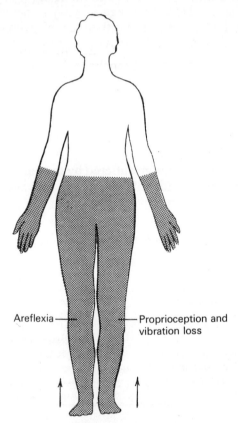

Areflexia —————————————— Proprioception and
vibration loss

Fig. 4.2. Subacute combined degeneration of the spinal cord.

Mononeuropathy

Sensory disturbance in the territory of a single peripheral nerve implies local damage to that nerve and is commonly due to entrapment neuropathies of the median or ulnar nerve in the upper limb or the lateral cutaneous nerve of the thigh in the lower limb. Such symptoms of a mononeuropathy are also seen with nerve infarction as in diabetes mellitus or the various arteritic diseases. In this situation it is not uncommon to find more than one peripheral nerve being involved when the syndrome is termed mononeuritis multiplex.

Investigations to identify such problems again include nerve conduction studies and EMG and in the case of mononeuritis multiplex a search for evidence of an underlying metabolic or inflammatory disease.

Radicular lesions

If the sensory symptoms relate to a dermatomal distribution rather than to a peripheral nerve distribution then the lesion has to lie in the plexus or root. The loss of sensation in the L4/5 or S1 dermatomes is commonly seen in the prolapsed lumbar disc syndrome whereas the C5, C6 or C7 dermatomes are commonly involved in cervical disc lesions. Numbness in the T1 distribution is rare but may occur with apical bronchogenic carcinoma and multiple root involvement is more commonly seen with diseases affecting the plexus.

With radicular lesions the relevant reflexes are lost and there are frequently motor symptoms and signs of lower motor neurone type.

The disease of shingles in which the dorsal root ganglion is involved with herpes zoster will characteristically cause a rash in dermatomal distribution frequently followed by hyperpathia or increased sensitivity in the same segmental region.

Cord lesions

Since, as has been described above, there is separation of the two types of sensory pathway within the spinal cord the cardinal feature of sensory disturbance due to lesions in the spinal cord is dissociation.

Posterior column lesions

The symptoms of loss of proprioception, band-like sensation of tightness and loss of vibration sensation are seen with damage to the posterior column. Such problems are most commonly seen in the lower limbs when they may reflect the presence of pressure upon the cord or the development of a plaque of multiple sclerosis in the posterior column. Occasionally the symptoms of such deafferentation are confined to both upper limbs due to lesions arising laterally in the cervical posterior column and this is strongly suggestive of multiple sclerosis (see Fig. 4.1). The picture, as has been mentioned above, is also seen in subacute combined degeneration of the spinal cord. The investigation will usually require examination of cerebrospinal fluid and probably myelography.

Suspended dissociated anaesthesia

The loss of pain and temperature sensation indicates a lesion affecting the spinothalamic tract and is most commonly seen with a central cord lesion in the cervical region. The pathology is commonly that of a syrinx or cord glioma resulting in damage to the crossing fibres shortly after they enter the spinal cord. Classic symptoms include a whole or half cape dissociated sensory loss usually associated with loss of cervical root reflexes and occasionally with both lower and upper motor neurone signs in the upper limbs (*Fig.* 4.3). Such symptoms usually indicate the need for myelography.

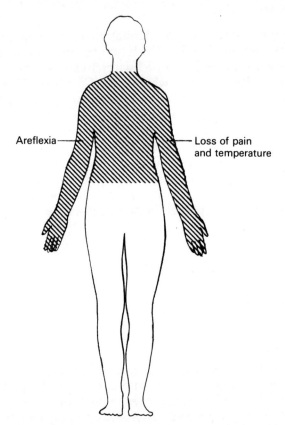

Areflexia — — Loss of pain and temperature

Fig. 4.3. Suspended dissociated anaesthesia. Central cervical cord lesion.

The loss of spinothalamic sensation in the lower limbs may be seen without posterior column loss in anterior spinal artery occlusion resulting in a cord infarct. These are usually associated pyramidal symptoms and signs in the legs and again myelography and examination of the CSF are indicated.

The loss of the sensation of pain is important in allowing the patient to suffer burns, cuts and grazes without awareness and even to allow subsequent infection of the lesions. Such trophic changes are important physical signs in the identification of a sensory lesion. In addition, the absence of pain can allow disorganization of a joint and consequent arthropathy—the so-called Charcot joint seen in syringomyelia in the upper limb and in diabetes mellitus and tabes dorsalis in the lower limbs.

Brown-Séquard syndrome

Damage to one half of the spinal cord as seen in multiple sclerosis, vascular lesions and some tumours causes the classic syndrome of spasticity and pyramidal weakness with brisk reflexes ipsilateral to the lesion, loss of proprioception and vibration sensation ipsilateral to the lesion and anaesthesia to pain and temperature on the contralateral side (*Fig.* 4.4). Although such a syndrome may occur with lesions other than structural it usually requires the investigation of myelography.

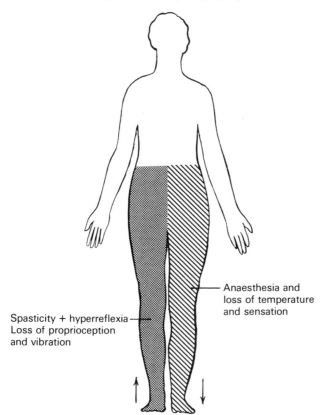

Anaesthesia and loss of temperature and sensation

Spasticity + hyperreflexia
Loss of proprioception and vibration

Fig. 4.4. Brown-Séquard syndrome. Right hemisection of cord.

Bilateral sensory loss

Lesions which affect the spinal cord and cause an evolving paraparesis are likely to result in bilateral sensory loss of all modalities in the lower limbs together with sphincter disturbance. Indeed, in the presence of a paraparesis it is often the sensory level in the dorsal dermatomes which identifies the precise level of the lesion. It is always necessary to remember that the neurological anatomical level suggests a structural pathology some segments higher. Thus the loss of sensation up to and including the tenth dorsal dermatome would imply a lesion at the level of the sixth or seventh dorsal vertebra (*Fig.* 4.5).

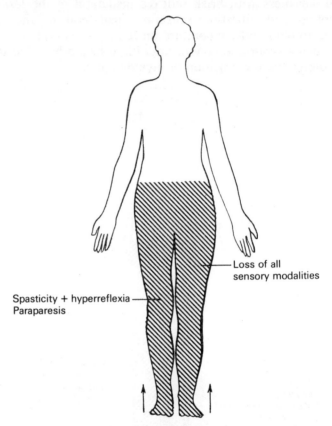

Loss of all sensory modalities

Spasticity + hyperreflexia
Paraparesis

Fig. 4.5. Evolving paraplegia. Spinal cord compression. Transverse myelitis.

Hemi-sensory loss

The loss of all modalities of sensation on one side implies a lesion above the medulla and up to the level of the thalamus. Above this level proprioception tends to be left intact and there is appreciation through poor localization of pain. The cause of hemi-sensory anaesthesia is usually vascular though it may occasionally be seen with cerebral tumour and rarely with multiple sclerosis. The investigation indicated would be a CT scan.

Cortical sensory loss

In some patients with apparent sensory disturbance testing the crude modalities of sensation is in fact normal. It may then be shown that the integration of this sensory information to enable the identification of objects by feel is affected and the lesion is then cortical in the parietal lobe contralateral to the problem. The symptom is termed 'agnosia' and is frequently seen in patients with sensory and/or visual inattention contralateral to the lesion. The presence of such abnormality would suggest the need for a CT scan.

Facial sensory loss

Sensation for the face is mediated by the three divisions of the trigeminal nerve; it synapses in the spinal tract of the trigeminal nerve and is then relayed in the thalamus to the cortex. Hemispheric lesions may cause sensory loss on one half of the face together with hemi-anaesthesia of the body and the cause is usually vascular or neoplastic. Lesions of the spinal tract of the trigeminal nerve may be associated with facial sensory loss, ipsilateral to the lesion and contralateral to anaesthesia in the body. The anatomical representation in the spinal tract of the trigeminal nerve is such that lesions in this area tend to cause sensory loss beginning around the mouth and spreading outwards.

Lesions of the trigeminal nerve itself tend to involve one or more divisions of the nerve and the division involved provides a clue to the site and nature of the lesion. Thus involvement of the first division of the trigeminal nerve implies a lesion in the anterior cranial fossa or orbit. Involvement of the first and second divisions together suggest the lesions lies in the cavernous sinus and the third division tends to be involved with lesions in the skull base.

The most objective of all sensory tests is the corneal reflex and it is the most sensitive indicator of damage to the first division of the trigeminal nerve.

Since sensory testing is so purely subjective, it is important to identify precisely the divisions of the trigeminal nerve and to remember that the first division supplies not only sensation to the face but to the scalp as far back as the vertex.

4.5 BLACKOUTS AND 'FUNNY TURNS'

The epidosic loss of consciousness or intermittent episodes of loss of awareness or abnormal behaviour are amongst the most dramatic and alarming of symptoms to be presented to the physician. The most important role of the doctor is to identify the cause of the attacks be they cerebral, metabolic, cardiovascular or hysterical and to apply the appropriate therapy. In all cases of disturbances of consciousness or awareness it is important to obtain a history not only from the patient but from someone who has witnessed the attack and to obtain details, usually from the patient's primary physician, of an antecedent or previous illness.

The epilepsies

As many as 2% of people may suffer a single seizure at some time in their lives and 1 patient in 200 will have epilepsy as defined by the occurrence of more than one seizure. Whilst the description by witnesses of a classic grand mal seizure or tonic–clonic attack with or without a prodrome, including convulsive movements, self-injury and incontinence and followed by drowsiness, confusion and headache, is so typical as to establish its nature, it must be remembered that epilepsy is a symptom and can reflect underlying cerebral or systemic disease.

Less typical attacks, particularly of partial epilepsy, may be much more difficult to diagnose. It is useful both in terms of determining further investigations and in deciding the most suitable treatment to attempt to classify by clinical and EEG findings the type of epilepsy. The most useful classification is based on the site of origin of the epilepsy:

1. *Generalized epilepsy*
    a. Petit mal
    b. Grand mal
2. *Focal epilepsy*
    a. Simple
    b. Complex
3. *Secondary generalized epilepsy*

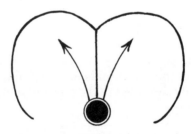

Fig. 4.6. Generalized epilepsy. Activity spreads bilaterally from a centrencephalic source.

1. *Generalized epilepsy (Fig.* 4.6)

The term 'generalized epilepsy' is retained for those people with previously termed subcortical or central epilepsy where instability in the diencephalon is believed to stimulate both hemispheres simultaneously and result in the seizure. No structural cause is found and the EEG is diffusely abnormal. Petit mal is a syndrome in childhood usually between the ages of 7 and 15 in which the child suffers episodes of loss of awareness often many times during the day and may have myoclonic movements. The EEG shows the characteristic 3 Hz spike-and-wave activity generalized and the most effective therapy is with valproate or ethosuximide.

Primary generalized grand mal epilepsy is most commonly seen in childhood or early adult life. Clinically the attack is a non-focal, tonic–clonic seizure and the EEG will show a diffuse and bilateral abnormality in a reasonable proportion of patients. Such seizures are most likely to be controlled with valproate, phenytoin or occasionally barbiturate therapy.

2. *Focal epilepsy* (*Fig.* 4.7)

Focal epilepsy indicates the presence of a focal hemispheric cause which may be insignificant in size and of long standing or may indicate the presence of a vascular lesion, a tumour, a focal infection, an abscess, head injury or a surgical scar. Rarely, focal signs may be seen in the context of generalized metabolic disease as in hypoglycaemia or hepatic failure when it presumably indicates some local vascular problem enhanced by the more general disturbance.

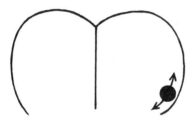

Fig. 4.7. Focal epilepsy. Activity in a lesion irritates the cortex locally.

If the lesion causing focal seizures lies in the frontal lobe then the symptom will be of focal motor seizures, in the parietal lobe focal sensory seizures and, rarely, lesions in the occipital lobe may cause visual disturbances. A complication arises with those focal attacks arising in the temporal lobe when the symptoms may be olfactory or gustatory causing the patient to lick or smack their lips or may involve disturbances of memory and awareness, *déjà vu, jamais vu* or absences. Rarely, formed visual hallucinations may occur and such phenomena can result in bizarre behaviour which can occasionally persist for hours. In general patients said to have developed 'petit mal' in adult life usually have absences occurring due to temporal lobe or complex partial seizures. This distinction is important since focal seizures of either simple or complex type are more likely to respond to therapy with carbamazepine or phenytoin than those agents used for genuine petit mal.

3. *Secondary generalized seizures* (*Fig.* 4.8)

The majority of major seizures developing in adult life are secondary generalized. There may be an indication of the underlying focus in that an attack may begin with a focal motor, sensory or temporal element and then rapidly progress to a tonic–clonic seizure. More rarely, focal motor or sensory seizures will develop into a generalized seizure by a Jacksonian march of the epilepsy as neurones along the homunculus are sequentially stimulated.

When generalized epilepsy can be shown to have arisen from a focal lesion therapy is most successful with the drug used for focal epilepsy such as carbamazepine or phenytoin. Sodium valproate is also occasionally used.

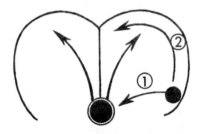

Fig. 4.8. Secondary generalized epilepsy. Activity from a focal lesion either initiates a seizure centrally (1) or spreads along the cortex (2) as a Jacksonian seizure.

The investigation of the epilepsies consists of obtaining an adequate history and performing an examination following which any suggestion of focal onset or signs makes formal investigation with an EEG and CT scan obligatory. If there is no suggestion of focal onset or signs then it is probably reasonable to perform an EEG and skull X-ray proceeding to a CT scan only if a focal abnormality is detected or if the management of the seizures proves difficult. Some authors suggest that all patients with epilepsy should be investigated with a CT scan but the yield of positive results in non-focal seizures is low and this ideal is not practicable in most hospitals. In cases of doubt as to the true nature of attacks, the newer techniques of EEG telemetry, video monitoring and 24-h EEG recording may be of considerable help.

Cardiovascular causes

The simple vasovagal attack or faint is usually identifiable from the history. There is a prodrome of light-headedness and swimming sensation in the head followed by a collapse from the standing position. The attack usually occurs when the patient is shocked or has been standing for some time in a warm environment often after taking a vasodilating agent such as alcohol. Sometimes a patient suffering a syncope may then go on to have an epileptic seizure raising problems in terms of diagnosis.

Micturition and cough syncope probably arise due to a Valsalva manoeuvre, the former usually being seen in someone who has recently arisen from a warm bed and is therefore likely to be vasodilated. They are usually relatively easy to diagnose though the problem of misdiagnosing such a loss of consciousness as epilepsy is not uncommon.

Cardiac causes of blackout are either due to obstruction to the outflow tracts, cardiac arrhythmias or pump failure. Obstruction to the outflow tract, most commonly seen with aortic stenosis or hypertrophic obstructive cardiomyopathy, should be diagnosed by clinical examination and confirmed by echocardiography. The problem of cardiac dysrhythmia may be difficult to identify but the technique of 24-h cardiac monitoring is a considerable help in this respect and both brady- and tachyarrhythmias can cause loss of consciousness. The possibility of a myocardial infarction resulting in pump failure should always be considered in the case of blackouts and is usually identifiable by performing an ECG.

Metabolic causes

Some metabolic problems such as renal or hepatic failure, anoxia and the exhibition or withdrawal of drugs may cause genuine epileptic seizures as part of their systemic disturbance. The underlying metabolic problem should be readily identifiable and such patients may of course still require conventional anticonvulsant therapy.

In children the possibility of hypoglycaemia or hypocalcaemia should always be excluded and in general hypoglycaemia, though uncommon, is a potentially dangerous cause of loss of consciousness which can easily be missed. The simple expedient of measuring the blood sugar in a patient who is unconscious should be one of the first estimations because once an intravenous line is established there is the risk of dextrose solutions being given and the chance of making the diagnosis may be lost.

Hysterical seizures

Although not common, seizures occurring in the hysterical patient or as a symptom of malingering do occur. Usually the circumstances in which the attack occurs provides a clue as to the diagnosis but whilst the classic hysterical patient may not be difficult to diagnose the patient with a few genuine seizures but many non-organic episodes grafted onto the underlying illness provides a particular problem. It is in this field that the EEG telemetry and 24-h EEG recording techniques are of most value. The identification of a normal EEG during an apparent seizure is the most important of all in excluding true epilepsy.

'Funny turns'

Episodes of abnormal feeling or behaviour occurring in a patient may reflect temporal lobe epilepsy or be due to posterior circulation vascular disturbance, psychiatric conditions and metabolic abnormalities. The diagnosis of such attacks is frequently difficult and it may be necessary to perform a therapeutic trial of anticonvulsant drugs in an attempt to establish whether or not there is a cerebral dysrhythmia to account for them.

Epilepsy and the law

With respect to driving, patients with seizures are ineligible to drive until they have had two years free from attacks or three years of only nocturnal episodes. The law is more stringent with heavy goods vehicle and passenger service vehicle licences in which a patient suffering a blackout after the age of five years is banned from ever holding such a licence.

Ideally, patients with epilepsy should not work in situations in which a blackout would cause danger to themselves or to others and they should inform their employers and thereby their employers' insurers of the problem.

There are few legal cases where the diagnosis of epilepsy is a successful defence from prosecution, one possible exception being in the case of shoplifting.

Status epilepticus

A fortunately rare but none the less frightening and potentially dangerous condition is status epilepticus when a patient either has continuous seizures or does not regain consciousness between episodes of frequent seizures. This may occur in a patient with previously diagnosed epilepsy when it may be precipitated by withdrawal, omission or overdose of therapy or by intercurrent events such as infection, trauma or systemic illness. It can also be the first manifestation of epilepsy when it may reflect an encephalitis, meningitis or a cerebral tumour, frequently frontal in site.

The management is first directed to the protection of the patient, the airway and circulation. Once this is achieved an attempt should be made to stop the seizures with intravenous therapy but as an intravenous site is established it is important to remember to withdraw blood for glucose and calcium estimations and possible other metabolic or drug evaluations. Most patients in status epilepticus will respond to intravenous benzodiazepine therapy with diazepam, lorazepam or clonazepam. If this is ineffective the use of an infusion of heminevrin should be used and if the seizures persist it is advisable to paralyse and ventilate the patient and control seizure activity with intravenous barbiturates or phenytoin. There is no place for the use of paraldehyde in the control of status epilepticus today.

Once the seizures are controlled background anticonvulsant therapy should be established or continued with intravenous phenytoin or oral carbamazepine or valproate. Investigations indicated once this resuscitation is achieved include formal haematological studies, metabolic investigations, EEG and possible CT scan and lumbar puncture.

Drop attacks

Sudden falls without loss of consciousness but resulting in trauma to the knees and face and usually occurring in the elderly are termed 'drop attacks'. The cause of them is unknown though they are probably not epileptic and may represent an episode of ischaemia in the posterior circulation. They do not usually persist for more than a few months or a year, occasionally respond to diazepam therapy and, provided that evident postural hypotension, posterior circulation ischaemia and basal ganglia disease are excluded they have a benign prognosis.

The narcolepsy syndrome

A rare tetrad of narcolepsy (inappropriate sleepiness), cataplexy (a collapse at times of emotion), sleep paralysis (a frightening syndrome of waking during the night and being completely paralysed) together with hypnogogic hallucinations (the feeling of there being something or someone just outside the field of vision as one drops off to sleep) is occasionally seen in the young adult. Narcolepsy itself is probably somewhat overdiagnosed but, in the true syndrome, responds to treatment with amphetamine, the sleep paralysis and hypnogogic hallucinations to imipramine and the cataplexy may be helped by anticonvulsant drugs.

4.6 STATES OF ALTERED CONSCIOUSNESS

Patients presenting with altered conscious levels may have diffuse or focal cerebral disease or a systemic abnormality which causes a degree of brain failure.

Confusion

Confusional states are most commonly seen in the elderly and are exemplified by those patients who appear awake and alert though often with disturbance of sleep pattern and who are disorientated in time, place and person. It is most commonly seen as the result of toxic conditions such as pneumonia or urinary tract infection in someone of advanced years who may also have a mild dementia. Characteristically such patients have a disturbance of memory and reasoning and management consists of the care of the patient often with adequate sedation and then the identification of the underlying abnormality be it cerebral as in stroke, meningitis, encephalitis or tumour or be it systemic as in the case of metabolic or infective conditions.

The differential diagnosis is of dementia which is usually of much slower onset and in which the history is diagnostic, and of dysphasia where the use of circumlocutions, paraphasias and neologisms, together with other evidence of focal dominant hemisphere disturbance, provides the most important clue.

Delirium

This is usually a subacute syndrome beginning with difficulty in concentration when it merges with confusion but evolving to cause irritability, tremor, insomnia and hallucinations. Patients often have a clouded mental state but remain physically restive and may even become aggressive. The syndrome is typified by the patient with delirium tremens following alcohol withdrawal and should always be considered in patients showing bizarre behaviour 2–3 days after being admitted to hospital. It may also occur in the presence of some fevers and with cerebrovascular disease in the elderly patient.

Both confusion and delirium are evidence of disturbed cerebral function and both may progress to stupor and coma.

Stupor

The patient who is drowsy but rousable and who will only respond to vigorous stimuli is said to be in stupor. This may reflect a diffuse organic pathology or be seen in the retarded depression of a psychiatric patient who will usually show catatonia—the maintenance of the limbs in any position into which they are put. Stupor may be seen as the early phase of coma but always suggests a diffuse rather than a focal cerebral pathology.

Coma

Since consciousness depends in part on the brainstem reticular-activating substance (the crude 'on-off switch') and in part on the cerebral cortex (the content of consciousness) it follows that focal structural disease in the brainstem or cerebral hemispheres may, by causing pressure, result in loss of consciousness and that diffuse disease as in anoxia, subarachnoid haemorrhage, metabolic abnormality or drug intoxication can all result in coma.

When faced with a comatose patient the physician should first protect the airway and circulation of the patient and then elicit a full and adequate history from others of the previous state and the onset of the coma. Following this the level of consciousness should be identified by reference to the

Glasgow Coma Scale testing verbal, eye opening and movement responses (*Table* 4.3). The examination of the brainstem reflexes and deep tendon reflexes follows in an attempt to identify the site of the lesion causing coma. In this way one should be able to identify coma without focal signs, suggesting the presence of a diffuse abnormality, coma with signs of hemispheric disturbance, suggesting a supratentorial mass lesion and resulting cerebral pressure cone and focal lesions within the posterior fossa resulting in brainstem pressure. A general examination may then show evidence of systemic infection, metabolic abnormality or drug intoxication.

Table 4.3 Glasgow coma scale

A. Eye opening	None	— 1
	Pain	— 2
	Voice	— 3
	Spontaneously	— 4
B. Motor	None	— 1
	Exterior	— 2
	Flexor	— 3
	Withdrawal	— 4
	Localizes	— 5
	Voluntary	— 6
C. Verbal	None	— 1
	Groans	— 2
	Inappropriate	— 3
	Confused	— 4
	Orientated	— 5

The progress of the conscious level of the patient as monitored by the Glasgow Coma Scale will make evident the need for continued support or investigation in that, if the patient is improving, no more than support is necessary but if the level of consciousness is deteriorating then a decision as to whether or not to investigate and then treat the abnormality revealed must be made. The types of investigation indicated range from routine haematological and biochemical studies through blood gas analysis to an EEG, CT scan and lumbar puncture.

The locked-in syndrome

A rare but important differential diagnosis of coma is seen in conditions causing damage to the ventral part of the pons. This most commonly occurs with vascular disturbance and in this condition the patient has no motor function other than the ability to blink and to move the eyes vertically. Despite this the sensorium is intact and it is imperative that the syndrome be recognized for the comfort and care of the patient. Most patients with the locked-in syndrome will die but occasional examples of recovery are recorded.

The vegetative state

Patients, typically after suffering an anoxic insult, may have diffuse cortical damage with an intact brainstem. They will then show spontaneous respiration and an active brainstem with roving eye movements and periods of sleepiness and wakefulness but without evidence of true cognition. This state may rarely show recovery after head injury but most medical causes of the persistent vegetative state carry a bad prognosis and yet the patient in a persistent vegetative state remains viable sometimes for many years.

Psychogenic coma

The apparent unresponsiveness of the hysteric or malingerer rarely causes problems in terms of differential diagnosis. Non-organic coma usually reveals itself by the bizarre circumstances surrounding its onset and can be identified by the simple expedient of performing the oculovestibular responses with ice cold water instilled into the external auditory meatus. In psychogenic coma this will result in nystagmus with the quick phase away from the stimulated ear.

Brain death

The identification of brainstem activity is the most important single feature in diagnosing brain death. Those vegetative functions including pulse, blood pressure, temperature and respiration together with corneal, pupillary and oculovestibular reflexes reveal the activity of the brainstem and hence the viability of the patient. If these reflexes are absent on two recordings approximately 24 h apart and provided that drug intoxication can be excluded, then brain death can be assumed to have occurred and support services may be withdrawn.

Dementia

Dementia implies a loss of intellectual faculties and tends to occur over a period of months or years. It may be suspected from the history and be confirmed by simple bedside psychometry including the testing of the orientation of the patients, their ability to calculate, their general knowledge and awareness of current events, their long and short term memory and their ability to handle conceptual thought. It may be formally analysed by psychometry and on occasion more than one examination may be needed to confirm the progressing nature of the problem. It must be differentiated from the retardation seen in some psychiatric syndromes particularly in depression which can give rise to a picture of 'pseudodementia'.

Senile and presenile dementia

These two syndromes are included together since there is increasing pathological evidence that they represent the same phenomenon and the distinction is merely an arbitrary one based on the age of the patient. By far the most patients showing this form of dementia have Alzheimer's disease with neuronal loss, neurofibrillary tangles and plaques demonstrated pathologically.

Such patients tend to present with a history of deterioration in memory initially and most profoundly for recent events and then later with the problems of dementia becoming more apparent to themselves and more particularly to their family and friends. Ultimately the patient with a dementia will become unable to be independent, untidy and careless with personal appearance and finally incontinent. Many patients will require institutional care at some time in their illness and, since the prognosis is so poor, reasonable investigation is indicated, certainly in the presenile group, to exclude the possibility of any other and more treatable conditions. The investigations indicated would include formal psychometry to establish the nature of the dementia, the assessment of vitamin B_{12} and folate, thyroid function and WR to exclude other causes, an EEG to exclude seizures, and then a CT scan to reveal the presence of cortical atrophy followed by lumbar puncture to exclude the unlikely possibility of a chronic meningitis.

There is no reasonable treatment for this condition though from time to time empirical therapy with high dose vitamin B_{12} and, more recently, choline chloride has been advocated. There is no evidence that the widely advertised preparations to improve cerebral blood flow have any effect on the outcome of this condition.

Vascular dementia

The diagnosis of 'hardening of the arteries' which was so common some years ago is now recognized to be an extremely unusual cause of dementia. Patients with hypertensive vascular disease do occasionally show a dementia due to multiple lacunes throughout the hemispheres but the diagnosis is usually revealed by a history from the patient's relatives of episodes of minor motor paralysis, speech disturbance or other focal neurological problems occurring over a period of years. CT scan on such patients may reveal multiple areas of low density throughout the hemispheres.

Other causes of dementia

It is imperative that more treatable forms of dementia be excluded before this terminal prognosis be made and, as has been intimated above, the most important of these include vitamin B_{12} deficiency, hypothyroidism and neurosyphilis. Occasionally patients with a chronic meningitis may present with dementia and even more rarely arteritis may present a similar picture. It is naturally important to exclude metabolic causes such as hypocalcaemia. intermittent hypoglycaemia, particularly in the elderly, and disturbances of electrolytes as in the inappropriate secretion of ADH.

One of the indications for performing a CT scan in patients with dementia is to exclude the unlikely possibility of a frontal or subfrontal lobe tumour in these patients and also to identify the possibility of a communicating hydrocephalus.

Normal pressure hydrocephalus

A rare condition which may arise spontaneously but which has been recorded after head injury, meningitis or subarachnoid haemorrhage is the development of ventricular dilatation without cortical atrophy and the presentation with a form of dementia. This particular syndrome tends to cause an apraxia of gait together with bladder disturbance and some patients have been recorded as responding well to the insertion of a ventriculo-peritoneal shunt.

Wernicke-Korsakoff syndrome

The presentation of a bizarre dementia with specific memory disturbance and confabulation often seen together with eye movement disturbances should always raise the possibility of a vitamin B_1 deficiency seen particularly in alcoholic patients but also in those with persistent vomiting or oesophageal obstruction. This syndrome responds well in a high proportion of cases to treatment with thiamine though a proportion of patients will remain demented and show no significant response.

4.7 DISTURBANCES OF SPEECH

Disturbances of speech and communication may occur with any condition causing diffuse cerebral damage resulting in confusion and delirium. It may also be seen as a more focal problem in some patients with dementia. Conversely, patients with focal lesions resulting in communication problems can sometimes be misdiagnosed as suffering from confusion or dementia but it should normally be possible to identify the genuine speech disturbances and to determine whether the problem lies posteriorly or anteriorly in the dominant hemisphere. It is also important to differentiate between those problems with speech which are due to hemispheric and usually cortical disease, namely the dysphasias, those which are due to problems with articulation, the dysarthrias, and those which relate to difficulties with phonation, the dysphonias.

Dysphasia

Disturbances of speech and language arising in the subcortical or cortical areas of the dominant hemisphere are termed dysphasia. The patient may be able to define the problem as knowing what they want to say but being unable to find the word. The medical clues as to the presence of dysphasia are the use by the patient of paraphasias of similar sound, as in using the word bread for head (phonemic) or of similar meaning as in using the word clock for watch (semantic) and circumlocution in which a patient may describe a pen as an 'object to write with' and neologisms when new words without meaning are coined.

The physician should make the attempt to identify and distinguish those patients with damage to the temporoparietal region of the dominant hemisphere who will have relatively fluent speech but with marked comprehension difficulties, the so-called sensory or receptive dysphasia from those patients who have great difficulty in saying words but have good comprehension, the so-called non-fluent, anterior or expressive dysphasia. The former is exemplified by the Wernicke dysphasia with a lesion in the temporal lobe and the latter by the Broca dysphasia where the lesion is frontal. The methods of testing such patients include asking the patient to identify objects and thereby checking their ability to name, having the patient repeat certain phrases or sentences and estimating their repetition, ordering the patient to perform simple tasks of gradually increasing complexity thereby testing comprehension and finally listening to the patient to evaluate their production of speech.

Once aphasia is identified the investigations to determine its cause comprise predominantly a CT scan and once the cause is established speech therapy may be offered in an attempt to improve the problem.

Dysarthria

Disturbances of articulation arise due to damage to the upper or lower motor neurones subserving speech, their cerebellar connections or the basal ganglia. The VIIth, Xth and XIIth cranial nerve nuclei are the ones involved in speech and are bilaterally innervated. Thus a single lesion in the hemisphere or internal capsule does not characteristically result in dysarthia.

Spastic dysarthria

Bilateral upper motor neurone lesions affecting the bulbar nuclei cause a spastic dysarthria usually associated with a spastic dysphonia. The problem may be seen in children with cerebral palsy and may occur in adults with multiple strokes, multiple sclerosis or motor neurone disease. The condition is part of the pseudobulbar palsy and may be associated with difficulties with swallowing and also with emotional lability.

Flaccid dysarthria

Damage to the lower motor neurones of the bulb results in a flaccid dysarthria and may be seen with lesions affecting the nuclei, cranial nerves, neuromuscular junction or muscle. Poliomyelitis and motor neurone disease are examples of conditions affecting the nuclei, diphtheria or post-infective neuropathies examples of nerve lesions and myasthenia gravis causing its typical fatiguing flaccid dysarthria, the most classic example of a neuromuscular junction abnormality. Although polymyositis may rarely cause a flaccid dysarthria due to muscle involvement such muscle disease is more commonly seen in oculopharyngeal dystrophy.

The flaccid dysarthria is also termed true bulbar palsy and in the case of motor neurone disease sometimes referred to as progressive bulbar palsy.

Cerebellar dysarthria

Lesions affecting the cerebellar connections of the bulbar nuclei may result in the characteristic slurring and stuttering ataxia dysarthria. This is perhaps most commonly seen in patients with multiple sclerosis though it may also occur in the cerebellar degenerations and after acute or chronic alcohol intoxication.

Extrapyramidal dysarthria

This comprises basal ganglia disease, classically Parkinson's disease, causes a monotonous and slow speech marked by akinesia and bradykinesia of the bulbar muscles.

Dysphonia

Most patients with dysphonia have a local laryngeal cause but the possibility of neurogenic dysphonia as seen in association with a spastic dysarthria or with lesions of the recurrent laryngeal nerve should not be forgotten. Patients who develop dysphonia after a unilateral recurrent laryngeal nerve lesion may appear to recover simply due to compensation by the other cord. A history of dysphonia should therefore be followed by the investigation of indirect laryngoscopy.

Dysphagia

Dysphagia is most commonly due to local problems in the pharynx or oesophagus but it can be one of the earliest symptoms of neurological disturbance. Classically dysphagia due to structural disease is worse with solids whilst that due to neurological disease is most apparent when attempting to swallow fluids. Such dysphagia may be seen in motor neurone disease, the myopathies and myasthenia gravis as well as in patients with a pseudobulbar palsy.

4.8 DISTURBANCES OF VISION

Disturbance or loss of vision is a dramatic and frightening symptom if it occurs acutely and yet may be almost unnoticed by the patient if the onset is sufficiently gradual. The speed of onset of visual loss and its pattern, be it monocular, binocular, homonymous or total, gives a clue as to the site of the abnormality. The formal assessment of vision in the patient includes determining the visual acuity with correction in each eye, establishing the size of the visual field followed by fundoscopy and assessment of conjugate and individual eye movements.

Monocular visual loss

The disturbance or loss of vision in a single eye identifies the lesion as lying anterior to the optic chiasm and may be due to abnormalities in the lens, aqueous or vitreous humours, retina or optic nerve. Slowly progressive visual failure raises the possibility of developing cataract, retinal or macular degeneration or glaucoma but it may indicate pressure on or growth in the optic nerve. Once ocular causes are excluded it is imperative that the optic nerve and chiasm be investigated possibly by visual-evoked responses and certainly by a CT scan through the orbit and anterior cranial fossa. Skull X-ray is relevant to show the presence of an abnormal pituitary fossa or calcification above the fossa and occasionally angiography or venography is necessary to identify the presence of a meningioma or a vascular lesion.

Acute visual loss in the eye may be due to ocular causes such as acute glaucoma but is more commonly the result of vascular or demyelinating lesions affecting the optic nerve or retina. The classic syndrome of amaurosis fugax with a shutter-like loss of vision in an eye presumed due to emboli from the carotid artery blocking the retinal circulation is transient, usually lasts for less than an hour and, though occasionally due to a migrainous vascular spasm, is more frequently indicative of atherosclerotic vascular disease. Subacute visual loss in a single eye often associated with pain on movement of the globe strongly suggests the possibility of retrobulbar neuritis and, though fundoscopy may be normal, the presence of a swollen optic nerve head is not uncommon which, when associated with visual loss, is indicative of papillitis rather than papilloedema.

Binocular visual loss

Disturbed vision in both eyes suggests the presence of a lesion at or behind the optic chiasm. Thus a bitemporal field defect suggests damage to the crossing fibres of the optic chiasm and may indicate the presence of a pituitary tumour, classically with the field defect beginning in the upper temporal quadrant and an abnormal pituitary fossa on skull X-ray, or a craniopharyngioma classically with the field cut beginning in the lower temporal quadrants and associated with the presence of calcification above the pituitary fossa on skull X-ray. Both of these lesions may be associated with endocrine defects.

Homonymous defects suggest a lesion in the optic tract or radiation, the former tending to cause hemianopia and the latter a quadrantanopia which, if inferior, suggests a lesion in the contralateral parietal lobe and, if superior, in the contralateral temporal lobe. Horizontal field defects occasionally occur and they indicate problems in the occipital cortex. Some clue as to the nature of the lesion causing the visual disturbance may be gleaned from formal charting of the visual fields on a Bjerrum screen by which a sharp edge suggests a vascular cause and a sloping edge a compressive lesion such as a tumour. In some patients though there may be no true visual field loss, inattention can be demonstrated by bilateral stimulation and this strongly suggests a parietal lobe lesion.

Bilateral total blindness is most commonly seen with cortical damage in the occipital region and may be associated with intact pupillary responses and even with denial of blindness by the patient in the so-called Anton's syndrome. Such problems most commonly occur with vascular lesions—frequently infarction in the posterior territory.

Most of the above discussion has related to patterns of visual loss but lesions at similar sites which are irritative in nature may cause positive visual phenomena such as flashes of light, stars and other similar phenomena which are most usually vascular in aetiology.

Double vision

The common symptom of double vision arises when the eyes are no longer maintained in their parallel axes. It may occur with local problems in the orbit, ocular muscle disease, problems affecting the neuromuscular junction, the nerves subserving ocular movement or in the brainstem. The cause is assessed by examination of the eye movement and by looking for evidence of proptosis or a skew deviation. Eye movements are formally tested both with respect to conjugate eye movements and also individual eye muscle movements.

Orbital disease

Structural orbital disease causing diplopia will usually be evident by the presence of a non-axial proptosis. Causes include tumour, primary or secondary, within the orbit, mucocele from frontal or ethmoidal air sinuses or from the antrum, dysthyroid eye disease and pseudo-tumour of the orbit. Pain is frequently present and the investigation of choice is a CT scan through the orbit.

Muscle disease

There are relatively few true muscle diseases which will affect eye movement. They are the oculopharyngeal dystrophies and the syndrome of ophthalmoplegia plus. The evidence of muscle disease is usually provided by an unusual distribution of external ophthalmoplegia, sparing of the pupillo-constrictor and pupillo-dilator muscles and the associated features of pharyngeal or facial weakness or, in the case of ophthalmoplegia plus, an atypical retinitis pigmentosa and other central nervous system signs.

Neuromuscular junction disease

The cardinal feature of diplopia due to disturbance of neuromuscular junction is that of fatigue. Ptosis and double vision may be absent or minimal in the morning and will develop increasingly through the day. The response to Tensilon is diagnostic of myasthenia gravis which condition may be confirmed by single-fibre EMG and the assessment of acetylcholine receptor antibodies. Both of these tests are, however, less helpful in the condition of ocular myasthenia than they are in generalized disease. Therapy may be symptomatic with pyridostigmine but the physician may need to revert to treatment with steroids, cytotoxics and thymectomy.

Nerve disease

In identifying the cause of diplopia due to damage or disease of the oculomotor, trochlear and abducens nerve it is necessary to test individual eye muscles in six positions (*Fig.* 4.9). The use of the cover test and identification of the distal or false image enables the physician to identify which muscle is paralysed in each direction of movement. In this way lesions

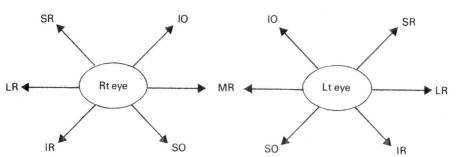

Fig. 4.9. Individual eye muscle movements. SR, superior rectus; LR, lateral rectus; IR, inferior rectus; MR, medial rectus; SO, superior oblique; IO, inferior oblique.

affecting the lateral rectus muscle can be attributed to disease of the VIth cranial nerve, the superior oblique to disease of the trochlear nerve and other eye muscle disturbances including those of pupillo-constriction due to damage to the IIIrd nerve.

Any of the three nerves may be damaged by lesions in the orbit, superior orbital fissure or anterior fossa, including the cavernous sinus. The IIIrd nerve is commonly damaged by a posterior communicating artery aneurysm and all three may be individually damaged by vascular lesions in the nerve trunk or nucleus in diabetes and hypertension. If the IIIrd nerve is damaged by pressure either due to an aneurysm or to a tentorial cone then the parasympathetic nerves arranged circumferentially around the IIIrd nerve are involved and the pupil will be fixed and dilated. In intrinsic or vascular lesions the parasympathetic supply may be specifically spared. Isolated

IVth nerve palsies are almost invariably vascular in nature and the VIth nerve is commonly involved in any intracranial mass lesion.

The precise nature of the lesion affecting the nerves involved in the eye movement may be determined by CT scan or angiography and CSF examination may be necessary to exclude the possibility of a basal meningitis.

Brainstem disease

Lesions in the brainstem may cause diplopia and frequently result in other abnormalities including nystagmus, other cranial nerve disturbance or evidence of long tract disease. Diplopia may be revealed as being intrinsic in origin by the presence of a skew deviation, the association of conjugate gaze palsies and problems with convergence. Most brainstem lesions are either vascular or demyelinating in origin though such ophthalmoplegias may be seen with brainstem gliomas and with rare postinfective demyelinating condition described by Miller Fisher and associated with areflexia and ataxia.

Conjugate gaze palsies

An eye movement disturbance without diplopia is seen in patients who are not able to look voluntarily in one or more directions. A horizontal gaze palsy is seen in hemisphere disease like stroke and may also occur in degenerative conditions such as progressive supranuclear palsy though in this condition and in Parkinson's disease vertical eye movements are more commonly affected. A tumour at the level of the quadrigeminal plate such as a pinealoma will cause failure of upgaze and may be associated with papilloedema in Parinaud's syndrome.

4.9 DIZZINESS AND DEAFNESS

One of the most difficult of all symptoms to evaluate is that of dizziness. The term may be used by the patient to describe a feeling of mild light-headedness which is rarely associated with a significant neurological cause, or to describe true rotational vertigo which is usually highly significant. Problems with both dizziness and deafness are most commonly due to endorgan disease and may need to be formally assessed by otolaryngeal investigations such as audiometry, caloric and tipping tests and examination of the external auditory meatus and drum.

Dizziness

The most important function to the physician in identifying the cause of disease is to help the patient to accurately identify the precise nature of the symptoms. Thus if patients are truly describing light-headedness then, although the cause may be either peripheral in the labyrinth or central in the brainstem, it is unlikely that a significant neurological cause will be found and it is usually assumed that such symptoms either reflect a minor posterior circulation disturbances or merely related to anxiety, tenseness or depression. If the patient is in fact describing a symptom of unsteadiness then, although again examination of the vestibular labyrinthine system is indicated, the cause is more likely to be visual, cerebellar or peripheral due to lack of proprioception in the limbs. When the patient is genuinely dizzy and especially if vertigo is described there is usually an organic cause which may be peripheral as in Ménière's disease or intermittent and postural as in benign positional vertigo or acute labyrinthitis. The association of deafness together with vertigo strongly suggests disease of the endorgan or auditory nerve, as in acoustic neuroma, when tinnitus is also a prominent symptom. Central or brainstem causes of dizziness and vertigo implies damage to the vestibular nuclei or their connections and is frequently associated with nystagmus and other signs of brainstem dysfunction.

Nystagmus of either horizontal phasic or rotatory type may be seen both with lesions of the peripheral labyrinth and with those affecting the brainstem. Vertical nystagmus is usually indicative of brainstem disease and the presence of significant nystagmus without the symptom of dizziness is invariably associated with central causes.

The side and site of the cause of the dizziness is usually detectable from the history, associated symptoms and signs but may require formal otological examination, including audiology and electronystagmography. The use of brainstem-evoked potentials is increasingly helpful in distinguishing between lesions of the nerve and stem, and electrocochleography and recruitment studies help differentiate stem disease from peripheral labyrinthine problems. In clinical testing of a patient with positional vertigo, one of the most useful tests is to tip the patient with the head turned towards the affected side. Observations are then made of the onset of dizziness and of any evident nystagmus. If vertigo and nystagmus occur immediately the tipping posture is adopted, and persist, then the disease is likely to be central in the brainstem but if the symptoms only begin after a few seconds and then fatigue follows and are not reproducible then the probability is that the lesion is peripheral.

The treatment of dizziness depends upon the underlying cause and it can be one of the most intractable of all symptoms. Symptomatically many patients will respond to treatment with Stemetil, Stugeron or Serc though others may respond to anxiolytics, antidepressants and even firm reassurance.

Deafness

Progressing deafness on one or both sides is usually a feature of otosclerosis, chronic middle ear infection or noise trauma. Acute loss of hearing, whilst occasionally due to middle ear disease including dislocation of the ossicle, is more commonly the result of an ischaemic lesion affecting the auditory nerve.

The simple clinical tests of Weber and Rinne enable a distinction to be made between conductive and sensory neural deafness and this may be reinforced by formal audiology and electrocochleography.

When nerve deafness occurs progressively the commonest cause is noise trauma but it is important to exclude compressive or granulomatous lesions affecting the auditory nerve. Usually mass lesions lying in the cerebello-pontine angle will also cause some involvement of the VIIth and Vth cranial nerves and acoustic neuroma is usually evident not only by the symptoms of deafness but also by that of persisting tinnitus.

The more acute forms of sensory neural hearing loss are usually vascular in aetiology though the possibility of congenital syphilis needs to be remembered as does that of exposure to certain ototoxic drugs in the course of treatment of intercurrent infections.

The investigation of the symptoms of dizziness and deafness is essentially directed towards the posterior fossa. The techniques already referred to of otolaryngology examination may well help to locate the site of the lesion but if the possibility of a cerebellopontine angle tumour, basal meningitis or a brainstem lesion exists then a CT scan is indicated followed most ideally by air meatography in which CSF is obtained for examination and air is introduced into the lumbar theca and allowed to flow into the cerebello-pontine angle. This technique is occasionally replaced by the use of contrast media cysternography and the whole may need to be followed by posterior circulation angiography. The techniques of brainstem-evoked responses are still undergoing assessment and modification but promise to be enormously useful in helping to detect the site of the lesion and therefore direct the type of investigations used.

4.10   SPECIFIC NEUROLOGICAL PROBLEMS

Cerebrovascular disease

Cerebrovascular disease is one of the·commonest causes of death and disability in the western world, ranking behind only myocardial infarction and neoplasm as a cause of death. The incidence of stroke is 200 per 100 000 per year and one-half of patients suffering strokes die in the original attack. The others suffer varying degrees of morbidity. The causes of cerebro-vascular disease may be reasonably considered under four major headings.

Embolic disease

Cerebral emboli are of varying size and origin. The most common site is probably from atheroma in the aorta, carotid and vertebral arteries. The emboli consist of debris from atheromatous plaques or small platelet-fibrin clots which are released into the circulation and cause occlusion of more peripheral vessels in the territory of the anterior, middle or posterior cerebral vessels or the basilar artery. Such emboli may be large enough to cause a stroke or more commonly cause a transient and completely reversible neurological deficit which, provided there is complete recovery within 24 hours, is designated a transient ischaemic attack (TIA). Patients suffering TIAs have a significantly increased risk of stroke of the order of 5% per year and their real importance lies not in the TIAs themselves but rather in the fact that they are warnings of potentially more serious cerebrovascular disease.

The cardinal features of emboli in the anterior (internal carotid) circulation are transient monocular blindness (amaurosis fugax), hemiplegia or hemianaesthesia and dysphasia. In the posterior circulation the symptoms are those of disturbances of vision in both eyes, dizziness, diplopia, dysarthria, dysphagia and motor or sensory symptoms in both hands or both legs. Posterior circulation disturbances involving the medial aspects of the temporal lobes may cause the syndrome of transient global amnesia in which the patient abruptly and usually transiently loses all access to memory.

Once TIAs are recognized, the cause should be sought and systemic problems such as anaemia, hypoglycaemia, hypertension, diabetes mellitus, syphilis and polycythaemia should be excluded. A neurovascular examination which includes assessment not only of the pulse and blood pressure and auscultation of the heart but also auscultation of the great vessels of the neck may then reveal the presence of a cardiac problem such as mitral or aortic valve disease, a prolapsing mitral valve or a cardiac dysrhythmia. Alternatively, there may be evidence of arterial disease revealed by the finding of bruits over the carotid arteries, subclavian vessels or orbits. A high ESR may suggest the presence of an atrial myxoma or of a generalized arteritis.

When the site of origin of the emboli has been determined further investigation is indicated and in the case of cardiac abnormalities two-dimensional echocardiography is the investigation of choice. In patients with arterial disease of the great vessels in the neck angiography may be indicated. It is, however, important to recognize that the procedure of angiography carries a risk to the patient and the new technique of digital vascular imaging may come to replace angiography. It should be obvious that angiography need only be considered for a patient in whom the possibility of surgical intervention is extant. At present the therapy indicated for TIAs remains questionable. The use of anticoagulation is established in heart valve and dysrhythmic causes and in the short term appears to reduce the risk of further TIA and stroke in patients with arterial disease. Longer term treatment with anticoagulation carries considerable risks to the patient and, except for those episodes arising in the posterior circulation, appears to have little benefit. The use of anti-platelet agents is advocated by many physicians and there has been a general agreement that acetylsalicylic acid is the most effective agent though this, too, is not without complications and further evaluation is necessary before it can be widely advocated.

The operations of carotid endarterectomy or vascular reconstruction are widely practised in certain countries for extracranial cerebrovascular disease but there remains considerable doubt as to their efficacy in reducing the risk of stroke. Perhaps the most important feature of TIAs is that, in general, they are indicative of a systemic vascular abnormality and, though patients with TIAs have an increased risk of stroke, they also have an increased risk of death from myocardial infarction.

Occasionally an embolus either from the left heart or a paradoxical embolus from the venous circulation may cause a completed stroke. The dilemma facing the physician then is that to use anticoagulation in an attempt to reduce the risk of further emboli carries the risk of potentially turning the original infarct into an haemorrhagic lesion and worsening state of the patient. In general, however, there is little doubt that long-term anticoagulation for emboli arising in the heart is the correct form of management.

Thrombotic

The majority of completed strokes are thrombotic in nature and arise due to the occlusion of a cerebral or extracranial vessel as the end result of atherosclerotic narrowing of the vessel. Such atheroma may be accelerated and made more extensive by associated disease such as diabetes or hypertension. Classically the thrombotic stroke will occur at times of relatively low cerebral blood flow and thus tends to occur during the night and is of course most common in the elderly patient. The stroke usually causes hemiplegia, hemianaesthesia and hemianopia together with, in dominant hemisphere lesions, aphasia. Strokes in the posterior circulation will of course cause disturbances of balance, dysarthria, dysphagia and diplopia and, if the dorsal brainstem is involved, may involve altered consciousness.

A completed stroke is defined as a neurological deficit due to a vascular cause lasting for more than 24 h. Some minor episodes may show considerable recovery within a few days or weeks but the more typical pattern is of a deterioration during the 48–72 h period after the stroke due to the development of cerebral oedema around the infarct followed by a 7–10-day period in which the patient is at risk of pneumonia, renal tract infection, deep vein thrombosis or bed sores. As previously mentioned, approximately half of all patients suffering stroke will die as a result of the insult. Death within the first few days is either due to extension of the original lesion or to the development of ischaemic cerebral oedema. At present there is no evidence that any form of medical therapy significantly affects the development of this potentially devastating complication. Though the use of steroids and low molecular weight dextran has been advocated, there is no evidence that it has any significant effect and whilst one might expect dehydration with diuretics and mannitol to reduce the amount of cerebral oedema, most patients admitted with cerebral thrombosis are already dehydrated and the risk of causing prerenal uraemia these usually elderly patients is considerable. Once the initial risk period is over, adequate nursing and physiotherapy together with the judicious use of antibiotics should prevent the secondary risks of infection, deep vein thrombosis and pressure sores.

In those patients who recover from thrombotic stroke, the majority will make their major improvement during the first 3 months and in this time physiotherapy, occupational therapy and speech therapy has the most to offer. There is no evidence that anticoagulation has any benefit in completed stroke and the physician's main role is to identify and correct problems which may have caused the initial insult and to help reduce resulting symptoms of spasticity and pain which may occur as a result of the stroke. The recent suggestion that revascularization in completed stroke may help recovery has no factual support at present.

Occasionally patients are seen in whom the stroke is still evolving. In this situation it is important to ensure that the lesion is due to thrombosis rather than haemorrhage and a CT scan and lumbar puncture may be helpful. If there is no evidence of haemorrhage then the use of anticoagulation with heparin may help to reverse the 'progressing stroke' and heparin should be continued for 7–10-day period followed by several months' treatment with oral anticoagulants.

Most thrombotic strokes are due to thrombosis in the arterial side of the circulation. A different syndrome occurs in patients who are dehydrated, who have local intracranial sepsis or who have general inanition in whom the possibility of venous sinus thrombosis needs to be considered. Thrombosis of a venous sinus is associated with intense headache, usually seizures and commonly the finding of bloodstained CSF at lumbar puncture. Venous infarcts are commonly haemorrhagic and, though the risks are not inconsiderable, the use of anticoagulation appears to give the most hope of improvement and recovery.

Haemorrhage

Intracranial bleeding may occur at several different sites within the head and each may result in a syndrome of stroke:

PARENCHYMAL

Bleeding into the parenchyma of the brain is almost confined to those patients with hypertension, a blood vessel malformation or a bleeding diathesis. The classic site for hypertensive parenchymal cerebral haemorrhage is from the small perforating arteries of the middle cerebral vessel. The stroke is usually abrupt, often occurring in the awake patient and usually associated with headache and occasionally loss of consciousness. The site of such haemorrhage may be demonstrated by CT scan and factors such as the age of the patient, the severity of the stroke and the site of the haemorrhage indicate whether or not angiography is indicated to show a potential arteriovenous malformation or berry aneurysm. Most patients with cerebral parenchymal haematoma may be managed conservatively and in those in whom the condition deteriorates sufficiently to warrant neurosurgical evacuation of the clot the prognosis is usually poor. If the patient survives the ictus the resorption of the haemorrhage occurs spontaneously and the advent of CT scan has enabled visualization of the considerable resorption and recovery that can occur. The greatest risk to the patient is of further bleeding or of the development of cerebral oedema and there is little evidence that any therapy other than the control of the blood pressure helps in this respect. Paradoxically over-zealous reduction in the blood pressure may actually cause a degree of relative cerebral ischaemia and make oedema worse.

SUBARACHNOID

The syndrome of subarachnoid haemorrhage has been discussed already and occurs when rupture of a berry aneurysm on the circle of Willis or an arteriovenous malformation releases blood into the subarachnoid space. The onset is usually dramatic with severe headache rapidly followed by occipital headache and occasionally coma. The cardinal features are the dramatic history, the finding of neck stiffness and a positive Kernig's test and the occurrence of subhyaloid haemorrhages on fundoscopy. Lumbar puncture will show bloodstained CSF which should always be centrifuged to demonstrate the presence of xanthochromia and to differentiate between true subarachnoid bleeding and a traumatic lumbar puncture. A CT scan may show the presence of subarachnoid blood and can even indicate the site of the bleed.

The investigation of choice is angiography but this should only be considered when the patient is fit for surgery. The presence of coma, confusion or a fixed deficit are relative contraindications to surgery since they usually indicate the presence of a degree of vasospasm. Some 25% of patients suffering subarachnoid haemorrhage will die of the original bleed and a large proportion of these patients do not even reach hospital. The true emergency is the apparently fit and healthy young adult with severe headache and signs suggestive of subarachnoid haemorrhage but without lowering of conscious level or focal deficit. The reason for the urgency is the recognized fact that 25% of patients will re-bleed between the seventh and tenth days after the initial ictus. Surgery is of dubious help in patients over the age of 65 years. Prior to undergoing surgery, which should be performed as early as possible, or in those patients who are to be treated medically the important points are to maintain the patient quiet and sedated and with an adequately controlled blood pressure. Most berry aneurysms are now accessible to surgery but many arteriovenous malformations because of their size or site remain unapproachable. The techniques of embolization by catheter under neuroradiological control may then be considered.

SUBDURAL

Classically after head injury but occasionally apparently spontaneously, patients may suffer deterioration in conscious level together with focal neurological signs both of which may fluctuate. The possibility of subdural haematoma then exists and is seen most commonly in the elderly and in alcoholics. Subdural haematomas arise from venous bleeding from the sinuses and classically cause their effects as a local space-occupying lesion. Once identified by CT scan they may be evacuated either by burr holes or by formal craniotomy with more complete removal. It should be remembered that not all subdural haematomas are symptomatic and therefore not all require surgical treatment.

EXTRADURAL

Skull fractures arising in the temporal region may damage the middle meningeal artery and result in the rapid accumulation of extradural blood. This is most commonly seen in children after relatively minor head injuries and is a neurosurgical emergency. The child's condition may deteriorate very rapidly and once the lesion is recognized surgical evacuation is obligatory.

Vasospasm

Cerebral vasospasm may occasionally be so severe and prolonged as to cause a cerebral infarction. This may be seen in patients with migraine in whom a completed stroke can occur and the recent evidence that patients having suffered migraine over many years may have evidence for cerebral atrophy on CT scan suggests that small cerebral infarcts may not be uncommon in the context of migraine.

Cerebral vasospasm is also believed to be the cause of focal deficits in the condition of hypertensive encephalopathy. Such patients, usually with accelerated hypertension, may present with headaches, confusion, focal neurological deficit and epileptic seizures. It is imperative that the hypertension be rapidly controlled and, though patients may make a complete recovery from this condition, permanent neurological deficits can also arise.

One other syndrome arising in this context of hypertension is that of lacunar strokes where small vascular lesions commonly arising in the perforating arteries are seen in association with Charcot–Bouchard aneurysms. Clinical syndromes produced by such minor strokes include the clumsy hand-dysarthria syndrome and pure motor hemiplegia and frequently such episodes can eventually result in the syndrome of the *état lacunaire* in which patients have basal ganglia disturbance, dementia and pyramidal signs or develop pseudobulbar palsy. The history of multiple episodes of minor stroke can usually be obtained from relatives of the patient.

Multiple sclerosis

In the western world multiple sclerosis occurs with an incidence of approximately 5 per 100000 per year and since the life expectancy is in excess of 20 years the prevalence of the disease is approximately 100 per 100000 in the population of the United Kingdom. Females are affected more commonly than males in the ratio of 1·7 : 1 and the commonest age of onset of the disease is between the 25th and 35th year of life. Multiple sclerosis characteristically has an acute relapsing and remitting course but, particularly in patients developing the disease later in life, may have a chronic progressive pattern. The lesions or plaques of demyelination occur scattered throughout the white matter of the nervous system and the symptoms which they generate depend upon the site of the lesion.

One of the most common sites is in the optic nerve when the syndrome of pain on movement of the eye, visual blurring or blindness arising over several days and lasting for weeks is characteristic of retrobulbar neuritis. Lesions arising in the spinal cord may cause either sensory or motor symptoms or disturbance of bladder function. The site at which the cord is affected will determine whether the symptoms are those of monoplegia, hemiplegia or quadriplegia and whether sensory symptoms are dissociate and which limb is affected. Lesions arising in the brainstem will tend to cause ataxia, diplopia, dysarthria and lesions in the hemispheres may cause disturbances of memory and dementia and rarely the symptoms of epilepsy.

The diagnosis of multiple sclerosis depends essentially upon the history of neurological disturbances scattered in time and place and confirmed by the examination. Cerebrospinal fluid examination will reveal a pleocytosis in a proportion of patients and an elevated level of gammaglobulin particularly of oligoclonal types in a further group of patients. Electrophysiological techniques such as visual evoked responses, brainstem-evoked responses and sensory-evoked responses may help to delineate the presence of scattered lesions throughout the neuraxis but there remains no absolute test for multiple sclerosis.

The cause of the disease is not known and there is to date no preventive or curative therapy. In acute attacks patients may be helped by the exhibition of steroids, particularly adrenocorticotrophic hormone which is usually given for a short course of approximately 4 weeks. Other steroids have been used and sometimes patients benefit from the prolonged alternate-day use of prednisone. Immunosuppressive agents are variously described as helping patients with multiple sclerosis and controlled studies of such treatment are presently being undertaken.

Symptomatic therapy is important in the management of the patient with multiple sclerosis. Spasticity is a common feature and may be helped by spasmolytics, pain can occur due either to spasticity, joint disease or to plaques arising in the sensory pathways and may be helped by analgesics, tricyclic agents or carbamazepine. Bladder symptoms are not uncommon and may respond to relaxant therapies but may require catheterization. Care of bowel and skin is also of importance. Physiotherapy, the provision of adequate aids and rehabilitation are amongst the most important points in management for the patient with multiple sclerosis.

Although multiple sclerosis is usually regarded as a disabling disease there is evidence that many patients do not become significantly disabled and there are recognized benign forms of it. The very variability of the illness creates difficulties for the physician in giving an accurate prognosis to patients and relatives and there is no simple rule as to how, what or when to tell the patient the likely diagnosis. It is imperative that this sort of decision be tailor-made for individual patients and depends upon many factors including the certainty of the diagnosis in the individual patient, the patient's particular circumtances and the relationship between the physician and the patient.

Evolving paraparesis

Though the syndrome of progressing weakness of both lower limbs has been dealt with in the section on movement disorders, the importance of progressing lower limb weakness with or without spinal pain together with the findings of a spastic paraparesis, sensory disturbance with a sensory level and evolving bladder and bowel disturbance is one of the true neurological emergencies. The dangers which can follow delay in diagnosing a progressing spinal lesion are such that whenever a paraparesis is suspected formal examination and consideration of the investigation are obligatory. It is advisable to remember that the finding of a paraparesis essentially excludes lesions in the lumbar spine and, though so frequently in this condition the lumbar spine is X-rayed, it is obvious that the most important parts of the spine to X-ray are the dorsal and cervical spine. If a spine lesion such as a collapse or metastatic deposit is revealed then no further investigation may be required and it might be adequate to treat the patient with local radiotherapy. However, the potential benefit from decompressing such a lesion is considerable and consideration should therefore always be given to myelography and surgery. If no lesion is detected on plain X-ray then it is important to proceed to a myelogram to identify the presence and site of any compressive spinal lesion.

Guillain–Barré syndrome

Although an uncommon neurological disorder, the usually benign nature of the Guillain–Barré syndrome together with its potentially lethal complications makes its assessment and management of importance. The syndrome is a demyelinating radiculopathy and peripheral neuropathy which follows viral infection and is usually reversible. The problem arises because the lower motor neurone problem of weakness and loss of reflexes can rapidly spread from the lower limbs to the upper limbs and muscles of the thorax and diaphragm. It is therefore important that any patient suspected of having a Guillain–Barré syndrome should be admitted to hospital and observed with particular attention being paid to the bulbar muscles and to the adequacy of respiration. Any problem arising in respiration should be managed by intermittent positive-pressure ventilation. The diagnosis is confirmed by the finding of a high protein with a normal cell count in the CSF and demonstration of slowing of conduction in the peripheral nerves and roots. Most physicians would still use steroids for patients with Guillain–Barré syndrome though the evidence for their effectiveness is not great. Recently, the suggestion has been made that patients might benefit from plasmapheresis but this technique is still undergoing evaluation.

Though some patients with Guillain–Barré syndrome are left with a permanent disability, the great majority will recover to a considerable extent and regain their independence.

FOR FURTHER READING

Adams R. D. and Victor M. (1981) *Principles of Neurology*. 2nd ed. New York, McGraw-Hill.

Bannister R. (1978) *Brain's Clinical Neurology*. 5th ed. London, Oxford University Press.

Walton J. N. (1982) *Essentials of Neurology*. 5th ed. London, Pitman.

5 Common Problems in Rheumatology

A. K. Clarke

5.1 INTRODUCTION

Something like thirty to forty million days are lost annually to British industry because of the rheumatic diseases. Back pain alone accounts for 5% of all absences from work and in certain groups in heavy industry may affect up to 80% of the work-force in a year. Rheumatoid arthritis affects 7% of all women over the age of 16 in Britain and osteoarthritis is at least twice as common; 12 000 children suffer from juvenile arthritis in Britain. This all adds up to an enormous burden for society to bear both in human and economic terms.

Not only are the rheumatic disorders important in their own right but research into the causation of them has led to considerable advances in our understanding of a wide range of chronic disease, while the 'Total Patient Care' approach to management has led to an improvement in rehabilitation services generally.

Many generalized diseases, ranging from simple viral infections like influenza to obscure immunological disorders like primary biliary cirrhosis, may present as arthritis. This means that it is always well worth taking a careful history and performing a thorough examination, especially if the arthritis has unusual features.

The history

It is important to ask about the involved joint, other joints, the general medical condition of the patient, as well as the past and family history and details of work and home conditions.

The patient should be encouraged to give the history in his own words and then any gaps should be filled by direct questioning. Among the details that it is important to elicit are the site of pain, its frequency, whether it is worse at any particular time of day, what is likely to precipitate it or make it worse, joint swelling, morning and immobility stiffness and loss of function. When considering distribution of the joint problem it is often worth asking about each individual joint or group of joints in the body, particularly if an inflammatory arthritis is suspected.

Care should be taken to ensure that the doctor and the patient are speaking the same language, especially when anatomical terms are used. The 'hip' to the layman often means the buttocks or outside of the thigh which is not where hip pain is felt.

Stiffness is very difficult to define but includes elements of pain, oedema in soft tissues and inflammation in joints. A patient almost invariably knows when he has stiffness but may be mystified by the term if he is free of it. Of particular importance is morning stiffness which is so characteristic of inflammatory arthritis. However, it is important to ask how long it lasts as stiffness lasting up to 5 or 10 minutes is commonly seen in osteoarthritis.

Enquiries about the general health and a systems enquiry are often extremely helpful in arriving at a diagnosis. Malaise accompanies severe inflammatory arthritis and depression is an important symptom in polymyalgia rheumatica. Special attention to the skin will help with psoriatic arthritis and Reiter's disease, while the eye is often involved in the seronegative arthritides.

Familial disease is frequent in rheumatic disease, especially in sero-negative arthritis, and an occupational and social history will assist greatly with rehabilitation.

The examination

It is rarely sufficient to examine just the complained-of joint or joints. Because so many generalized diseases can present with rheumatic complaints a careful examination of the skin, chest and abdomen may reveal the true cause of the problem. In any patient with a neck or back pain, a neurological examination is mandatory.

Referred pain is common and hence no complaint of pain in the arm is complete without examining the neck or pain in the leg without examining the back. A particularly common catch is for hip disease to present as knee pain and the hip always needs special attention when pain occurs in the knee.

Joint examination is not difficult but does require a little practice. The individual joint should first be inspected and note made of swelling, deformity and discoloration. The muscle bulk around the joint should be inspected. Palpation will reveal tenderness, the presence of fluid and other causes of swelling, and increase in temperature. Fluid is most easily found in the knee by eliciting a patellar tap or, when less fluid is present, the 'wipe sign'. In this, fluid is forced into the joint cavity by firm pressure on the thigh towards the patella and the back of the other hand is firmly stroked against the medial side of the knee (*Fig.* 5.1). If fluid is present it will produce a visible bulging which in turn can be forced to the medial side.

The range of the joint should then be assessed to reveal its functional ability and limitation by pain. Conventionally, the range of movement of a joint is assessed in relation to the anatomical position, i.e. standing (or lying) with the arms by the side, the palms turned to the front and the legs straight. It is useful to record range of movement by goniometer, especially if serial measurements are being made to assess treatment, or by eye. The normal ranges of movements for the major joints are given in *Table* 5.1.

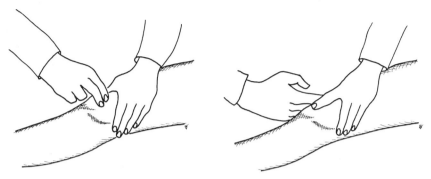

Fig. 5.1. The 'wipe sign'.

Table 5.1. Range of movements of normal joints

Cervical spine	Flexion 45°	Extension 45°
	Rotation 60°	Internal flexion 45°
Shoulder	—with scapula fixed	
	Flexion 90°	Abduction 90°
	—with scapula movement	
	Flexion 180°	Abduction 90°
	Extension 50°	
	Internal rotation 90°	External rotation 90°
Elbow	Flexion 135°	
Wrist	Extension 70°	Flexion 90°
	Radial deviation 20°	Ulnar deviation 45°
Hip	Flexion 135°	Extension 30°
	Abduction 50°	Abduction 15°
	Internal rotation 45°	External rotation 45°
Knee	Flexion 150°	
Ankle	Dorsiflexion 20°	Plantar flexion 45°
	Inversion 50°	Eversion 10°

Whenever possible the examination should include some form of functional assessment, especially if the hand is being considered. Often the most deformed rheumatoid hand will be able to perform complex and skilled movements. Similarly, walking should be assessed in any lower limb problem.

If the assessment of the patient is being done to judge progression or improvement with therapy then objective measurements may be important. This is an area of controversy and many clinicians believe that the best guide is to ask the patient how he or she is getting on but simple measurements such as joint range, grip strength, pain levels assessed on a four-point scale, walking time, etc, may well have a place.

Radiology

After the history and clinical examination, radiology is perhaps the most important part of the diagnostic process. Special radiological examination will be referred to later but plain radiographs of the hands, feet, pelvis and knees will reveal the features of many of the rheumatic disorders. Erosive changes, sacroiliitis, calcification in the menisci, periosteal reaction and many other features will be revealed by these simple views. However, there is little purpose in the obvious rheumatoid patient in taking radiographs of, say, a painful shoulder, unless surgery is contemplated, as little is likely to be seen that will modify therapy. Also it is important to remember that in the spine, degenerative change is the rule rather than the exception and the detection of cervical or lumbar spondylosis does not itself necessarily explain symptoms.

Special investigations

Rheumatology is essentially a clinical specialty and the special tests, if adhered to slavishly, will often mislead. Hence back pain and a raised urate is not gout, nor is the finding of a positive latex test proof of rheumatoid arthritis. The tests will be referred to later in the context of the various conditions but it is important to recognize the limitation of tests in the locomotor disorders.

Psychological aspects

Pain is a very individual thing. This is especially true with back pain. Rarely do patients present who are malingering although back pain is reputedly often used as an excuse to get off work for the midweek football match! Back pain sufferers often are involved in compensation cases and they will not, as a rule, get better until their cases are settled. Similarly, the psychological effects of the chronic pain and disability of rheumatoid cannot be over-estimated, especially in the young housewife or the manual labourer who is likely to lose his livelihood. The ankylosing spondylitic often looks very well but chronic back pain, stiffness and malaise may be very demoralizing, especially if it elicits no sympathy. Fear of crippling disease may cause depression which is often unwarranted.

5.2   OSTEOARTHRITIS

Degenerative disease of the joints is the commonest of the locomotor disorders. The impact of osteoarthritis of the hip on orthopaedic practice in the UK, especially since an effective operation has been available, has been enormous. It can affect practically any joint in the body, including the spine (where it is usually referred to as spondylosis).

Osteoarthrosis or osteoarthritis?

This condition was originally called osteoarthritis but over the past twenty years or so the tendency has been to call it osteoarthrosis indicating that it is a degenerative condition rather than inflammatory. However, recently a number of workers have produced good evidence to suggest that inflammation may well be present, particularly in the hereditary form of the disease, and osteoarthritis is again a respectable term. Both terms are acceptable.

Clinical features

Osteoarthritis (OA) can be primary or secondary. In both cases the symptoms are the same, i.e. pain, loss of function and immobility stiffness. In the primary condition, so-called generalized nodal OA, more than one joint is usually involved.

Initially the pain is on use, with rest producing relief although night pain, particularly in OA of the hip or knee, can be particularly troublesome. However, resting does produce a penalty, immobility stiffness. Thus getting up from a chair can be particularly difficult for up to 5 min until the sufferer gets going. Loss of function may be consequent upon pain or mechanical disruption of the joint.

In the secondary form of the disease, the history will reveal previous injury or disease in the affected joint. In the primary condition there will be complaints, not only of major joint problems, often a hip or knee, but also other joints, especially in the hands. The patient may have noticed the growth of Heberden's nodes on the distal interphalangeal joints, often accompanied by pain during the active growing phase, and pain in the bases of the thumbs, although it may be poorly localized and be described as pain in the wrist.

Referred pain has been emphasized previously but is particularly important in OA. Whenever a patient complains of knee pain, careful enquiry about the hip should be made. The hip is a region of the body that is often misinterpreted by the patient. When he mentions the hip it is well worth enquiring exactly where he means as it often transpires that the part complained of is the buttock or even low back. Hip pain is in the groin and radiates down the front of the thigh to the knee. It rarely goes beyond the knee but quite often no pain is experienced in the groin at all.

A family history, especially on the female side, of Heberden's nodes, is a frequent finding in primary OA.

Examination

In the primary condition Heberden's nodes will frequently be found on the distal interphalangeal joints, and less commonly, Bouchard's nodes on the proximal interphalangeal joints. As a rule they are hard, bony lumps proximal to the joint but sometimes they are quite inflamed and may obviously contain fluid. With the continual growth of the cysts there is often deformity of the terminal phalanges.

The other joint commonly involved in the hand is the first carpo-metacarpal joint at the base of the thumb. It characteristically produces a 'square' hand and the joint is frequently very tender.

Hallux valgus is frequently seen in the feet, especially in women, the deformity being encouraged by unsuitable footwear.

The major involved joints should, of course, be carefully examined, and this should include a functional assessment, including walking in lower limb involvement. When the knee is the major joint complained of, the hip above should be very carefully examined. Fluid may well be present, especially in OA of the knee and its presence should be noted.

General examination does not reveal any special features but obesity is a frequent aggravating problem and, in patients who may require surgery, fitness for anaesthetic should be assessed.

Investigations

Blood tests are unhelpful. Apart from the exclusion of inflammatory arthritis in doubtful cases, and the measurement of haemoglobin prior to surgery there is little justification for routine tests.

Radiology is more helpful, first to confirm the diagnosis and secondly to assess progress, especially if surgery is contemplated. Radiographs of the hands in the primary nodal variety of the disease will reveal the true nature of the Heberden's nodes, that is bone cysts, rather than the erosions of rheumatoid arthritis. Also, there is no periarticular osteoporosis. Frequently there will be gross degenerative changes in the first carpometacarpal joint.

Again it is important to emphasize that if there is knee pain, then a pelvic radiograph to assess the hip is essential as it may well be the true site of the pain. In secondary OA of the hip there is usually wear where one would expect, that is on the superior surface of the head of the femur but in the generalized nodal disease wear tends to be much more uniform and can be confused with rheumatoid. Osteophytes, which represent attempts at repair, are commonly seen around the affected joint.

When examining radiographs of the spine in spondylosis it is important to remember that osteophytes and disc space narrowing are common but do not necessarily parallel clinical symptoms. The same is true of peripheral joints and hence the radiographs must be interpreted in the light of the clinical findings.

If fluid is present in a joint, it should be withdrawn for examination and to help relieve the symptoms of pain and loss of function that a large effusion can cause. The fluid in OA is, as a rule, clear, glairy, pale yellow in colour and exhibits the 'string' sign, that is it has the consistency of thin golden syrup and does not form drops if allowed to run out of the syringe. The fluid should be examined for crystals, infection and cell count (this being very low in OA).

Management

MEDICAL

Once the diagnosis has been established, this should be communicated to the patient. Most are afraid that they are suffering from rheumatoid arthritis, a disease which the public regards as inevitably crippling. An explanation that this is not the case but that this is the more benign and often self-limiting type of joint disease can greatly help many patients. If the problem is one of predominantly hand disease in generalized nodal OA then firm reassurance that the painful Heberden's nodes will settle can be given, although any deformity is likely to remain. However, if major joints are involved then it is important to be more cautious, although it is reasonable to point out that with proper supervision most of the symptoms can be controlled or even completely relieved.

Particularly with lower limb disease, weight reduction will be beneficial in the obese. Patients do not normally appreciate that muscle action in such activities as walking and running can multiply the body weight many times and transmit it through vulnerable joints such as the hip, knee and great toe.

Physiotherapy has a part to play in building up muscle groups around damaged joints, improving gait patterns and improving general physical fitness. However, this therapy must be active and the application of heat, ice, etc. without active exercise after is without value, other than as a very short-term palliative and is almost certainly a waste of patient's and therapist's time.

In lower limb disease a walking stick carried in the opposite hand to the diseased side can greatly relieve weight through the damaged joint and limit pain, as well as giving added confidence when walking out of doors, particularly on rough ground.

Drugs have an important part to play. Simple analgesics, such as paracetamol or aspirin are often very effective but they can be replaced by the non-steroidal anti-inflammatory drugs (NSAIDs) such as indomethacin. The NSAIDs are very helpful, especially as they tend to be longer acting than analgesics and help with immobility stiffness.

There is seldom a place, if ever, for strong analgesics and usually it is unjustified to use steroids except for the occasional local injection. Repeated steroid injections seem to cause accelerated joint destruction but can be particularly helpful in the painful first carpometacarpal joint or in the knee when there is a large effusion present.

SURGICAL

Because of the relative self-limiting nature of OA, coupled with fairly normal bone structure, surgery has a major role to play in the management. Some joints are more suitable than others for surgical attack. The best example is hip replacement which is highly successful in most cases and will usually allow a return to full activities. The removal or replacement of the trapezium to relieve the pain in first carpometacarpal OA rarely leads to any functional loss. Knee surgery is, perhaps, disappointing when compared to the hip but osteotomy to re-align the load-bearing surfaces or joint replacement have their place.

It is of great assistance to the orthopaedic surgeon if patients who are referred for surgery are properly medically assessed, especially as far as fitness for anaesthetic is concerned. As well as the assessment, obese patients should be urged to lose weight and smokers to stop. Preoperative physiotherapy to build up muscle groups around the target joint, can be extemely helpful in speeding rehabilitation but must be active. The use of heat lamps and other passive methods has no place here.

With new surgical techniques and aggressive rehabilitation the period of immobility following orthopaedic surgery is minimized today. However, some patients are either not medically fit or may refuse surgery and in these cases, especially where pain is the major problem, referral to a specialist pain clinic is often worthwhile. Here techniques such as nerve block and the use of transcutaneous nerve stimulators can greatly help. Physiotherapy may give temporary relief but the temptation to give prolonged courses of palliative treatment must be resisted as it is wasteful of professional time and of minimal lasting benefit, except psychologically, a benefit which is probably better satisfied by such things as luncheon clubs!

5.3   RHEUMATOID ARTHRITIS

Rheumatoid arthritis (RA) is extremely common with a prevalence of 4% in the adult population of Britain. It is nearly twice as common in women as in men and men often suffer from the more usual systemic complications of the disease. The popular view of RA is that it is an inevitably crippling disorder but this is far from the truth. The majority of cases are quite mild and modern treatment will prevent the worst ravages of the disease in all but the most severe cases. When the diagnosis is made these points should be emphasized to the patient as fear of the disease may be worse than the disease itself, and the resigned attitude that the patient will just have to learn to live with it should be strongly resisted by patient and doctor alike.

Clinical features

RA can affect any joint in the body and presentation may be variable. A number of typical presentations, however, are worth listing.

POLYARTHRITIS

This is the classic presentation with a symmetrical small-joint arthritis, affecting hands and feet and then spreading to involve other joints. The first complaint is usually pain in the feet on walking, the patient often describing the pain as a sensation like a pebble in the shoe, or walking on glass. However, it is not until the hands are involved that most patients will consult their medical attendant. Typically it is the metacarpophalangeal (MCP) and proximal interphalangeal (PIP) joints that are involved, together with the wrists. The complaint usually takes four forms. The first is of pain, which is well localized to the affected joints. Secondly, there is marked stiffness, usually worse in the mornings, lasting anything from a few minutes to all day depending on the severity of the attack. The next complaint will be of swelling, often of the wrist and dorsal surface of the hand, as well as the MCP and PIP joints. The last complaint is of loss of function, particularly while stiff. Teapots may be dropped, buttons be impossible to do up and tasks like shaving take much longer. The loss of function may be aggravated by the carpal tunnel syndrome, a frequent accompaniment of RA.

LARGE-JOINT ONSET

About a quarter of cases will present as pain, swelling and stiffness of one or more large joints, most frequently the knees and then the shoulders. RA is one of the most important differential diagnoses in monoarthritis of the knee, for instance, and may occur spontaneously or following trauma. Any traumatized joint that does not settle as expected with appropriate treatment may turn out to be the site of the first attack of RA and it may be many months before a more widespread picture appears.

PALINDROMIC RHEUMATISM

A palindrome is a word which spells the same backwards as forwards, such as madam. Palindromic rheumatism is so called because the attack is short-lived and after it subsides there is no clinical evidence of the disease. It is uncommon but is such a striking presentation that it is worth mentioning. The attacks can come at any interval but usually are seen every 2–8 weeks. They usually last from 2 to 48 hours and during this time there is marked pain in the joints, and swelling and stiffness. It may just be two or three joints or it may be a quite striking polyarthritis. In some patients the attack may be so short-lived that they are unable to see their medical attendant and there is a tendency to disbelieve them. Many patients continue to get attacks like this, but in about half the disease progresses to more typical RA.

EXTRA-ARTICULAR PRESENTATION

Occasionally the disease will start with minimal joint symptoms. Thus the first notice of the disease may be a ganglion, especially around the wrist, or carpal tunnel syndrome. Rarely, it may present as a severe systemic illness, with fever, lymphadenopathy and peripheral oedema. About 10% of patients diagnosed as having polymyalgia rheumatica turn out to have RA.

No matter how the disease presents, the outcome is hard to predict. There are a number of rules of thumb, but in each individual the disease is personal to him or her and this is the reason why the management of RA requires such attention to detail. Of a hundred patients *presenting to hospital* about 25% will go into full remission, 60% will follow a variable course with remissions and relapses and about 15% will have a fairly progressive course. The more explosive the onset, paradoxically, the better the prognosis and this is especially true in the over-70s in whom a sudden severe attack often goes into complete remission within a year to 18 months. Bad prognostic signs include insidious onset, early erosions on radiography, strong seropositivity and early nodules. It is well known that pregnancy will produce a remission and that a relapse, often severe, can occur within 3 months of delivery.

A number of diseases mimic RA, but most are strictly self-limiting, such as rubella arthritis, and hence it is not really safe to make a diagnosis of RA until the symptoms have been present for at least 3 months.

Examination

In a case of suspected RA, all the joints should be examined, including the spine. A general medical examination is also necessary. Affected joints will, as a rule, be visibly swollen with overlying erythema, and some deformity such as ulnar drift in the fingers, may be present. Loss of muscle bulk should be noted. The joints are tender and palpation will reveal soft-tissue swelling, which feels quite boggy, and the presence of fluid, especially in the knee, may be detected. Moving the joint may produce crepitus and tests of function, such as grip strength in the hand or walking time for lower limb movement are useful and recordable measures. Watching the patient undress may be the most revealing part of the examination!

Special attention should be made in the joint examination to the metatarsophalangeal (MTP) joints. Tenderness is not only suggestive of the diagnosis but can be functionally disastrous, especially if callus formation is prominent. The neck requires careful attention. The hips also should be carefully examined, especially in sexually active women as sexual problems are common but often overlooked. The temporomandibular joints can often be painful but the pain is usually self-limiting and surgery is rarely required.

In the general examination, the single most important sign is the nodule. It is pathognomonic of the disease. Typically it occurs at sites of pressure and the commonest site is the extensor surface of the forearm just distal to the elbow, or in the walls of olecranon bursae. Other sites include overlying the Achilles tendon, the occiput and in tendon sheaths, especially in the flexor tendons of the hands, which can result in 'triggering', where the fingers will not extend beyond a certain part and then suddenly snap open.

Other points to note on general examination include pallor, as anaemia is common, palmar erythema (liver palms), lymphadenopathy and nailfold lesions. These are small infarcts around the nail bed and are due to vasculitis. The spleen may be enlarged in Felty's syndrome (*see below*). Pleural and pericardial effusions may be found, as may the fine crepitations of fibrosing alveolitis.

Examination of the eye will occasionally show episcleritis and by performing Shirmer's test, in which strips of filter paper are placed under the eyelids, the dry eyes of keratoconjunctivitis sicca (Sjögren's syndrome) may be revealed.

Neurological examination will frequently reveal the carpal tunnel syndrome. Much less commonly a sensory neuropathy or mononeuritis multiplex will be revealed. With neck involvement tetraparesis can occur. This may be a very difficult diagnosis to make as it usually occurs in advanced cases and assessing strengths in badly deformed hands or trying to elicit a Babinski response in a foot with gross hallux valgus may be virtually impossible.

Investigations

RA is essentially a clinical diagnosis but investigations may assist with the difficult cases and may help with assessing prognosis, progression of disease and response to treatment.

The blood count can be revealing. Anaemia is almost invariable in active disease, with a haemoglobin between 9·5 and 11·0 g/dl. The anaemia is normochromic and normocytic and if tests for iron levels in the body are performed, it becomes obvious that it is not due to iron deficiency. Although the serum iron may be very low the total iron binding capacity is in the normal range and bone marrow examination will show plentiful iron stores. The haemoglobin will rise spontaneously if the disease comes under control. Because many of the drugs used in the treatment of RA can cause gastric erosion or peptic ulceration, a superadded iron deficiency picture, however, can occur.

The white cell count is usually normal. If it is raised then the possibility of septic arthritis should be remembered as this is common in RA, and a very low neutrophil count may be seen in the rare complication of Felty's syndrome. These patients are particularly liable to infection and may succumb. Much of the problem appears to be due to destruction of the white cells in the spleen, and splenectomy may produce quite dramatic improvement.

The platelet count is often raised in active disease and, like the low haemoglobin, can be used as an indication of disease activity. Counts of 1 000 000/ml are not unknown but there is rarely any platelet dysfunction.

The erythrocyte sedimentation rate (ESR) is usually raised as are acute phase reactants of various kinds and the plasma viscosity. These are non-specific tests and do not always mirror clinical progress. Some patients seem to have a raised ESR permanently even though the disease is quiescent. However, it is probably one of the best ways of assessing the disease.

Rheumatoid factor is thought of as a specific test for RA. It is a complex, as a rule, of IgM produced in response to other IgM molecules circulating in the blood, although IgG rheumatoid factor is found. Various tests are available to test for it, including the slide latex test, which is entirely a qualitative test, the tube latex and sheep cell agglutination tests, which are serial dilution tests, and nephalometry, which is an absolute measure of the quantity present. Serial dilution tests are particularly difficult to interpret and should always be viewed with caution, especially if the progress of the disease is being assessed. It is also important to realize that as a test it is fairly non-specific; 10% of the normal population have positive tests as do 20% of people over the age of 75. It may also be positive in some systemic illnesses, such as acute bacterial endocarditis. Therefore, a few aches and pains plus a positive rheumatoid factor do not add up to RA and a negative test does not preclude the diagnosis.

Apart from the rheumatoid factor, other immunological tests are worth considering. The antinuclear antibody (antinuclear factor) is not specific for systemic lupus erythematosus but may be present in any disease in which there is considerable cell destruction. A positive antinuclear antibody is a poor prognostic factor in RA. Immunoglobin levels can be used to assess progress especially if they are initially elevated, but they are generally disappointing.

Of the biochemical tests, apart from the iron tests mentioned above, the alkaline phosphatase is the only one of interest. It is frequently elevated in active RA and, like the haemoglobin, platelet count and ESR can be used to monitor disease activity. It would be tempting to think that this elevation was related to bone destruction but the alkaline phosphatase is derived from liver. However, severe liver dysfunction is virtually unknown.

If joint fluid is present it should be aspirated. A number of tests can be performed. The most important is bacterial culture because septic arthritis is more common in RA than in normal joints. Cell counts are worth doing. Over 95% neutrophils is indicative of infection. If the diagnosis is in doubt, then polarized-light microscopy is necessary to exclude crystal deposition disease. Also, the phagocyte, the typical cell of RA, may be seen. Other tests include protein counts and rheumatoid factor.

If pleural effusion is present this should be tapped, first for symptom relief and secondly for diagnostic purposes. The most significant finding in pleural fluid is a very low glucose level in the absence of infection.

In many respects the radiological examination of the patient is the most useful investigation available. As a diagnostic test, the hands and feet give the highest yield. The earliest signs are soft-tissue swelling (although one hardly needs a radiograph to show this!) and periarticular osteoporosis; next, erosions are seen. Strictly these are breaks in the cortex of the bone and usually occur at the point where the synovial membrane is affixed to the bone, i.e. a little removed from the joint surface itself. The feet are usually first involved, although any appearances in the first MTP should be ignored because of the very considerable trauma to which this joint is inevitably exposed. The ulnar styloid is frequently involved early, despite the fact that it does not articulate with anything. This is an evolutionary curiosity as the bone with which it articulates in the monkey's hand has been lost but the synovial remnant remains. Large cysts may occur beneath a joint surface, so-called geodes from the geological term, and these may suddenly collapse causing quite gross deformity of the joint. With more advanced cases subluxation and total loss of bone definition may be seen.

There are two examples when special radiographs are worthwhile. The first is with the neck where flexion and extension films may be necessary to exclude odontoid peg and vertebral body slips. The second is the use of arthrography to outline the joint. It is particularly helpful in the diagnosis of the ruptured knee joint with leakage into the calf (*see below*). It is a very easy technique which can be performed in any X-ray department.

The other special investigation which sometimes is of value in RA is nerve conduction times in carpal tunnel syndrome, other suspected entrapments and peripheral neuropathies. Because the combination of a joint and a neurological problem can be so disabling and also because of the difficulty of distinguishing them clinically, conduction studies should always be performed when severe loss of hand function is found.

Complications

The many rare complications are outside the scope of this book but the more frequent ones, especially those that have serious clinical significance, are worth listing. A number have already been referred to in passing.

Anaemia is frequent but should not be regarded as a serious complication unless the haemoglobin falls below 9·0 g/dl. It is usually normochromic and normocytic but iron deficiency can occur through gastrointestinal bleeding associated with the use of antirheumatic drugs.

Rupture of the extensor tendons in the hands occurs when the tendon sheaths are extensively involved with the disease. The medial fingers are involved first, as a rule. Tendon rupture should be regarded as an emergency because the proximal end will retract up into the arm rapidly if fixation is not achieved. However, this process can be slowed and sometimes even reversed by the use of a splint to hold the dropped fingers in extension.

The ruptured knee joint is an important diagnosis to make as the physical signs are identical to those of a deep vein thrombosis in the calf. When the joint ruptures fluid rich in liposomal enzymes is forced into the tissue of the calf with the sudden onset of pain, swelling of the calf, with tenderness and a positive Homan's sign. The clue to the diagnosis is the sudden onset coupled with the previous history of joint disease. An arthrogram will confirm the diagnosis but should be performed within 24 h of the incident as the site of rupture tends to heal rapidly.

Neurological complications of various types are seen and can be life threatening. The commonest, as mentioned earlier, is carpal tunnel syndrome. The most serious neurological complication is tetraplegia or tetraparesis from the cervical spine involvement. Surprisingly, disease occurring in the C1–2 level is relatively benign but the major problems occur with vertebral subluxation at the C4–5 or C5–6 levels. The other major group of neurological complications relate to vasculitis affecting the small blood vessels supplying the nerves, the vasa nervorum. In its most benign form this will produce a peripheral neuropathy of the glove and stocking type. However, mononeuritis multiplex or very widespread mixed sensory and motor neuropathy, which has an extremely poor prognosis, is seen occasionally.

Vasculitis affects not only the nerves but can affect many other organs; of these, the most important is the skin. Apart from the nailfold lesions which herald vasculitis, ulceration, usually of the lower legs, is seen. These ulcers are painful and indolent.

Keratoconjunctivitis sicca (Sjögren's syndrome) is a common association of RA. It produces drying of the various mucosal surfaces, most noticeably the eyes, which become itchy and red. The mouth may also be dry, making it difficult to eat food unless it is moist and the vagina may also be low in secretions making sexual intercourse difficult.

A rare but fatal complication of RA is amyloidosis. The waxy fibrils are produced in a number of chronic suppurative disorders, in multiple myeloma and, in primary cases, spontaneously. The material is laid down in many organs of the body and can cause renal and cardiac failure. The finding of protein in the urine should alert the clinician to the possibility, especially in the longstanding rheumatoid. The diagnosis can be confirmed on a rectal or renal biopsy.

Management

It is convenient to divide up the management of RA into drug therapy, physical methods of treatment, and surgery but it must be emphasized that the management is a matter of attention to detail and also of a team approach. Just prescribing drugs or operating on one or more joints will not solve the many problems that the established RA sufferer has.

DRUGS

The use of drugs in RA can be divided into three groups, i.e. simple drugs, second-line agents and local therapies. The simple drugs fall into two groups, although there are obvious overlaps. The first one is simple analgesics. As with all analgesic prescribing the mildest agent that will control the pain should be used. Paracetamol still has a place but other drugs such as diflunisal (Dolobid) appear to be useful. Despite recent criticism dextropropoxyphene and paracetamol mixtures (Distalgesic) is a drug which many RA patients find useful and often it is difficult to find an adequate substitute. Strong analgesics do not play any part in the management of RA and are, in any case, usually ineffective.

The other, more important, group of simple agents are the non-steroidal anti-inflammatory drugs (NSAIDs). There is a vast range of these now available and it is beyond the scope of this work to list them all and comment on the individual merits and demerits. What follows is a brief outline of some of the most commonly used agents in the group, together with a strategy for their use.

Aspirin in its various forms is the longest lived member of the NSAIDs. It has one major drawback and that is that relatively large quantities of the drug need to be taken. Thus an average male will need to take four 300 mg tablets four times a day. Preparations like benorylate (Benoral), a chemical combination of aspirin and paracetamol, can overcome this by having a longer half-life and by the mode of presentation (a liquid rather than tablets). All NSAIDs have side-effects, of which those associated with the gastrointestinal tract are the commonest. Aspirin is, of course, no exception and minor bleeding from the stomach is the rule. Major gastric erosions are, however, uncommon.

Indomethacin (Indocid) is the widest used NSAID. It comes in a variety of presentations. The 25 mg and 50 mg capsules give flexibility of dosage. Many drugs, including NSAIDs, are recommended in a dosage of, say, one three times a day. These sorts of recommendations take little or no account of the size of the patient or the severity of the symptoms he is experiencing. One of the commonest faults in prescribing NSAIDs is to give too small a dose and then change to another agent without trying an increase in the first agent. The other side of the coin is to prescribe a drug in a dosage that not only relieves symptoms but produces unacceptable side-effects. Here, the correct thing to do is to give a lower dose. If indigestion is a problem then thought should be given to the time of the drug consumption. NSAIDs should be taken after meals or even with meals. Indomethacin is a potent cause of peptic ulceration and it might be thought that giving the drug by another route might obviate this. However, the ulcerogenic properties appear to be systemic rather than localized. Therefore, suppositories will not necessarily protect against this. Indigestion, however, is likely to be lessened and suppositories are long lasting and may be useful for helping morning stiffness, if inserted before going to sleep. However, many patients do not like using suppositories. If the patient has finger problems they are difficult to get out of the packet and to insert. They can cause local irritation of the rectum and some patients cannot retain them. Their use has very largely been superseded by the introduction of a 75 mg slow release capsule (Indocid-R) which seems to have most of the virtues of suppositories with none of the vices.

Apart from its gastrointestinal side-effects, indomethacin also produces a significant number of central nervous side-effects, either headache or dizziness. This may cause problems with driving or operating heavy machinery. These side-effects are commoner in elderly patients.

If side-effects or lack of efficacy occur then another agent from the NSAID list should be substituted. Among the agents which are commonly used, naproxen (Naprosyn), flurbiprofen (Froben), piroxicam (Feldene) and diclofenac (Voltarol) might all be tried, in reasonable doses, for two weeks at a time to see which suits the patient best. If indigestion is a real problem then agents such as ibuprofen (Brufen) or fenbufen (Lederfen) might be considered. Constipation worries some patients and here mefenamic acid (Ponstan) might be helpful.

Apart from the gastrointestinal and central nervous side-effects mentioned with indomethacin, skin rash is common in NSAIDs and may well limit the use of potentially useful members of the group, such as feprazone (Methrazone). The use of phenylbutazone (Butazolidin) is rarely justified because of the risk of fatal blood dyscrasias.

There is nothing to be gained by giving more than one NSAID at a time, mainly because of the strong protein binding of most of these agents which results in competition for the binding sites. This protein binding also leads to the necessity to take care as far as anticoagulant therapy is concerned but a number of agents such as diclofenac (Voltarol) and fenbufen (Lederfen) have virtually no interaction and are quite safe to use, although the possibility of bleeding from the gut should be remembered. Even highly protein bound agents such as naproxen (Naprosyn) can be used as long as careful monitoring of the prothrombin time is undertaken for the first 2 or 3 weeks of the initiation of treatment.

It is probably best for the non-specialists to become familiar with the use of four or five NSAIDs and stick to those. If adequate control of the symptoms cannot be achieved in this way then expert help should be sought.

There are now a number of second-line agents available. These can be defined as drugs which modify disease but which do not produce immediate relief of the symptoms. Although it is probably best for a rheumatologist to initiate treatment with these agents all practitioners coming into contact with patients on them should be familiar with the principals underlying their use. Second-line agents should be employed when there is evidence of progressive disease or serious complications which are not controlled by simple agents alone. Pain or loss of function alone is not sufficient and it must always be borne in mind that almost without exception these are dangerous drugs and should only be used when the disease is sufficiently severe. In many respects the best criterion is the progression of erosive changes on radiography. Steroids will be mentioned here only to be dismissed. Steroids have little or no place in the routine management of RA other than as a localized injection (*see below*). Side-effects are almost inevitable and the risk of skin breakdown, Cushingoid features and osteoporotic collapse are so great that they cannot be justified. It is often tempting to give a small dose for a few days or weeks, but almost inevitably the patient remains on them for ever.

Antimalarials have been under something of a cloud in recent years because of the possibility of eye damage but recent reappraisal shows that there is little evidence of retinal damage if the dose is kept below 300 mg daily. Regular eye checks are not necessary, nor should courses be restricted to 18 months or 2 years as has previously been stated. Of the second-line drugs, the antimalarials are probably the least effective but their safety may well make them the drug of first choice in, say, the young housewife.

Gold is the oldest of the second-line agents still in use and is probably the most useful, especially in early disease. It is potentially very toxic and may cause extremely unpleasant skin rash, nephrotic syndrome, and fatal bone marrow suppression, either neutropenia or thrombocytopenia. Hence, regular blood counts, urine testing and enquiries about the skin need to be made, preferably weekly during the induction of treatment and then monthly in the well-established regimen. It has one major advantage over the other second-line treatments in that the patient has to be seen regularly by the doctor or nurse and hence compliance and surveillance are easier. It is the only agent that is of use in seronegative RA. The usual way to give gold is to start with two or three test doses of 10 and 20 mg over a week or so to check that early allergic reactions do not occur and then to give 50 mg weekly until clinical control of the disease occurs, which is usually between 400 and 600 mg. Dosage can then be cut to 50 mg monthly. Gold should *not* be given in courses, but if working successfully continued ad infinitum. The dose regimen does not have to be adhered to rigidly; however, if a flare occurs the frequency can be increased and in some patients a much lower maintenance dose, e.g. 20 mg a month can be tried. Patients should be warned that they will not gain immediate benefit from the injections and that the NSAIDs will need to continue.

D-penicillamine is probably the best drug in advanced disease. It has most of the drawbacks of gold as far as side-effects are concerned and care has to be taken with blood counts and urine testing. The nephrotic syndrome usually does not occur until 6–12 months after the commencement of treatment and is usually reversible, if treatment is stopped, although proteinuria may persist for months. When the drug was first introduced relatively large doses were recommended. However, this approach produced a high incidence of unacceptable side-effects and the policy of 'go low, go slow' has increased acceptability often with much lower doses being necessary to control the disease. Hence a normal starting dose is 125 mg daily and this is then increased at the rate of 125 mg per day every 4–6 weeks until the disease comes under control. This may result in doses as low as 250 mg daily being used. There is no point in dividing the doses. It should be taken on an empty stomach if possible as this will increase absorption. As with gold the patient must be warned that the effects will not be immediate and that NSAIDs will need to be continued.

Immunosuppressants have found some favour. Azathioprine (Imuran) has been shown to be about as effective as gold. It is usually given in a dosage of 2·5 mg/kg/day in divided doses. The major problem with the drug is that it is a potent suppressor of the bone marrow and regular checks must be made of the peripheral blood. However, should suppression occur, simply stopping the drug is usually sufficient treatment. Within 24–36 h the marrow will have recovered and the drug can be reintroduced at a slightly lower dosage within a few days without harm. Patients again must be warned about the slow onset of action. Cyclophosphamide, chlorambucil and methotrexate have all been used but are really quite toxic and should be supervised by an experienced specialist.

Local drugs fall into three groups. The first are the rubs which act as counterirritants on the skin. They give good symptomatic relief to some patients, but, of course, have no long-lasting effect. The second group are intra-articular injections. For all practical purposes these are steroids. The agents used are microcrystalline preparations which are suspended in an aqueous medium. When injected the crystals cover the surface of the joint and its lining and very slowly dissolve, delivering the agent where it will be most effective. With one or two noticeable exceptions, like the hip, the injection is easy. It should be done with a sterile, no-touch technique but does not require a full theatre procedure. It can be done quite safely in the clinic, surgery or patient's home. Any fluid present in the joint should be removed for laboratory investigation and for the relief of symptoms, and it is usually helpful to mix the steroid with some plain local anaesthetic to produce immediate pain relief, the steroid not usually working for 24–48 h. Injections can be repeated but there is a real risk of hastening cartilage and bony degeneration if repeated too often and it is best not to inject any single joint more than three times in a 12-month period.

The last group of drugs are the topical agents for keratoconjunctivitis sicca. For the dry eyes, artificial tears can be used liberally, hypromellose being the usual preparation used. The mouth is much more difficult but the use of tart things, such as lemon to stimulate salivary flow, together with the advice to drink plenty of fluids with a meal will help. For the lack of vaginal secretions, a simple lubricant such as KY jelly can be of great assistance.

PHYSICAL TREATMENTS

The management of RA is never complete without an adequate programme of physical treatment. This must be tailored to the individual patient's needs. Every rheumatoid patient should have the opportunity to seek the advice of an occupational therapist and physiotherapist. Simple measures may be all that are required. Hence, the advice to keep as active as possible and to keep the weight under control is essential for all sufferers. Very painful joints, however, should be rested, using splints if necessary. Splinting may be resting or active to allow the patient to continue with their daily activities.

The technique of joint protection should be taught to the patient by a therapist. This involves teaching the patient to minimize damage to joints by doing such things as sitting with the hands flat on the knees to prevent flexion deformities and filling a kettle with a jug. An extension of this is a full Activities of Daily Living Assessment by the occupational therapist and the provision of suitable aids to help with those activities which are difficult. There is a vast range of aids and appliances now available but they need to be selected to the patient's individual needs.

All patients should be taught a programme of loosening-up and muscle strengthening exercises to do at home. These can be helped by simple measures such as soaking in a hot bath first thing in the morning. Heat can be applied to stiff joints in a number of other ways and there is little to choose between them. The hot water bottle may be the simplest and easiest method to use. Inflamed joints should be cooled using ice but heat and cold only give temporary relief and it is the active exercising which really provides the long-term aid. When more formal physiotherapy is required this again should be active. There is nothing lasting in such techniques as short-wave diathermy and such modalities should only be used to facilitate the more active treatment. Hydrotherapy is particularly useful as initially gravity can be eliminated and then graded exercises can be introduced using the resistance of the water to increase the effort needed to perform them. It is important to try and evaluate the results of treatment by proper assessments such as muscular strength and joint ranges but it is also important to place the therapy in context. There is no point in expending considerable amount of effort on teaching the patient to walk a few steps if the best functional approach would be to provide a wheelchair and teach sliding transfers.

The social worker will often have an important part to play in the management of RA. Help may be needed with such things as welfare benefits, rent, etc but the social worker will be able to assist in more complex problems such as interpersonal relationships and with helping the patient to come to terms with his or her disease.

If employment is giving problems, then the help of a Disablement Resettlement Officer (DRO) should be sought. The DRO is to be found at the Job Centre. The DRO will offer advice even if the patient is unlikely to be permanently disabled. If permanent disability does occur then there are considerable resources available to the DRO, including assessment, placement and financial facilities.

SURGERY

The orthopaedic surgeon has an important role especially in the management of advanced disease. If there is any question that surgery might help them an opinion should be sought. It is better to be told that an operation is not necessary than to miss an opportunity to help the patient. It is beyond the scope of this book to review fully the whole of orthopaedics in RA but one or two points are worth making.

Hand surgery is specialized and it must always be remembered that the important thing about the hand is function, not appearance. A proper functional assessment is undertaken before considering surgery. Carpal tunnel release is a simple and effective method of relieving the unpleasant paraesthesiae in the hands.

The hip is a satisfactory joint to operate on as is the forefoot. Surgery to the knee, shoulder and ankle is less satisfactory and operations like elbow replacement have over the years proved disappointing.

The cervical spine should be stabilized if there is evidence of spinal cord compression or severe pain in the presence of instability. It is major surgery but the complications of neck disease are so severe that the risk is usually justified.

Before a patient is sent for surgery, it is of great assistance to the surgeon if a full medical assessment is undertaken, if the patient is urged to lose weight if obese and if the physiotherapist has instructed the patient in exercises designed to strengthen the muscles around the target joint so as to speed rehabilitation.

5.4 SERONEGATIVE ARTHRITIS

Although it is quite possible to have rheumatoid arthritis with a negative rheumatoid factor, there is a group of chronic arthritic conditions which are consistently seronegative and which have specific features. Recently, the discovery of a distinct genetic predisposition has strengthened the idea that these are a clearly associated group of disorders. The group consists of ankylosing spondylitis, Reiter's syndrome, psoriatic arthritis and the arthritis of inflammatory bowel disease. In all these conditions there is a considerable excess in the prevalence of the tissue-typing antigen, HLA B27. The prevalence varies but in ankylosing spondylitis it occurs in 95%. However, it must be stressed that 8% of the normal population carries the antigen and only 10%, at the most, of the B27 carriers will never contact a B27 related disease. Therefore tissue-typing patients with obscure arthritis is not likely to be helpful.

Ankylosing spondylitis (AS)

This is a disease which effects about 1 in 200 men in Great Britain. In most hospital series there are 10 men to every woman, but the prevalence in women is probably much higher although its manifestations may be milder and less classic than in men. It usually occurs in the third and fourth decades of life, but because back pain is so common, it may not be recognized until much later in life. The history is one of back pain and stiffness which is usually worse in the morning or after a period of immobility. Initially the pain is likely to be in the low back but it will later affect the cervical spine, which is when many patients first take the trouble to complain to their medical attendant. Occasionally, peripheral arthritis may be the presenting feature and involvement of the manubriosternal joint leading to chest pain may cause patients to seek advice.

Apart from back symptoms, fatigue is the major complaint. It comes on as the day goes by and can be more debilitating than the arthritis itself. The other common symptom is that of the red sore eyes due to anterior uveitis.

Examination will reveal the diagnosis in the vast majority of patients. It is important to strip the patient down to the underpants so that the back movements can be properly observed. It is perfectly possible to touch the toes if the hips are mobile, even with a totally stiff spine. The doctor should stand behind the patient and ask him or her to touch the toes (with the knees straight!), extend the back and then laterally flex right and left. In all but the mildest cases of AS one or more of these movements will be restricted. Placing the fingers of one hand on the vertebral spine during flexion will allow the examiner to see if the vertebral bodies are moving in relationship to one another.

With the patient lying down it is possible to test for active sacroiliitis. The object is to spring the pelvis by applying pressure and seeing if pain is produced. There are a number of methods described but three simple ones are: (a) applying pressure directly to the two joints in turn with the patient prone, (b) applying pressure to the sacrum, again with the patient prone, and (c) applying pressure over the greater trochanter with the patient lying on his side. However, the tests may be negative, even in active disease and are not particularly reliable.

Chest expansion, however, is a good guide. The patient should be standing, with the hands behind the head and the tape measure applied around the chest at the nipple level. Although chest expansion diminishes with age in normal people, it should be in excess of 6 cm in the young adult male and anything below 4 cm is definitely abnormal. Neck movements should be carefully assessed and peripheral joints, especially the hips and shoulders, examined.

The eye should be examined for the presence of iritis. Small black specks on the back of the cornea, so-called keratic precipitates, may be found using the ophthalmoscope and are evidence of old iritis. Examination of skin may reveal psoriasis (see below). Although it may be obvious, a careful search in the umbilicus, natal cleft and hair may reveal small patches of psoriasis. Although aortic valve disease is uncommon, it is always worth listening for an early diastolic murmur.

The only investigation of value in diagnosis is the radiograph. It is difficult, if not impossible, to make a diagnosis of AS in the absence of radiological changes in the sacroiliac joints. The earliest changes are widening of the joint with sclerosis and erosive change. Gradually fusion will occur leading finally to total obliteration of the joints. The best view to take is a straight AP of the pelvis, special views rarely adding to diagnostic precision. By taking the whole pelvis, the hips can also be examined and other typical radiological signs looked for. These include erosions in the public symphysis, osteitis along the iliac crests and pubic rami and the presence of syndesmophytes in the lower lumbar spine.

Adolescent sacroiliac joints frequently look very abnormal on radiography and then the clinical features must be relied on, although sometimes a bone scan may be helpful.

Radiographs of the lumbar spine will reveal changes in moderate to severe cases but it is perfectly possible to have a completely stiff back clinically without any changes in the vertebrae. Contrary to popular belief, the disease does not start in the sacroiliac joints and spread up the spine. The first vertebral involvement is usually between D10 and L2. The vertebral ligaments become ossified producing the characteristic syndesmophytes. Other radiological signs on the lateral views include squaring of the vertebral bodies and erosive changes in the bodies themselves, the so-called Romanoff lesions.

The ESR and other non-specific measures of disease activity may not be abnormal in AS and give little useful information about the severity of the disease or its progress. Anaemia is uncommon.

As stated previously, testing for the B-27 antigen has little to recommend it as a diagnostic tool and should only be done for research purposes.

Treatment falls into three groups. The first, and most important, is physical. The preservation of good posture, a good vital capacity, and a good range of movement, especially in the neck, are the main aims of physical treatment. Patients should be encouraged to do the daily exercises which the physiotherapist has shown him. Apart from the regular, formal exercises, general physical fitness should be encouraged. Swimming is a particularly beneficial form of activity.

The next group is drug treatment and this is confined, except in rare cases, to the non-steroidal anti-inflammatory drugs such as indomethacin and naproxen. Usually fairly modest doses of these drugs can be given and will control pain and morning stiffness very adequately. Iritis can usually be treated with topical application but in very severe cases, which should be under specialist care, oral steroids may be necessary.

Surgery is the last form of treatment and is mainly confined these days to hip replacement but spinal osteotomy may still be required in the neglected case. This is heroic surgery and should only be undertaken by experienced spinal surgeons.

Radiotherapy acquired a bad reputation because it has been shown that AS patients treated with it suffer a 10-fold increase in the incidence of leukaemia. However, techniques have improved considerably and occasionally there may be a place for this form of treatment, particularly for a peripheral, painful joint such as a shoulder.

Psoriatic arthritis

Arthritis complicates psoriasis in about 10% of cases. Apart from the chance coincidence with rheumatoid arthritis, as both are very common disorders, there are three forms of arthritis seen in association with psoriasis.

All are seronegative and have distinctive features. The first is ankylosing spondylitis. There appear to be no specific features of these patients that distinguish them from the normal spondylitic patient.

The next variety seen is the mild polyarticular form. Clinically it resembles rheumatoid arthritis but has a number of differences. The most striking is the involvement of the distal interphalangeal joints in both hands and feet, often accompanied by psoriatic nail dysplasia. The digits may well assume a sausage-like appearance. There is moderate morning stiffness. However, the disease rarely causes more than a moderate annoyance in what is already an annoying disorder. Symptoms can usually be controlled simply with the use of non-steroidal anti-inflammatory drugs but in those cases which are more troublesome gold is remarkably effective (for treatment regimen see under rheumatoid arthritis, *above*). Often when the skin improves the joints get better and vice versa.

The most serious form of arthritis, however, is the so-called mutilans variety. As the name implies, it can be devastating, with many joints throughout the body being badly destroyed by the relentless disease. Finger joints may totally disappear, with considerable shortening of the digit, leading to the 'opera-glass' finger which can be lengthened and shortened like a telescope. Gross deformity with loss of function is common and the involvement of the neck, in particular, may lead to spinal cord compression. Many of the patients with this type of arthritis can also have a very severe psoriasis of the geographic or even 'homme rouge' variety. Although non-steroidals are needed to control pain, second-line agents are the rule. Gold may be efficacious but methotrexate, which treats both skin and joints, also has a definite place. Steroids should be avoided as any attempt to stop the drug or even lower the dose usually cause a severe relapse of the skin disease. These patients should be under specialist care.

Reiter's syndrome

This is the best described of the so-called reactive arthritides, some of which will be described in more detail later. The majority of patients with Reiter's syndrome are B-27 positive individuals who then are exposed to either non-specific urethritis or dysentery. The post-dysenteric form may lead to several cases presenting simultaneously. The dysentery may be of practially any bacterial type but some outbreaks produce far more cases in susceptible people than others. The complete syndrome consists of arthritis, eye involvement, usually sterile conjunctivitis, skin or mucosal lesions and a urethral discharge, even if the disease is post-dysenteric. The arthritis is variable in presentation. It may be sacroiliitis, a large joint monoarthritis or a symmetrical polyarthritis. Planter fasciitis and Achilles tendinitis are also common. Radiographs of the heel may reveal an exuberant, fluffy calcaneal spur or erosions at the insertion of the tendo Achilles. The skin lesions can be very variable. Typically they look like guttate psoriasis and may occur on the soles of the feet or palms producing a characteristic keratodermia blennorrhagica. Other lesions include circinate balanitis on the end of the penis and similar lesions on the musocal surfaces of the mouth. The urethral discharge may not be very obvious but can be distinguished by the so-called two-glass test in which the first specimen of urine voided in the morning is passed half into one glass and half into the next. If urethritis is present the specimen in the first glass will be noticeably cloudier and may contain small 'threads' not present in the second.

Usually the attack will come on 2 or 6 weeks after the precipitating cause. The condition often only presents with two or three features, the skin lesions being the least common. Attacks last anything from a few days to indefinitely. Total remission can occur, only to recur if further non-specific urethritis or bowel infection is encountered. A few cases are relentless and can lead to a destructive peripheral arthritis or classic ankylosing spondylitis.

Treatment consists of physical methods of pain relief and mobility together with non-steroidal anti-inflammatory drugs for symptom relief. In venereally acquired cases tetracyclines may help. In relentless cases, gold may have a place but it is advisable to seek specialist help.

The arthritis of chronic bowel disease

Both ulcerative colitis and Crohn's disease may be complicated by arthritis. In B27 positive individuals this is likely to be ankylosing spondylitis, especially in ulcerative colitis. It is interesting that the sex ratio in these cases complicating bowel disease is about equal, rather than much higher male prevalence of uncomplicated ankylosing spondylitis. The other type of arthritis is a large joint mono- or pauciarticular arthritis, often affecting the knees. Unlike the AS, the large joint arthritis is likely to improve when the bowel disease is quiescent, while removal of the affected bowel surgically will cause the large joint disease to improve but, again, not the AS.

The treatment of the AS is the same as classic AS (*see above*) but the large joint disease may be treated by local measures including physiotherapy and joint injection. The arthritis will also respond to primary treatment of the bowel, including steroids, immunosuppressants and, as stated above, surgery to the bowel.

5.5 CONNECTIVE TISSUE DISEASES

It is beyond the scope of this book to describe in detail the whole range of the fascinating but rarer connective tissue diseases. However, certain of them are sufficiently common, and liable to occur in general medical practice, to warrant attention. Also, with more sophisticated diagnostic tests they are being more readily identified, especially the milder cases.

Systemic lupus erythematosus (SLE)

SLE is now recognized with greater frequency than previously, thanks to the ready availability of the antinuclear antibody test (ANA) and tests for DNA. The older LE cell test is tedious and unreliable and is now obsolete.

The classic disease is a serious condition but rarely seen. Clinical features include skin rash, arthritis, general malaise, neuropsychiatric involvement, serositis and renal failure. Any age can be affected from adolescence up. The black races are more prone to the disease and it appears to be commoner in hot, sunny climates. The skin rash is photosensitive and not infrequently produces a butterfly distribution on the cheeks and across the bridge of the nose. A variety of other rashes are seen, especially on exposed parts of the skin. Hair loss, or frank alopecia, is common. The arthritis is curious. Pain is often the most prominent feature with very few objective signs. Any patient who complains of severe joint pain with no obvious synovitis should be screened for SLE. Where more obvious signs are present there is likely to be a symmetrical peripheral polyarthritis which is usually non-erosive and non-deforming. However, especially in blacks, marked swan-necking of the fingers may be seen and very rarely a deforming and non-erosive arthritis is seen, so-called Jaccoud's arthritis.

General malaise with anaemia and fever are frequent in classic disease. The anaemia may well be haemolytic. The most confusing and difficult group of symptoms in classic disease are neuropsychiatric. These can range from depression to frank psychosis and from mononeuritis multiplex to stroke. These complications are rheumatological emergencies. The real difficulty with them is to decide the best form of treatment which will be discussed below.

Serositis may present as pleural or pericardial effusion and, rarely, ascites. The pleural effusion rarely gives trouble but the pericardial effusion may, especially if there is concomitant carditis.

Renal involvement is very serious and is a common cause of death. A range of histological appearances are seen on renal biopsy and all known cases of SLE should be screened at intervals to ensure that renal damage is not occurring. Apart from the blood urea and creatinine, it is worth measuring the creatinine clearance at least once at the beginning of the disease and also the C4 levels as these may be low in the presence of active renal disease.

However, this florid disease is relatively uncommon and much milder disease is being increasingly recognized. Among the manifestations that may present are persistent Raynaud's phenomenon, marked arthralgia without much in the way of synovitis, non-specific skin rashes and general malaise.

Screening for autoantibodies in patients with rather indefinite symptoms is worthwhile.

The florid disease may be life-threatening and requires vigorous, expert management. The mainstay of treatment remains steroids. Quite large doses may be necessary and additionally immunosuppressives may be required. However, it must be emphasized that the prognosis is much better than was originally thought, the neuropsychiatric and renal complications being the most sinister. The implication of this is that in the absence of these complications, and especially in mild disease, steroids may not be required and may only be necessary in very small doses. Chloroquine remains a useful and safe drug and should be used as a steroid sparing agent. In the mild case it is reasonable to use one of the non-steroidal drugs to control symptoms. As long as careful follow-up is arranged for these patients the prognosis is now relatively good.

Dermatomyositis and polymyositis

These are uncommon disorders characterized by muscle pain, weakness and tenderness and, in dermatomyositis, a variety of skin rashes some of which are typical.

Dermatomyositis occurs at two distinct ages, in childhood and in middle life. In childhood the disease manifests itself as a marked rash, muscle weakness and later calcinosis. The rash includes collodian patches on the knuckles, increased capillary loops in the nail beds, heliotrope rash on the eyelids and a profuse erythematous rash, with vasculitis on the rest of the body. The weakness may be marked and will put the child off its legs. The simple tasks may become impossible and the respiratory muscles may become involved. The prognosis is generally good but the treatment does require fairly large doses of steroids and these may in themselves cause morbidity. However, the onset of calcification, subcutaneously and in muscles, can cause considerable disability in later life. In middle life the muscular problem may be more obvious, the rash forming a less prominent part. Muscle weakness occurs mainly in proximal muscles. Calcinosis does not occur in adults. Malignancy is *not* associated with the juvenile disease nor with disease in young adults but it may be seen more frequently in adults over the age of 50 and in this group some screening should be undertaken to ensure that malignancy is not the underlying cause. Polymyositis is the same condition except that there is no rash present. However, it does not appear to occur with any frequency in children.

Apart from the clear-cut clinical features, there are three investigations that are worth doing. The first is to measure the creatinine phosphokinase (CPK). The muscle enzyme is increased in the blood when there is considerable muscle breakdown but it is not invariably elevated. Electromyographic studies may show the characteristic polyphasic units and other features. However, the definitive investigation is muscle biopsy. This should be done from a clinically affected muscle, although the quadriceps is the muscle of choice. Care should be taken to avoid areas that have been sampled by the electromyographic needle. The sample should be carefully transported to the laboratory, closely following the instructions of the histopathologist about collection. Among the appearances seen on the microscope, the finding of large numbers of inflammatory cells in and around muscle fibres are characteristic.

Treatment is usually with steroids in both adults and children. If an underlying malignancy is found, then treatment of this may well lead to the suppression of the muscle and skin disease. Recently, immunosuppressives have been used in conjunction with, or instead of, steroids, methotrexate being the most favoured. However, immunosuppressives should be used with the utmost caution in children because of the risk of malignancy and sterility.

Polyarteritis nodosa (PAN)

PAN is uncommon but is a serious condition that may present in a number of ways which means that a wide range of departments may come into contact with it. The basic underlying process is, as the name implies, a vasculitis which affects arteries of all sizes throughout the body. The skin may be affected by painful nodules or by livido reticularis, a purplish net-like rash, usually in the legs. Renal failure, infarction of the bowel and mononeuritis multiplex are severe complications. Polyarteritis may be accompanied by eosinophilia and by patchy consolidation in the lungs. A deforming arthritis can occur and rarely rheumatoid arthritis can progress to PAN. The Australia antigen has been isolated in a number of patients suffering from this condition, suggesting that it may be virally induced.

Treatment requires quite large doses of steroids, with immunosuppressives added. The renal failure may require long-term dialysis or renal transplantation.

Scleroderma

Scleroderma is a curious condition of the skin and other organs which can present in a number of different ways. These include the highly localized forms, such as morphoea seen in children, in which there is gross skin atrophy with atrophy of the underlying tissue leading to marked growth problems. However, more commonly it presents as localized scleroderma affecting the skin of the extremities only, as the so-called CRST syndrome or as full blown progressive systemic sclerosis (PSS). However, the clinical features overlap so much that these are a spectrum of disease rather than distinct entities. In its simplest form there is marked Raynaud's phenomenon with tethering of the skin and fingers which may extend up the hand and forearm. The progression tends to be slow. The skin of the face may become involved and the mouth become small. As the skin gets tighter, contractions of the fingers and other joints may occur. The CRST syndrome includes not only Raynaud's phenomenon (R) and tightening of the skin of the fingers, syndactyly (S), but also calcinosis (C) in the fingers on radiography and telangiectasia (T) on the face and extremities. This variant is fairly benign but may have systemic involvement. This involvement is typically of the gut, lungs, heart and kidneys. The oesophageal involvement is common, even in the CRST syndrome and leads to difficulty in swallowing food with regurgitation. The disease may spread to involve the whole gut, however, in PSS. The pulmonary involvement leads to gross diffusion block with carbon dioxide retention. The cardiac involvement leads to cardiac failure while renal involvement, which can be fulminant, can cause rapid anuria. Keratoconjunctivitis sicca is an almost invariable accompaniment of the condition.

The diagnosis is essentially clinical but investigations can help considerably. The ESR may be normal or raised. Autoantibodies are often present. Antinuclear factors, usually the speckled variety, are often present and the recently characterized centromere antibody seems to be fairly diagnostic. A barium swallow will reveal the characteristic dilated oesophagus while lung function tests will reveal the diffusion block. Biopsy of the involved skin will show thickening of the collagen with a marked paucity of the skin appendages.

Treatment is highly unsatisfactory. Established disease is virtually untreatable but there is evidence to suggest that fairly aggressive therapy with steroids or penicillamine may help in the very early stages. If severe peripheral vascular disease complicates the Raynaud's then there may be a place for medical or surgical sympathectomy.

Mixed connective tissue disease (MCTD)

MCTD, or overlap syndrome, is a recently recognized, relatively benign, condition with features of the number of the connective tissue diseases. It was first differentiated from SLE and scleroderma by the characterization of certain antibodies, particularly the extractable nuclear antigens (ENA). The typical features are mild myositis, skin changes similar to scleroderma, a non-deforming arthritis, like SLE, and occasional internal organ involvement. Renal involvement is rare but does occur. The antinuclear antibodies are often positive and this is an important diagnosis to make because of the relative benign nature of the condition.

5.6   CRYSTAL DEPOSITION DISEASE

Gout was the first well characterized arthritic condition. Hippocrates was familiar with it and was well aware of some of its aetiological features, noting that eunuchs, menstruating women and prepubertal boys do not get gout. It is also a disease that has a rather humorous image but in reality is extremely distressing and potentially lethal. The disease is caused by crystals of sodium urate forming in joints and other tissues. In recent years the effects of other crystals, especially calcium pyrophosphate and hydroxyapatite, have been recognized, as they too can cause arthropathy.

Gout

Gout is said to be the most painful condition known to man. Primary gout tends to be familial and is associated with elevated serum uric acid levels. As mentioned above it is not seen, as a rule, in prepuberty in males and before the menopause in females. Secondary gout is occasionally seen, complicating such diseases as severe psoriasis or leukaemia, conditions associated with high tissue turnover. The reason for this is that urate, in the human, is the end-point of purine metabolism. Other mammalian species possess the enzyme uricase which converts the urate, which is relatively insoluble, to allantoin which is highly soluble and which is rapidly cleared by the kidney. In man this enzyme is not found and hence anything which pushes up the urate levels will cause the urate to come out of solution and cause a clinical attack of gout, or the laying down of crystals in tophi or in the kidney.

Traditionally, gout was precipitated by over-indulgence in food and drink and this is still a fairly frequent occurrence, especially in patients with high serum uric acids between attacks. However, it is fairly frequent to see attacks following surgery, myocardial infarction and especially diuretic medication. Diuretics are certainly the commonest cause of the first attack of gout today.

Presentation

Gout presents in three major ways: 1. Acute gout. 2. Chronic tophaceous gout. 3. Renal failure.

ACUTE GOUT

Clinically the attack occurs in one or other great toe, in the metatarsophalangeal joint, so-called podogra. The onset is rapid, over a couple of hours, and the pain is such that the weight of the bed clothes cannot be borne. The joint is exquisitely tender, swollen and red. Unlike the infected joint, the overlying skin is quite dry and shiny. Although the great toe is the commonest site, the knee, wrist and elbow are all commonly involved. Curiously, the shoulder is hardly ever the site of acute gout. Unless drugs are taken to relieve the symptoms the attack will drag on for up to a week or more.

CHRONIC TOPHACEOUS GOUT

In the chronic disease, acute attacks may still occur at regular intervals, but urate tends to be laid down in the tissues, especially in and around joints.

These tophi can cause bone erosions and sometimes the subcutaneous variety can ulcerate through the skin, exuding the urate as chalky material. The other classic site is in the external pinna of the ear. These are quite small and can be confused with sebaceous cysts. Sometimes huge deposits can be found in olecranon bursae. The rate of deposition varies from patient to patient. In those with rapid deposition there is the real danger of urate stone formation in the kidney and renal failure.

RENAL FAILURE

This is the rarest presentation of gout. Occasionally a patient will be seen with either primary or secondary gout who minimizes their joint symptoms, especially if it is chronic tophaceous disease, and is found to have renal failure. The urate causes not only stone formation but also tubular damage. If renal damage is discovered in a gout sufferer then long-term treatment is invariably indicated.

Non-gout

Aches and pains and a raised uric acid do not constitute gout. Gout can only be diagnosed in the presence of clear-cut clinical features, together with the demonstration of urate in either joint fluid or tophi. Hyperuricaemia is common, especially after the introduction of diuretic therapy. Although hyperuricaemia increases the chances of getting classic gout, it is far from inevitable and hyperuricaemics are entitled, like the rest of us, to get low back pain, tennis elbow, etc. Certainly the presence of hyperuricaemia without chronic or repeated acute gout is *not* an indication for treatment with, say, allopurinol. There is no real evidence that such treatment protects against renal failure or heart disease.

Fluid examination

As stated above, the finding of urate crystals in joint fluid confirms the diagnosis. If a joint contains fluid it should be removed, which is therapeutic in itself, and there is a lot to be said for replacing the fluid with intra-articular steroid which will help to rapidly abort the attack. It is essential that the fluid is examined not only for crystals but also for infective agents.

The fluid should be examined with a polarizing light microscope that has a rotating stage and the facility to interpose a first-order red filter. With the poles crossed, urate crystals show up as brilliant thin spindles, often intracellular, and the interposition of the first-order red filter shows that the crystals are negatively birefringent, in that they change from yellow to blue when the stage is rotated, with the crystals initially parallel to the plane of the compensator.

Treatment

ACUTE ATTACKS should be treated with high doses of a potent non-steroidal anti-inflammatory agent such as indomethacin (300 mg first day, 200 mg second day and then 150 mg daily until the attack has entirely subsided). Alternatively, colchicine can be used in the dosage of 0·5 mg hourly until either the attack subsides or gastrointestinal intolerance occurs. The latter is more usual and really limits the usefulness of this drug. The affected joint should be rested and fluids encouraged. If possible, precipitating causes, such as diuretics, should be removed. If diuretics have precipitated the attack, and in the elderly, phenylbutazone should be avoided as it is a potent cause of fluid retention and it is also in the elderly (especially women) that the idiosyncratic blood dyscrasias occur.

If fluid is present it should be aspirated and steroids instilled to abort the attack.

Aspirin can be used but must be given in large doses of 16–20 tablets a day and as such is best avoided as smaller doses are urate retaining and may prolong the attack.

Allopurinol has *no* place in the treatment of acute attacks as it can make the whole episode worse by mobilizing urate stores in the body.

CHRONIC TREATMENT is best undertaken by the use of allopurinol. Such treatment should only be commenced when the acute attack has entirely subsided and then should only be contemplated when acute attacks are occurring reasonably frequently (say more than twice a year) or when tophaceous deposits are evident.

Side-effects with the drug are rare, the most troublesome being skin rash. It is usual to start the treatment at 100 mg daily, building up by each increment. The normal dosage is usually 300 or 400 mg daily. It need not be given in divided doses. For the first 8 weeks or so of treatment it is important to give either a small dose of colchicine (0·5 mg b.d.) or a non-steroidal anti-inflammatory agent in modest dosage (say indomethacin 25 mg t.d.s.) to prevent an acute attack occurring as urate is mobilized from body stores. If an acute attack does occur, it should be very vigorously treated as above and the patient should have the reason for the attack explained and be encouraged to continue treatment. He should also be encouraged to continue treatment when the urate is normal and tophi have disappeared as the condition will inevitably return when the drug is stopped.

The drug works by blocking xanthine oxidase that converts xanthine, which is highly soluble, to urate which is not. Although xanthine crystals are laid down in muscle on this treatment there is no evidence that this is harmful.

Occasionally, patients will be seen who will either not tolerate allopurinol or who produce so much urate that allopurinol alone is insufficient. If this happens then a uricosuric agent such as probenecid can be used. These drugs work by blocking the tubular reabsorption of urate and their action is enhanced by a high fluid intake.

Dietary restriction is rarely necessary in gout these days but in patients with very high urate production, moderation in the intake of purine-containing foods is advisable and the help of a dietitian is well worth seeking.

Calcium pyrophosphate deposition disease (CPPD)

Calcium pyrophosphate (CPP) is a normal intermediary of calcium metabolism in the body. For reasons that are not entirely clear it may build up in abnormally high concentrations in joints to give a condition which can be very similar in its manifestations to gout, or even be mistaken for septic arthritis, so-called pseudogout. In such attacks, which are mainly seen in the knee, wrist and shoulder, a large tense effusion will be present. Aspiration, together with steroid injection, is symptom-relieving and will also enable the fluid to be examined under the polarizing light microscope. CPP crystals are rhomboids and are positively birefringent with the first-order red filter.

The radiographic appearances are characteristic. Calcification will be present in the affected joint, as well as in other sites (chondrocalcinosis articularis). In the knee the menisci and the hyaline cartilage will be affected and calcification is also seen in the triangular ligament in the wrist, the pubic symphysis, the femoral and humeral heads and occasionally in the intervertebral discs.

Apart from the acute attacks, there is a more chronic form associated with degenerative changes in the affected joints, effusion and occasionally gross destructive disease. Symptomless chondrocalcinosis is common and increases with age. Because of this there is debate as to the role of CPP in degenerative disease of the joints.

The CPPD is rarely associated with more generalized metabolic disorders. These are haemochromatosis and hyperparathyroidism and it is worth screening patients with CPPD for these two conditions as they are treatable and potentially serious.

Unlike gout, there is no specific enzyme inhibitor to affect the production of CPP and therefore treatment has to be symptomatic. As stated above the acute attack should be treated with aspiration and injection, supplemented by oral non-steroidal drugs such as indomethacin. Colchicine is nowhere near as effective in pseudogout as it is in gout itself. In the chronic form of the disease, non-steroidal agents, in conjunction with physiotherapy to strengthen the muscle groups around the affected joint or joints, is the treatment of choice. Severely damaged joints may require surgery.

Ochronosis

Ochronosis, or alkaptonuria, is one of the inborn errors of metabolism in which homogentisic acid is deposited in cartilage and other sites. It is due to the absence of homogentisic acid oxidase, a defect which is inherited as an autosomal recessive gene. Homogentisic acid is a black pigment and it will stain the sclerae of the eyes and the superficial cartilages in the external ear. It is also laid down in the intervertebral discs and causes them to lose fluid and become leathery—they are literally tanned. This process takes many years and will not manifest itself clinically until the fourth or fifth decade of life. The patient will then complain of persistent backache which is often resistant to normal treatment.

Radiographs will reveal marked calcification in the discs. If a urine sample is allowed to stand in the light for several hours it will darken and go black.

Treatment is unsatisfactory. There is no adequate way to compensate for the enzyme defect and by the time the condition has become symptomatic the damage will have been done. Therefore, physiotherapy to strengthen the muscles, advice about general physical fitness and analgesic or non-steroidal anti-inflammatory drugs are the treatments of choice.

Hydroxyapatite deposition

Hydroxyapatite is also an intermediary of calcium metabolism. The crystals of this compound are tiny and are barely visible on light microscopy. They are implicated in the aetiology of osteoarthritis but are present in quite large deposits in some cases of periarticular disease, of which painful arc syndrome is the commonest. This is discussed further, in the chapter on soft-tissue conditions.

5.7   INFECTIVE ARTHRITIS

Infection can result in arthritis either due to direct involvement of the joint by the organism or as an immunologically based response to a systemic episode. As such this group of disorders worldwide is the largest group of arthropathies. However, in a book of this scope, the discussion will be confined to those commonly seen in the Western industrialized societies.

Direct involvement by the organism

This can be conveniently divided into septic and non-septic arthritis.

Septic arthritis can be caused by practically any bacterium which affects the human body. Certain circumstances will make infection more likely. These include trauma, especially if there is bleeding into the joint, pre-existing arthritis, especially inflammatory, and the presence of a metallic or plastic implant. Direct invasion of the joint by puncture is uncommon, except as a complication of orthopaedic surgery, most cases being from haematogenous spread. Commonly encountered organisms are staphylococcus, strepto-coccus, gonococcus (but *see below*) and pneumococcus. Gram-negative bacilli are also seen as complications of septicaemia.

The diagnosis is made by first having a high index of suspicion to the possibility. Infected joints are extremely painful and hot. As a rule they occur as a monoarthritis but multiple joints may be affected, especially in the debilitated patient or in rheumatoid arthritis. Usually the patient is febrile and toxic but some arthritics who are being treated with steroids will have these systemic expressions of the sepsis suppressed. The joint will be distended and fluid should be aspirated and sent for culture *before* treatment is commenced. A useful quick test is to have a cell count, with differential, done on the fluid. Although many conditions will have a raised white cell count, if the neutrophils total more than 95 per cent then infection is very likely. The peripheral blood count will reveal a leucocytosis and the ESR will be raised. Blood cultures should be performed as these may be more help than the joint fluid examination itself. Radiographs will not, as a rule, be of assistance, as the bony changes take several weeks to develop but the joints should be radiographed as a base-line. If there is a joint replacement present, infection will be suggested either by evidence of loosening or by doing a bone scan. If there is a discharging sinus at the site of previous surgery, then a sinogram should be performed to ensure that there is no connection with the underlying joint.

Treatment consists of first resting the joint and giving adequate analgesia. If the patient is toxic, liberal fluids and general nursing measures are indicated. The joint will have been aspirated for diagnostic purposes and this will be therapeutic, especially if the joint is aspirated to dryness. It is rarely necessary to lay open the joint formally but repeated aspirations are of value in removing the infected material. If possible the use of antibiotics should be withheld until the cultures and sensitivities are known from the laboratory. However, if the patient is very ill then broad-spectrum antibiotics should be given parenterally. It is sensible not to chop and change the antibiotics unnecessarily and if there is any doubt the opinion of the microbiologist should be sought. Assuming that clinical improvement occurs, treatment should possibly continue for 6 weeks with careful follow-up for several months after.

Non-septic arthritis is usually due to tuberculosis although atypical microbacteria, mycoplasma, etc. are occasionally seen, especially in immunosuppressed or debilitated patients. Tuberculosis is becoming a little more frequent again. It is seen not only in immigrant populations who are known to have an altered response to the tubercle bacillus, but also in the indigenous population. It can affect practically any joint, although the spine (Pott's disease) is amongst its commonest manifestations, while tuberculosis is one of the few diseases that attacks the sacroiliac joint, apart from the seronegative arthritides.

Typically the infection spreads across the joint space (or disc in the spine) affecting the bones on either side. This contrasts with metastatic disease in which the joint space is preserved. Unlike septic arthritis, the patient will not be so ill but night sweats may be present, together with weight loss and reduction of appetite. Although there may be some swelling of the joint, it will not usually be as grossly inflamed as a septic arthritis. Aspiration is again the investigation of choice, the fluid needing to be cultured for acid-fast bacilli. The ESR will normally be raised, the chest radiograph may show evidence of active or old disease and radiographs of the joints will show the involvement of the joint space. If no growth is obtained and the Mantoux test is strongly positive, then culture of the bone marrow may be worthwhile.

Treatment is the standard antituberculosis therapy. The introduction of rifampicin has simplified this, especially in combination with isoniazid and streptomycin. Although streptomycin can usually be stopped within 3 months of the commencement of therapy, the other two agents need to be continued for at least 18 months in established bone or joint disease.

Reactive arthritis

Perhaps the commonest group of inflammatory arthritic conditions are those in which inflammation occurs in joints in response to infection but without the organism being actually in the joint itself. The model for this is rheumatic fever but a wide range of other organisms, especially viruses and organisms found in the bowel, can be responsible. In simple terms, there is an infection to which the body mounts a response. The resulting antibodies can either attack the joints because of molecular similarity between the organism of the body constituents, or from complexes which are filtered out by the synovial membrane, causing localized damage. The disorders in this group are, by the nature of things, self-limiting although further attacks may occur with re-exposure to the organism.

Rheumatic fever is a condition of the joints, heart and occasionally the brain, which is due to certain strains of the β-haemolytic streptococcus. At one time it was common but the changing characteristics of the organism, together with the widespread use of antibiotics in upper respiratory tract infection, has made it a comparative rarity. Even prior to the introduction of penicillin it was occurring in older children and tends now to be seen in adolescents and young adults. The history is one of sore throat followed weeks later by the onset of a severe arthritis which has the characteristic tendency to flit from joint to joint. Practically any joint may be affected with swelling, loss of function and severe pain. The patient is ill with fever and malaise and there may be erythema marginatum which is characteristic. Endocarditis is much less frequently seen now but may present as cardiac failure or a gross murmur which may change with the passage of time. Chorea, due to the involvement of the basal ganglia, is now rarely, if ever, seen. Apart from being severe and flitting in nature, there are two comments worth making about the arthritis. The first is that despite its severity it only very rarely given rise to permanent damage to the joint. Secondly, if aspirin is given the flitting nature of the arthritis is lost, the joints affected at the time of the exhibition remaining affected until the attack subsides. Apart from the clinical features there are some aids to diagnosis. If antibiotics are not used, the streptococcus may be found persisting in the throat swab, or on the throat swabs of clinical contacts. The antistreptolysin titre (ASO) in the blood will be elevated and may even be shown to rise, although the ASO may be elevated in any patient who has had a recent streptococcal infection. In the later stages of the disease the ASO titre may actually fall towards a more normal level. This can cause confusion. A tense swollen joint should be aspirated to exclude sepsis. Radiography of the joint is unrewarding but a chest radiograph may show evidence of cardiomegaly. Electrocardiography may reveal evidence of subclinical disease of the heart. Unless there is a persistent streptococcal infection there is little point in giving penicillin. The treatment of the arthritis is with rest and high-dose aspirin which will halt the fever and pain. In the absence of heart disease, there is no necessity to restrict mobilization once the pain has started to settle. The heart disease needs treating with rest, anti-failure drugs and occasionally emergency valve replacement if gross endocarditis occurs.

Viral arthritis can occur in response to almost any organism but a number occur with sufficient frequency to be worthy of special mention. The best known example is rubella. Some epidemics are characterized by a fairly high rate of arthritis, while others may be free of this complication. The arthritis comes on several weeks after the infection itself as a rule. As rubella can be a very benign, even silent, infection, the patient may not associate the viral illness with the severe widespread polyarthritis that follows and a careful history should be taken. The arthritis looks exactly like acute rheumatoid arthritis, with a symmetrical, peripheral polyarthritis, with considerable swelling and morning stiffness. However, the rheumatoid factor test is usually negative and there are no nodules or radiographic changes. Rubella antibody titres will usually be high. The attack lasts 6–8 weeks and then usually completely subsides without any sequelae. Treatment is with high dose aspirin or a non-steroidal agent and with rest of very painful joints.

Viral hepatitis commonly presents as arthralgia and in hepatitis B a fairly florid synovitis can occur in which Australia antigen–antibody complexes have been identified. Influenza frequently includes arthralgia in its symptom complex. The common cold and other minor viral illnesses involving the upper respiratory tract may present with pains in the joints. Although no clear genetic patterns have been established, it would appear that a proportion of the population are 'arthriticky' by nature and will get arthralgia or even frank synovitis in response to a whole range of viral and other illnesses.

Reiter's syndrome has been referred to above in the section on seronegative arthropathies but it is worth just underlining that this is a classic example of a reactive arthritis, following either dysentery or non-specific urethritis, usually in HLA B27-positive individuals. The sexually transmitted type in particular will tend to recur if further infection occurs.

Although as stated above, gonococcal arthritis may be septic, over half the cases seen are reactive, although curiously evidence of gonococcal septicaemia in the form of skin lesions is frequent. As with other forms of reactive arthritis the initiating infection may not be obvious, especially in women, in whom the diagnosis can be notoriously difficult. The arthritis affects one or two joints initially although it can be more widespread. An effusion can occur but will be sterile, even with meticulous technique with the fragile organism. However, the gonococcus may well be grown from the black necrotic skin lesions which occur, often on the hands, and which can easily be missed, and from blood culture. Urethral and rectal swabs are important but the gonococcal fixation test in the blood is virtually useless, although tests for syphilis, which may accompany the gonococcus, should always be performed. The treatment is that of gonorrhoea. Resistant strains of the gonococcus are beginning to appear but high-dose penicillin, with probenecid, is still the most useful treatment. The joints should be treated on their merits, with immobilization, aspiration and injection, non-steroidal anti-inflammatory agents and physiotherapy.

5.8 BACK PAIN

Of all the locomotor disorders affecting modern man, back pain is the commonest, least understood and socially most important. The investigation is often unrewarding, the treatment of doubtful value and the patient's satisfaction limited. Some of the more obvious clinical syndromes will be listed here, including those affecting the cervical and dorsal spines, together with a suggested schedule of investigation, and with treatments as and when appropriate. It must be appreciated, however, that at the time of writing there are still a large number of backs of somewhat indefinite nature which do not necessarily fit into any convenient diagnostic category and which it is virtually impossible to conveniently investigate.

When faced with a patient with back pain the real problem is to sort him or her into one of a number of different categories. The first step is to ask if the pain is acute or chronic. If acute, is it related to trauma, is it a recurrence of a previous long term problem, is it associated with neurological signs, or is it associated with systemic illness? If it is chronic, is it getting better, or getting progressively worse, does it wax and wane, or is it associated with more widespread disease? The age of the patient is also important to consider, as some conditions, such as Paget's disease of bone or prolapsed intervertebral disc, occur at fairly specific times of life. It is important, therefore, to take a careful history and to examine the patient fully, particularly if the pain is persistent.

The lumbar spine

Acute trauma can lead to disc rupture, vertebral fractures and ligamentous damage. The usual cause is faulty lifting technique although direct trauma can occur. The important diagnosis to exclude at this time is an acute prolapsed intervertebral disc. This used to be a very popular diagnosis but careful analysis has shown that only about a quarter of acute back lesions are disc related. The ruptured disc leads to protrusion of the nucleus pulposus which in turn leads to either nerve root pressure or, if the rupture is central, to corda equina damage. In disc prolapse, nerve root signs are invariable. The exact findings are shown in *Table* 5.2. With corda equina involvement there may be either corda equina claudication, which resembles normal vascular claudication but in younger patients with normal leg arteries, or as acute retention of urine, a rheumatological emergency.

Table 5.2. Lumbar root symptoms and signs

Root	Area of pain	Muscle weakness	Jerk involvement
L1	Upper lumbar area, groin and buttock	—	—
L2	Lower lumbar area and upper buttock, upper thigh	Psoas	—
L3	Front and inner aspect of thigh to knee	Quadriceps	Knee
L4	Outer thigh and calf to foot	Tibialis anterior, Extensor hallucis longus	—
L5	Down back of leg to foot—'classical sciatica'	Extensor hallucis longus, peronei, gluteus medius	Ankle

The classic symptom is sciatica, i.e. pain down the back of the leg, made worse by coughing and sneezing and by straining at stool, and accompanied by paraesthesiae in the leg. Straight leg raising is grossly reduced and the pain is persistent.

However, 'sciatica' can occur with little or no reduction in straight leg raising and no neurological signs. There has been a tendency to ignore these patients as malingerers but this type of pain is referred pain from paraspinal structures, such as ligaments, and is quite genuine. It is obviously much less serious than prolapsed disc but can still be very disabling. Referred pain of this type can be relieved by proper treatment of the underlying back problem.

If the back pain is an exacerbation of a previous back problem, then the history should differentiate between old disc or ligamentous problems and ankylosing spondylitis (*see above*).

A number of serious conditions present as acute back pain and should be borne in mind, especially if the acute attack does not subside as most cases do. In the younger patient infection, including tuberculosis, may occur. In the older patient secondary deposits from internal malignancy, especially breast, prostate, lung, thyroid and kidney, need to be excluded as does osteoporotic collapse, multiple myeloma and Paget's disease of bone. Shingles can produce acute pain, both in the spine and radiating into the dermatomes, the rash sometimes being quite inconspicuous.

In the chronic case, it is important to exclude the serious causes such as ankylosing spondylitis and then try to differentiate the more benign conditions, as treatment is dependent on making an accurate diagnosis. Although many female patients with back pain are referred to gynaecologists and abdominal surgeons, internal disease rarely causes persistent back trouble. In patients with benign pain a number of possible causes can be differentiated. Simple clinical examination will help. Scoliosis will suggest degenerative disease (lumbar spondylosis), pain on extension is indicative of posterior facet joint disease and trigger spots will be found in ligamentous involvement.

There is a residue of patients who have persistent pain but in whom the symptoms seem out of proportion to their signs. If certain signs are present then it is likely that the patients have psychological problems which need treating. One of these so-called inconsistent signs is not sufficient to suspect a psychological cause but three or more are highly suggestive. The first is axial pressure, that is pressure on the head with the patient standing. This should not produce pain in the back. The next is to get the patient to stand with the hands held against the top of the thighs and to rotate the body at the hips. This should not cause pain in the back as it is not being moved. In patients with reduced straight leg raising it is possible to sit up with the legs straight, in front, nor should the pain persist with the knee flexed. Also grossly reduced straight leg raising with apparent severe pain in the absence of neurological signs is inconsistent.

Investigation of back pain depends upon the clinical state of the patient. In the overwhelming majority of acute cases no investigation is necessary as the patient's symptoms will settle with rest and analgesics alone. It is only when symptoms persist that tests are necessary. The ESR is a useful screening test that, if raised, will alert the doctor to serious disease. An increased alkaline phosphatase suggests bone problems and, in the male, a raised acid phosphatase is seen in prostatic carcinoma. Plasma electro-phoresis, and demonstration of Bence-Jones protein in the urine will identify multiple myeloma. Radiographs of the spine can be a little confusing and should be done mainly to exclude serious disease such as secondary deposits, infection, osteoporosis and Paget's disease. The majority of the population have evidence of degeneration both of bone and disc on radiography and even quite gross deficits such as disc degeneration, the massive osteophytes of hypertrophic vertebral hyperostosis or spondylolysis may be symptom-free. In particular, there are, as a rule, no radiographic signs of acute disc prolapse, the loss of disc space not being evident for many months after the acute episode. It is the clinical features that are the most important.

Bone destruction on radiography can be for a number of reasons. Osteoporosis will give considerable thinning of the bones generally with anterior wedging. Malignant deposits will be visible initially in the pedicles and when the vertebral bodies collapse the disc spaces will be preserved. By way of contrast, infection will involve the disc space. The single dense vertebral body is likely to be due to Paget's disease of bone, myeloma, a sclerotic bony secondary, or rarely, a haemangioma.

If disc protrusion is suspected, then myelography should be contemplated. However, this should not be undertaken unless there is a firm commitment to surgery if a positive result is found. As a rule water-soluble dyes are used these days, so-called radiculography. Bone scan is an extremely useful technique in patients with persistent pain in whom a serious cause is suspected, especially secondary deposits, but in whom no radiological evidence is available.

Treatment obviously depends on the cause. Ankylosing spondylitis and infection are dealt with above. Malignant disease will require specialist treatment but decompression, when nerve and spinal cord pressure occurs, radiotherapy and chemotherapy all have their place. Osteoporosis is difficult to treat but spinal braces, anabolic steroids, hyaline cartilage extracts (Ossopan), female hormones and analgesics are all regularly used. Maintaining activity and a positive calcium balance is always advisable.

For the acute back problem, including the prolapsed disc, analgesics and rest, followed by active exercises, especially those aimed at strengthening the abdominal muscles, and careful instruction in the proper use of the back, remain the best method of treatment. Weight loss and an improvement in general physical fitness will also be beneficial. Most patients will respond to this regimen but if there is a delay, hydrotherapy, Maitland's manipulations, local steroid and epidural injections all have their place. Local injections are particularly helpful with ligamentous and posterior facet problems. Only very rarely is surgery necessary and then only after full investigation has shown evidence of a definite remedial lesion that is causing symptoms, like a prolapsed disc with nerve root pressure. Palliative treatments like short-wave diathermy have little or no place. Corsets act in two ways, first by restricting flexion and extension and secondly by holding in the anterior abdominal wall. Both of these can be achieved by physiotherapy and corsets are, therefore, rarely necessary, but in heavy manual labour they can be beneficial. In patients with an unidentifiable psychological cause for their symptoms, antidepressants or formal psychiatric help are worth pursuing.

The dorsal spine

Many of the conditions that affect the lumbar spine also cause problems in the dorsal spine. Thus osteoporosis, spondylosis, ankylosing spondylitis and secondaries are all seen. Pain may be in the back or may radiate round the body to produce girdle pain. This may be mistaken for pleurisy, indigestion or cardiac pain but the clue to the true origin is its reproduction by rotating the dorsal spine. Scheuermann's disease, a form of osteochondritis of the spine, attacks adolescents.

Degenerative disease producing pain in the dorsal region is often harder to treat than in the lumbar region, but physiotherapy, especially Maitland's manipulations, can be helpful. It is far harder to get a corset to control the pain in the dorsal spine but the use of one incorporating a brassière in the female may be of use.

The cervical spine

Pain in the neck is one of the commonest reasons for patients consulting their doctor. A number turn out to be due to acute infection of the upper respiratory tract with gross lymphadenopathy but the majority are due to cervical spine problems. Typically the pain affects not only the neck but radiates into one or both upper limbs, or into the occiput and even across the top of the head and into the frontal region. Paraesthesiae in the upper limbs are common and weakness of various muscle groups may be evident if there is nerve root involvement (*Table* 5.3). Long tract signs can be present and it is mandatory to check the Babinski response in any patient complaining of neck pain.

As with the rest of the spine, the major diseases are ligamentous, spondylosis, ankylosing spondylitis, and the serious conditions like secondaries and infection. However, there are a number of specific conditions that are not seen lower down. Rheumatoid arthritis commonly affects the neck, as does juvenile chronic arthritis (*see below*). Acute wry neck or torticollis is an acute ligamentous problem of the neck which responds well to manipulations.

Cervical spondylosis is extremely common. Most people over the age of 30 have radiological changes consistent with this diagnosis and most people get symptoms from time to time but few have permanent problems. Nerve root involvement by osteophytes is uncommon and transverse myelitis leading to tetraplegia is rare, despite quite severe changes on radiography.

Many patients with neck pain also have tenderness along the tops of the shoulders with the finding of hard nodules. This in the past was called fibrositis and the diagnosis was generally discarded, but a reappraisal recently has led to the definition of a syndrome which is now called fibromyalgia. The essential elements are pain in the neck, 'fibrositic' nodules, pain in the upper limbs and sleep disturbance. This last named problem appears to be at the heart of the matter. If the sleep disturbance is corrected by the use of an antidepressant such as doxepin (Sinequan) then the symptoms will often disappear. Just giving hypnotics, which do not allow

Table 5.3. Cervical root symptoms and signs

Root	Area of pain	Muscle weakness	Jerk involvement
C2	Occiput, spreading over the top of head to forehead	—	—
C3	Neck, including jaw and cheek	—	—
C4	Shoulder and supraclavicular and suprascapular areas	—	—
C5	Deltoid area and lateral side of arm	Spinati, deltoid, biceps	Biceps, brachioradialis
C6	Front of arm and lateral portion of hand	Biceps, supinator, wrist extensors	Biceps
C7	Hand, especially index, middle and ring fingers	Triceps, wrist flexors	Triceps
C8	Medial portion of hand and forearm	Finger and thumb flexors, thumb extensors and abductors	—
T1	Medial portion of arm	Intrinsic muscles of hands	—
T2	Medial portion of upper arm and axilla, upper pectoral and mid-scapula regions	—	—

natural sleep to occur, will not help. It is worth mentioning that as part of this syndrome and in other patients with neck problems, initial symptoms may be felt in the arms, often presenting as bilateral painful shoulders, tennis elbow, or even carpal tunnel syndromes.

Investigation of the neck is as for the lumbar spine but it is worth getting flexion and extension radiographs taken to ensure that there is no vertebral slip leading to spinal cord compression.

As with the lumbar spine, analgesics and physiotherapy form the mainstays of treatment. However, collars can be useful. There is no evidence that one collar is better than another nor is there any evidence that the standard collars available will prevent movement of the cervical spine. However, they are undoubtedly symptom-relieving in many cases.

5.9 SOFT-TISSUE CONDITIONS

Many patients present with ill-defined soft-tissue lesions which tend to be ignored but which can give great distress. There is a tendency to put little credence on any condition for which there are no radiological or blood changes but a tennis elbow in a carpenter can make it impossible for him to follow his trade and a capsulitis of the shoulder can prevent sleep and lead to chronic disability. When faced with a patient with a soft-tissue condition, it is important to exclude an underlying spinal problem or a more generalized arthritic condition. Rheumatoid arthritis may well present as painful shoulders or as a carpal tunnel syndrome.

Many soft-tissue conditions are due to problems at the enthesis, the junction between bone and tendon. Inflammation occurs in any movement which applies stress at the site and will result in pain and prolongation of the inflammatory problem. Investigations are usually negative. Treatment is usually by the use of steroid injection, rest, analgesics and physiotherapy.

Fibromyalgia has been mentioned in the section on cervical spondylosis. It is generally associated with sleep disturbance and can be controlled with antidepressants.

The painful shoulder is very common. A number of distinct clinical syndromes are seen. The painful arc syndrome occurs when there is inflammation in the supraspinatus tendon. Pain occurs when the shoulder is abducted in the range 30°–120° and in the same range when the shoulder is brought back to the side. Radiography will often reveal a calcific deposit in the tendon, both the deposit and the pain disappearing when the tendon is injected with steroids.

Perhaps the commonest shoulder lesion is non-adhesive capsulitis or periarthritis. In this condition the full range is preserved, although full voluntary movements may be limited by pain. Although there may be a history of trauma, at least half the cases seem to arise spontaneously. Night pain is characteristic with considerable sleep disturbance. As a rule the condition will not improve until the night pain goes. Internal rotation is usually the most painful movement on examination. The most effective treatment is intra-articular steroid injection, which can be repeated once or twice. Night pain should be relieved by the use of adequate doses of an analgesic, or, preferably, a non-steroidal anti-inflammatory drug such as indomethacin. The joint should be kept mobile *within* the limits of pain. If mobility is not maintained then an adhesive capsulitis, or frozen shoulder is likely. Too vigorous exercising, especially while night pain persists is likely to perpetuate the lesion almost indefinitely. Physiotherapy should, therefore, be given with caution but can be most helpful in the later stages, especially if any limitation of range has occurred.

Frozen shoulder is much less common. It can be very painful, with night pain. The range of movement is limited throughout although elevation of the arm and internal rotation are the most annoying. Treatment should be aimed at relieving the pain, first by the use of drugs and local steroid injection and then mobilization. Night pain is again the limiting factor. Physiotherapy, including hydrotherapy, is essential to regain range of movement. The condition can take many months to settle and there is frequently a residual loss of range.

Tennis elbow, or lateral epicondylitis, and golfer's elbow, or medial epicondylitis, are annoying, painful conditions. The epicondyle is tender and any stress on the muscle insertion, such as pronation and supination of the arm against resistance will produce pain at the epicondyle down into the forearm. Forearm pain may be the most prominent feature. The lesion may follow a blow but more usually is seen after constant, repetitive movements which stress the insertion. If bilateral disease is seen it is worth checking that the cervical spine is not the seat of the problem. Treatment is best done by local steroid injection. This may need to be repeated several times. Recurrence is frequent and really resistant cases may require surgical intervention.

Carpal tunnel syndrome has been mentioned elsewhere. Most cases are idiopathic but it may be the presenting feature of rheumatoid arthritis, myxoedema and acromegaly. It is commoner in women and is often more pronounced just prior to menstruation, due to premenstrual fluid retention. It can also be extremely troublesome in pregnancy. Typically the patient complains of painful paraesthesiae in one or both hands which spares the little finger. The patient is woken at night by the symptoms and finds relief by hanging the hand out of the bed. On examination there is blunting to pin-prick and light touch in the median nerve distribution (i.e. the palmar surface of the thumb, index and middle fingers, and half of the ring finger). There may be wasting of the thenar eminence with weakness of the abductor pollicis brevis, the only muscle innovated by the median nerve distal to the carpal tunnel. The weakness is demonstrated by getting the patient to lay the hand flat on the desk and then raise the thumb vertically towards the ceiling against resistance. Steroid injection may give temporary relief and night splints may help. However, carpal tunnel release is a simple operation and it should be recommended in all but the mildest cases and is mandatory when there is muscle wasting.

De Quervain's stenosing tenosynovitis is a painful condition of the wrist in which abduction of the thumb causes pain along the lateral border of the wrist and lower forearm. It is due to inflammation of the tendon covering of the long abductor of the thumb. On examination the pain can be reproduced by abduction of the thumb against resistance and crepitus felt overlying the tendon. The majority of cases can be cured by a steroid injection into the vicinity of the tendon. Persistent cases are invariably relieved by surgical release.

The medial ligament of the knee is frequently painful, especially in obese women. The complaint is one of pain in the knee, especially on walking. A localized area of tenderness is found on the medial side of the knee. Steroid injections are extremely effective in testing this condition.

Achilles tendinitis may complicate Reiter's syndrome and rheumatoid arthritis or can occur spontaneously. There is pain in the back of the heel made worse by plantar flexing the foot against resistance. The condition must *not* be treated by using steroid injection as rupture of the tendon is a frequent complication. Ultrasound, non-steroidal anti-inflammatory drugs and immobilization in plaster-of-Paris are the treatments of choice.

Painful heel, or plantar fasciitis, may also complicate Reiter's syndrome, as well as the other seronegative arthropathies. However, it usually occurs as an isolated problem. There is little correlation with the presence of plantar spurs on radiography. The heel is tender, either on the plantar surface or to one side. Walking aggravates it. Ultrasound is worth trying in the very early case. In established disease, steroid injection is helpful. This should be given from the side of the foot, not through the plantar surface as this route is extremely uncomfortable. A sorbo rubber pad, with a hole cut out in the shoe corresponding to the most tender area, can be symptom relieving.

Pain in the forefoot, metatarsalgia, is the earliest presentation of rheumatoid arthritis. Again it may occur spontaneously. March fracture, usually of the third or fourth metatarsal bone, can give rise to persistent pain and can be excluded on radiography. Some cases are due to neuromas occurring in the webspace of the toes. However, most cases appear just to be related to minor ligamentous and periarticular inflammation. Treatment is aimed at relieving pressure on the joints. A metatarsal dome support carefully positioned in the shoe so that the weight is taken on the metatarsal shafts is highly effective but the insoles are relatively bulky and a size larger shoe is usually required. Any persistent case of metatarsalgia should be carefully screened for rheumatoid arthritis.

Of all the soft-tissue conditions the one which needs the most careful attention is polymyalgia rheumatica. It is a disease of middle to late life rarely occurring before the age of 55. The history is one of morning stiffness, often quite profound, which may last for many hours but tends to wear off as the day goes on, occurring around the shoulders and, less commonly, around the buttocks and upper thighs. Mild synovitis is fairly frequent but depression is virtually universal. As a number of cases progress to temporal, or cranial, arteritis, it is always advisable to look for tender temporal arteries without pulsation, and tenderness in the occiput. Enquiry about visual disturbance is important as sudden loss of vision is one of the most serious complications of this condition. The muscles may well feel tender and often a story of fatiguability is given. The ESR is almost invariably raised, often to very high levels. Care should be taken to exclude rheumatoid arthritis, presenting predominantly as pain in the shoulders.

Treatment is with oral corticosteroids. Relief from all the symptoms including the depression, usually occurs within the first 24 hours, often after the first tablet. In doubtful cases a so-called steroid sandwich can be given. The sandwich consists of ascorbic acid given three times a day for a week, the prednisolone 5 mg three times a day for a week and then the ascorbic acid again. There will be no improvement in the first week, dramatic relief in the second, and a gradual relapse in the third.

If temporal arteritis is suspected the daily dose of prednisolone should be 30 mg in divided doses, but in straightforward polymyalgia rheumatica 15 mg a day is usually sufficient. The ESR and the absence of morning stiffness will show the effectiveness of treatment and after a fortnight or so the dose can be reduced, first in 2·5 mg increments until a dose of 7·5 mg a day is reached and then by 1 mg increments, the reduction usually being at fortnightly to monthly intervals. Many patients can be managed on 5 mg or less a day although it is uncommon to be able to completely stop steroids, even after many years.

5.10   JUVENILE ARTHRITIS

Although arthritis is usually considered to be a problem of later life, there are a number of distinct conditions occurring in childhood that are worthy of mention. There have been problems with nomenclature in the past but there is now a general agreement that what was previously called Still's disease or juvenile rheumatoid arthritis should be called juvenile chronic arthritis (JCA). JCA is *not* rheumatoid arthritis in children, having a number of distinct differences. As well as JCA there are a number of other conditions which can present as arthritis in childhood.

Juvenile chronic arthritis (JCA)

JCA occurs in three distinct forms. All are seronegative. By convention, to be JCA the condition needs to be present for over 3 months and to have started under the age of 16 years.

The first variety is systemic. This tends to occur in the younger age group (under 8). The child is ill, feverish, there is a fairly characteristic red, slightly raised but faint rash, and lymphadenopathy. The arthritis may be a fairly minor component. Over half the cases will have splenomegaly while hepatomegaly and pericardial effusion are less common. This variety can be a very serious illness. Stunting of growth is common. With the passage of time the arthritis is likely to become more prominent.

The polyarticular variety occurs mainly in the under-8s as well. Joints commonly involved include the hands, knees, feet and cervical spine. Considerable pain, swelling and deformity can occur. The deformity may be made worse by growth inequalities.

The last variety is the pauciarticular onset type. This, by definition, means that there are four or less joints involved within 3 months of onset. The commonest target joint is the knee. The importance of this variety lies in the serious complication of chronic iridocyclitis. The onset is insidious and the first symptom may well be reduction in vision. Therefore, it is important that all children with pauciarticular JCA have a full slit-lamp examination every

3–6 months. The eye involvement is much more likely if the antinuclear antibody is positive.

All three varieties of JCA have a reasonably good prognosis, although in the systemic type amyloidosis can occur and is usually fatal, and some patients with pauciarticular disease, apart from getting the eye disease which can lead to blindness, seem to add on joints relentlessly with the passage of time and become considerably crippled. For the majority of patients, however, it is possible to be optimistic about the outcome, although in males a number will go on to have ankylosing spondylitis (*see below*).

Investigations are of limited value. A rheumatoid factor test should be done, especially in the older child, to exclude rheumatoid arthritis (*see below*). In pauciarticular disease, the antinuclear factor is worth doing to help identify the patients most at risk from eye disease. Radiographs will show not the erosions of rheumatoid disease but periostitis in the early stages. Slit-lamp examination of the eye is essential in the pauciarticular disease.

Treatment demands some attention to detail and, as a rule, there should be a referral to the specialist centre. Aspirin still remains very useful for most cases. Sufficient should be given to relieve fever and pain, although care should be taken not to cause aspirin toxicity in very young children.

The newer non-steroidals are now establishing a place. Naproxen, in suspension form, appears to be particularly helpful. In very active disease steroids are still an essential part of treatment. Given daily they cause stunting of growth which is particularly unfortunate in a disease which already has growth problems. However, alternate-day dosage goes a long way to stop this problem. Obviously the smallest dose possible to control symptoms should be used. Local injections, used with care, are helpful.

Physiotherapy and occupational therapy play central roles in the management of JCA. Children are much more likely to guard painful joints and they need great encouragement to keep muscle groups strong and joints mobile. Splintage of painful joints, help with activities of daily living and advice about careers are essential parts of the occupational therapist's role. Education leading towards a more intellectual type of employment is important. Surgery can be very helpful in the reconstruction of damaged joints and in particular one would mention hip replacement in girls entering a sexually active phase.

Apart from JCA a number of other conditions occur in childhood. Rheumatoid arthritis does start under the age of 16. These patients usually present over the age of 12 and are seropositive. The prognosis is poor with a long, usually unrelenting, course.

Ankylosing spondylitis can also start in childhood. These patients look exactly like JCA. Back pain and stiffness are not complained of until late adolescence, even if the disease has been present for some years. There is a much more peripheral picture and the radiographs of the sacroiliac joints are not helpful as the adolescent joint nearly always looks roughened and widened, even in the absence of disease. Therefore, in males with JCA the possibility of ankylosing spondylitis should always be kept in mind.

Back pain in children is, as a rule, sinister and requires much more vigorous investigation than in an adult. The cause often turns out to be due to infection or malignancy of various kinds, including leukaemia. Leukaemia can also present as joint pain, especially around the knee, due to a 'green tumour' deposit in the bone adjoining the joint.

Other haematological diseases can present as joint problems in children. These include haemophilia and Christmas disease, in which the recurrence of haemarthrosis can be the most serious complication of the disease, and sickle-cell disease, in which bone infarcts close to joints may simulate arthritis.

Because properly managed JCA and the other arthritic disorders of childhood do so well and as the consequences of mismanagement are so disastrous every child with one of these conditions should be seen at least once by a rheumatologist or paediatrician with special experience in these disorders.

FOR FURTHER READING

Boyle A. C. (1980) *A Colour Atlas of Rheumatology*, 2nd ed. London, Wolfe Medical Books.

Currey H. L. F. (1980) *Mason and Currey's Clinical Rheumatology*, 3rd ed. Tunbridge Wells, Pitman.

Dieppe P. A., Bacon P. A., Banji A. N. et al. (1982) *Slide Atlas of Rheumatology*. London, Gower Medical Publications.

Golding D. N. (1982) *A Synopsis of Rheumatic Diseases*, 4th ed. Bristol, Wright.

Hughes G. R. V. (1979) *Connective Tissue Diseases*, 2nd ed. Oxford, Blackwell Scientific Publications.

Jayson M. I. V. (1980) *The Lumbar Spine and Back Pain*, 2nd ed. Tunbridge Wells, Pitman.

Kelley W. N., Harris E. D., Ruddy S. et al. (1981) *Textbook of Rheumatology*. Philadelphia, Saunders.

McCarty D. J. (1979) *Arthritis and Allied Conditions*, 9th ed. Philadelphia, Lea & Febiger.

Moll J. M. H. (1980) *Ankylosing Spondylitis*. Edinburgh, Churchill Livingstone.

Wright V. (ed.) (1982) *Topical Reviews in Rheumatic Diseases*, Vol. 2. Bristol, Wright.

6 Common Haematological Problems

I. W. Delamore

6.1 INTRODUCTION

Iron-deficiency anaemia represents approximately two-thirds of all patients referred to a haematology clinic. Many systemic diseases will be seen in such a clinic since they result in haematological abnormalities which are relatively easily detected in the blood because it is the body tissue most easily biopsied. This section will deal in more detail with the common anaemias such as iron deficiency and megaloblastic anaemia, but other less common disorders will also be discussed particularly where they throw light on the general principles of investigation and management.

As in all branches of medicine, history is of vital importance. It should be determined whether the symptoms of which the patient complains have been of slow or sudden onset and the general features of anaemia such as paraesthesiae, ankle swelling, headaches and lethargy, have been distinguished from features which point to a specific cause of the anaemia such as dyspepsia or malaena in iron-deficiency anaemia, glossodynia in megaloblastic anaemia and pruritus in polycythaemia rubra vera. Hypermetabolic states with night sweats and weight loss must be distinguished from other causes of such symptoms, e.g. septicaemia. A careful drug history is always important but particularly in haematology where toxicity may result in various types of anaemia, e.g. aplastic anaemia, haemolytic anaemia or other disorders such as thrombocytopenia and agranulocytosis.

If bleeding does occur it is necessary to determine the nature; petechial haemorrhages or a purpuric rash may be due to thrombocytopenia, bleeding from mucosal surfaces to a platelet or a vascular defect and ecchymoses and haemarthroses to a coagulation disturbance. In an inherited bleeding disease there is usually a positive family history and a history of bleeding episodes since early childhood, but local lesions must be excluded, especially where bleeding from the alimentary or genitourinary tract is concerned. A family history is also required if there is suspicion of an inherited red cell enzyme deficiency giving rise to haemolytic anaemia, and in autoimmune diseases such as pernicious anaemia where there may be an association with other autoimmune diseases in other members of the family.

Chronic disorders, e.g. haemophilia or leukaemia, frequently give rise to serious social and psychiatric effects. Many patients when first asked to see a haematologist automatically assume that they have a serious disorder and such patients should be reassured if no such disorder exists, but if their suspicions are confirmed, the situation should be fully explained together with the possibilities of modern-day therapy. No patient should be left without hope but nor should he or she be left in ignorance.

Much can be learnt from routine clinical examination. For example, cervical lymphadenopathy frequently poses a diagnostic problem but infective glands are small and tender whereas malignant glands tend to be non-tender, larger and of a firmer consistency. The nature of splenomegaly can often be determined by accompanying clinical findings such as the presence or absence of lymphadenopathy in lymphoid disorders of the blood, or the presence of spider naevi in hepatic disorders. The size of the spleen is also important; for example, huge splenomegaly extending down to the left iliac fossa suggests chronic myeloid leukaemia or myelosclerosis but is rarely seen in polycythaemia rubra vera or cirrhosis of the liver, while any degree of splenomegaly would almost certainly exclude a diagnosis of idiopathic immune thrombocytopenia. The full clinical appreciation of disorders of the blood requires a wide knowledge of general medicine since diseases of almost any system in the body may result in haematological abnormalities and the proper investigation of blood disorders involves a wide range of disciplines including medical biochemistry, histopathology, microbiology, virology, radiology and nuclear medicine. In almost every instance it must be remembered that a simple diagnosis of anaemia, thrombocytopenia, granulocytopenia or splenomegaly is insufficient and the underlying cause must be determined.

Much of haematology is now very specialized and as such does not fall within the scope of this book but brief mention will be made of disorders which are best treated in special centres.

Summary

1. Disorders of the blood frequently reflect disease in some other system of the body and a wide knowledge of general medicine is required.

2. The history must include a careful questioning about drugs ingestion and a detailed family history.

3. Full use must be made of all the diagnostic facilities available in a large district hospital. A sternal puncture or iliac crest puncture in order to obtain bone marrow for examination is a minor procedure and should not be thought of as a barrier to further investigation; in the hands of a skilled operator most patients tolerate such procedures with the minimum of inconvenience and discomfort. If the disease falls into one of the rarer categories of blood disorders it may be necessary to refer the patient to a special centre for further management.

4. Many serious and longstanding blood disorders are accompanied by social and psychiatric complications.

6.2 HAEMOPOIESIS

The morphology of the most primitive blood-forming cell is unknown but it is usually designated as a multipotent stem cell which is capable of

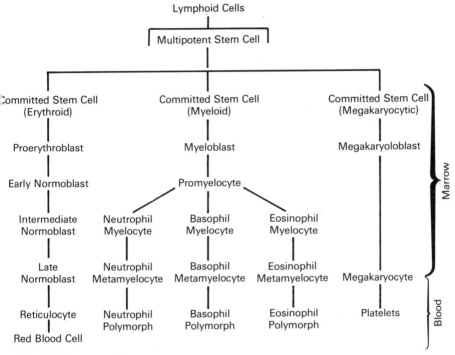

Fig. 6.1. Haemopoeisis.

self-replication and of giving rise to cells which are committed to produce one or other cell line: the so-called committed or unipotent stem cells. The cell lines predominating in any particular site seem to be related to the micro-environment, so that while the granulocytic, megakaryocytic and erythropoietic cell lines predominate in the bone marrow, lymphoid cell lines flourish in spleen and lymph nodes. A schematic representation of haemopoiesis is shown in *Fig.* 6.1.

Erythropoiesis is under the control of the hormone erythropoietin whose production is controlled by the kidney, which responds to anoxaemia, e.g. from anaemia, with a resultant increase in the level of circulating erythropoietin, and this in turn speeds up erythropoiesis at all stages. Other factors necessary for red-cell formation are vitamin B_{12} and folate, iron, protein, vitamin C and trace elements such as manganese and copper. Deficiency of any one of these might result in anaemia.

6.3 ANAEMIAS

Common anaemias are listed in *Table* 6.1. In determining the type of anaemia, two critical indices are the mean corpuscular volume (MCV) and

Table 6.1. Some causes of anaemia

Normocytic, normochromic MCH 27–32 pg MCV 80–100 fl	Microcytic, hypochromic MCH 27 pg MCV 80 fl } or less	Macrocytic MCV 100 fl or more
Anaemia of chronic disorders	Iron deficiency Blood loss, e.g. gastro-	Vitamin B$_{12}$ deficiency: Pernicious anaemia
Malignancy	intestinal lesions	Gastric resection
Rheumatoid arthritis	Menorrhagia	Disease or resection of
Chronic inflammation	Increased demands	lower ileum, e.g.
Collagen disease	Dietary inadequacy	Crohn's disease
Uraemia		Sprue
	Thalassaemia	Blind-loop syndrome
Endocrine deficiency		Jejunal diverticulosis
Addison's disease	Sideroblastic anaemia	
Hypopituitarism and	Primary	Folate deficiency
hypothyroidism	Secondary	Coeliac disease
	Pyridoxine deficiency,	Malnutrition
Haemolysis (*see Table* 6.2)	alcohol, antitubercu-	Increased demands, e.g.
	losis drugs, lead	pregnancy, rheumatoid
Aplasia	poisoning, chloram-	arthritis, malignancy
Idiopathic	phenicol, malignancy	
Drugs		Haemolysis
Radiation		
Viruses (hepatitis)		Anticonvulsants

Normal values: Mean corpuscular haemoglobin (MCH) = 27–32 pg; mean corpuscular haemoglobin concentration (MCHC) = 32–35 g/dl; mean cell volume (MCV) = 80–100 femtolitres (fl); haemoglobin (Hb) = 12·8–17·2 g/dl for men, 11·7–16·3 g/dl for women; red blood cells (RBC): 4·5–6·5 × 10^{12}/l for men, 3·9–5·6 × 10^{12}/l for women.

the mean corpuscular haemoglobin (MCH) levels, both of which are accurately measured by electronic counters in current use.

Hypochromic anaemia

The three major components of the haemoglobin molecule are iron, haem and globin. Anything which gives rise to deficiency of any one of these may produce hypochromic anaemia, i.e. iron deficiency, deficiency of haem synthesis (sideroblastic anaemia) and reduced globin chain synthesis (thalassaemia).

Iron-deficiency anaemia

In the adult, average iron losses amount to about 1 mg/day from the gut, skin, hair and nails. In menstruating women there is a further loss of 0·6 mg/day. Iron absorption does increase in iron deficiency to above the normal absorption of about 10% of the ingested dose, but menstruating women need at least 16 mg of elemental iron in the diet per day. During pregnancy demands may increase considerably and can on occasions be as much as

4–8 mg/day during the third trimester. Worldwide, iron deficiency is the most common type of anaemia of all and it is particularly common in women of child-bearing age. The major causes are shown in *Table* 6.1. Inadequate iron intake alone or in combination with blood loss from menstruation or other sites is the major factor. Other factors include impaired iron absorption, as in coeliac disease, or reduced absorption of ingested inorganic iron, as in chronic atrophic gastritis with achlorhydria. Iron losses from desquamated cells containing ferritin may also be increased in these two conditions.

Hypochromic anaemia of infancy is not uncommon and is due to prolonged milk feeding, particularly in low birth weight babies, because such babies have reduced iron stores.

A rare cause of iron deficiency is seen in adolescent males, where increased requirements of iron for growth can occasionally be responsible. It should, however, never be diagnosed until other causes have been excluded. An even more rare cause is atransferrinaemia, which results in an inability of the blood to transport iron for red-cell formation.

Clinical features

These are those of anaemia plus symptoms specifically due to a deficiency of iron, together with those related to the underlying cause. The symptoms of anaemia may affect almost any system in the body and consist of dyspnoea on exertion, lethargy, dizziness, paraesthesiae, headache, insomnia, anorexia and dyspepsia, palpitations and occasional angina of effort. On examination there is pallor of the skin and mucous membranes; tachycardia, cardiomegaly and functional systolic murmurs are common. In severe cases oedema of the ankles and basal crepitations may be present.

Features indicative of iron deficiency consist of chronic atrophic glossitis (50% of cases), koilonychia (20%) and an oesophageal web in the postcricoid region (5–10%). The Plummer–Vinson syndrome consists of dysphagia, glossitis and anaemia.

Investigation

The blood count shows anaemia with a low MCV and a low MCH; hypochromic red cells are present on the blood film and the bone marrow shows a normoblastic reaction. The serum iron is low and total iron binding capacity is raised, giving a transferrin saturation level of 16% or less. Serum ferritin levels are reduced and stainable iron in the bone marrow is absent. A diagnostic itinerary for iron-deficiency states is shown in *Fig.* 6.2.

Management

The most important aspect of management is to determine the cause. It is particularly important not to miss malignant disease of the alimentary tract.

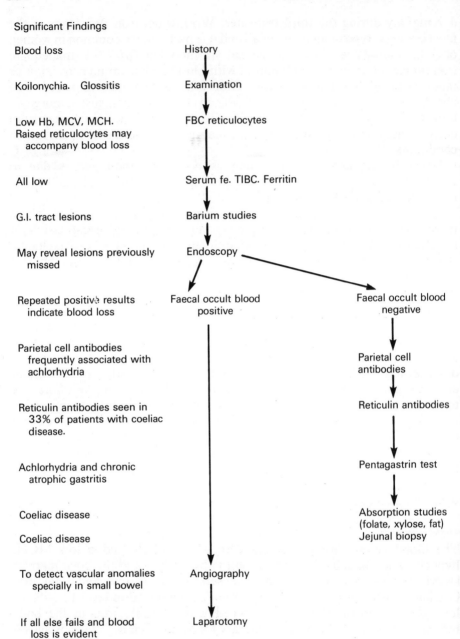

Significant Findings

Blood loss	History
Koilonychia. Glossitis	Examination
Low Hb, MCV, MCH. Raised reticulocytes may accompany blood loss	FBC reticulocytes
All low	Serum fe. TIBC. Ferritin
G.I. tract lesions	Barium studies
May reveal lesions previously missed	Endoscopy

Faecal occult blood positive — Faecal occult blood negative

Repeated positive results indicate blood loss

Parietal cell antibodies frequently associated with achlorhydria — Parietal cell antibodies

Reticulin antibodies seen in 33% of patients with coeliac disease. — Reticulin antibodies

Achlorhydria and chronic atrophic gastritis — Pentagastrin test

Coeliac disease — Absorption studies (folate, xylose, fat)

Coeliac disease — Jejunal biopsy

To detect vascular anomalies specially in small bowel — Angiography

If all else fails and blood loss is evident — Laparotomy

Fig. 6.2. Stepwise investigation of iron-deficiency anaemia.

Iron therapy should usually be given by mouth. It is given in the form of ferrous salts. Many such preparations are available but the cheapest, and probably the best, is ferrous sulphate 200 mg three times a day after food. Almost all of the preparations available are in fact effective and they include ferrous gluconate, ferrous fumarate and ferrous succinate. Proprietary liquid preparations may occasionally be necessary but they are expensive. Vitamin C supplements are not necessary and slow-release preparations are probably best avoided since very occasionally they are not well absorbed. There is usually a delay of a week before any rise in haemoglobin is seen and then it rises at the rate of 1 g/dl per week. Treatment should be continued for 2–3 months after the haemoglobin has returned to normal in order to replenish body stores.

Parenteral iron therapy is occasionally necessary but should only be given when strict indications are present. These are true intolerance to oral iron, failure to comply with oral therapy, inflammatory lesions of the alimentary tract, malabsorption of iron as in disease of the small intestine, or after partial gastrectomy and an inability to replenish iron stores at a sufficient rate by mouth when blood loss is heavy. Contrary to the belief of many, the response to parenteral iron is not quicker than that to oral iron. There are two main preparations: sorbitol–citric acid complex (Jectofer) and iron–dextran complex (Imferon). Jectofer may be given intra-muscularly in a dose of 1·5 mg of iron per kg of body weight daily, and about 250 mg of iron are required to increase the haemoglobin level by 1 g/100 ml of blood; the total dose should not exceed 2·5 g. It is contraindicated in patients with renal or hepatic disease and in those with active urinary tract infection. Intramuscular injections may be associated with pain and staining of the skin and occasional systemic reactions with fever, headache, vomiting, arthralgia and lymph-node enlargement. Urticaria and broncho-spasm have also been reported. Such reactions are fortunately very rare and seldom serious.

Imferon is rarely given intramuscularly because of local pain and is usually given as a total dose infusion. It is unnecessary in the majority of cases and is used infrequently because of the incidence of 1 or 2% systemic reactions. Most of these reactions are mild and occur immediately with flushing, headache, cough, pain in the chest, back or abdomen, lacrimation, photophobia, nausea, vomiting or bronchospasm. Hypertension, cyanosis, oedema and urticaria with arthralgia and lymphadenopathy have been reported. These reactions can be minimized by administering the drug slowly, but preliminary skin testing is of no value. The drug may be given undiluted but it is recommended that it should be administered in 5% dextrose saline solution; 150 mg are required to raise the haemoglobin concentration by 1 g/dl.

In addition to determining the cause of the anaemia, steps should be taken to prevent further blood loss and the patient should be placed on an iron-rich diet. This will not, however, obviate the need for iron therapy.

Sideroblastic anaemia

This arises from a deficiency of haem synthesis, either congenital or acquired.

Clinical features

There is a hereditary form of the disease which is X-linked (occurring in young males but transmitted by females) and is often pyridoxine-responsive. It is more often acquired either in primary form or associated with underlying diseases such as myelofibrosis, myeloid leukaemia, alcoholism, lead poisoning or drug therapy, e.g. isoniazid (see Table 6.1). In the primary acquired type the condition is often benign with a life expectancy of 10 years or more, but is important to follow such patients carefully because underlying malignant conditions may eventually become manifest.

Investigations

The anaemia may be mild in some cases. It is of the hypochromic type with a low MCH and low MCV, but the MCV may be raised in some of the acquired forms. There is no evidence of iron deficiency and the serum iron is usually elevated with a normal TIBC and serum ferritin level. The bone marrow shows iron stores to be normal and the diagnostic finding is that of ring sideroblasts, i.e. erythroblasts with siderotic granules arranged in a ring form around the nucleus. There may be associated changes of concomitant folate deficiency which is also reflected by a low serum folate.

Management

In many cases, the anaemia is not severe and no specific therapy is required. It is customary to try the effect of pyridoxine, particularly in the congenital types, and while they may fail to respond to small doses of pyridoxine, they sometimes respond to larger doses, e.g. 500 or 600 mg/day. Those patients who are folate deficient should be given folic acid supplements in a dose of 5–10 mg daily. In a selected group of patients, iron overload becomes a problem and venesection has been recommended in such patients, assuming that the anaemia is not very severe. It is a difficult form of therapy to manage in anaemic patients but may occasionally be beneficial. Where possible the underlying cause should be sought and treated.

Conclusion

Sideroblastic anaemia is a rare form of refractory anaemia which presents with hypochromic cells in the peripheral blood but the patient is, in fact, iron replete. Rarely, it is due to an inherited anomaly but more commonly it is acquired and underlying causes such as drugs and malignancy should be sought.

Thalassaemia

Thalassaemia syndromes are found in many parts of the world but are very common in Cyprus and those countries bordering the Mediterranean. They represent a group of disorders in which the synthesis of either α chains or β chains of the haemoglobin molecule is reduced. In α-thalassaemia there is a defect of α chain synthesis and in β-thalassaemia there is a defect in β chain synthesis.

Clinical features

In β-thalassaemia trait the heterozygous state results in a low MCV and a low MCH with an increased proportion of HbA$_2$ on electrophoresis. The haemoglobin level is normal or only slightly reduced and no treatment is required. The homozygous state results in severe anaemia with a large increase in fetal haemoglobin in the red cells. Bone marrow expansion results in bone deformities and thinning of the bones which may fracture. Wasting and fever are often present and multiple blood transfusions eventually lead to iron overload which may affect cardiac, hepatic and endocrine functions. In classic β-thalassaemia, anaemia becomes apparent 3–6 months after birth. There is progressive enlargement of liver and spleen as a result of red-cell destruction.

While there are only two functional β globin genes, there are four functional α globin genes. Patients with α-thalassaemia may have three, two or only one functional gene (those patients which inherit no functional genes do not survive and die of a condition known as Hb Bart's hydrops fetalis syndrome). The MCV and MCH become progressively reduced as the number of functioning genes is reduced and those patients with only one functioning gene have a large excess of β chains which form HbH. Such patients have the features of chronic haemolytic anaemia.

Investigations

In β-thalassaemia minor (trait) there is a low MCV and MCH but little or no anaemia and no evidence of iron deficiency. A raised level of haemoglobin A$_2$ is usually present, i.e. above 3·5%. If two subjects with this condition marry, there is a 25% chance of their offspring having thalassaemia major, but this can be prevented by antenatal diagnosis and abortion. Half of their offspring will be carriers.

In β-thalassaemia major there is severe hypochromic anaemia. Other features in the peripheral blood include a high reticulocyte count, circulating normoblasts, target cells and basophilic stippling of the red cells. Haemoglobin electrophoresis shows an almost complete absence of haemoglobin A which is replaced with haemoglobin F. The HbA$_2$ level is normal or only slightly raised. Haemoglobin chain synthesis studies show a marked reduction in β chain synthesis.

Alpha-thalassaemia trait is usually associated with little or no anaemia but the MCV and MCH may be reduced. There is no abnormality on haemoglobin electrophoresis and a marked reduction in α chain synthesis is required to make the diagnosis.

Management

Alpha- and beta-thalassaemia traits require no specific therapy and they run no particular risk as a result of their disorder. β-Thalassaemia major on the other hand presents a major therapeutic problem. These children are usually severely anaemic and the correct management is to give blood every 4–6 weeks in sufficient quantity to maintain the haemoglobin level above 8 g/dl. This usually means about two to three units every month. Because of the high red-cell turnover, regular folic acid supplements are required in doses of 5 mg daily and iron chelating agents to prevent iron overload from repeated blood transfusions. Desferrioxamine in a dose of 2 g is added to each unit of blood transfused and more recently this drug has been administered in a daily subcutaneous dose of 1–4 g over 8–12 h, by means of a syringe driver which can be attached to the patient's body. As much as 200 mg of iron may be excreted in the urine daily by this means and it is usually enhanced by the addition of vitamin C in a dose of 200 mg a day. The precise dose is titrated against the urinary excretion of iron to obtain the maximum therapeutic effect. Splenectomy may be needed to reduce hypersplenism but this is usually withheld until the patient is over 6 years old because of the increased risk of infection following such a procedure, but pneumococcal vaccine or prophylactic penicillin following the operation help to reduce the risk.

Conclusion

Patients with the thalassaemia syndrome in the heterozygous state may superficially appear to be iron deficient but further investigation clearly demonstrates that the hypochromia is not associated with iron deficiency. It appears that the outlook for patients suffering from β-thalassaemia major may be vastly improved as a result of modern forms of iron chelation, but it is still too soon to be sure.

Other abnormalities of the haemoglobin molecules such as structural defects found in sickle-cell anaemia have not been discussed and the reader should refer to more specialised textbooks for information on these disorders.

Megaloblastic anaemia

This type of anaemia is due to abnormal DNA synthesis as a result of impaired pyrimidine or purine synthesis. Deficiency of vitamin B_{12} or folate is usually the cause, but other causes such as specific enzyme deficiencies and drugs may be responsible in some cases. Vitamin B_{12} is found only in foods of animal origin such as liver, fish and dairy produce and combines in the stomach with intrinsic factor which is secreted by parietal cells. The vitamin is absorbed in the lower ileum and once in the portal blood, is carried by transcobalamin II (TC II) to the bone marrow and other tissues for utilization. Minimal daily requirements amount to 1–2 μg. Folate, on the other hand, is found not only in animal foods such as liver, but also in green vegetables and yeast. It is absorbed through the upper part of the small intestine and the daily requirements amount to 100–200 μg. The causes of megaloblastic anaemia are listed in *Table* 6.1. The commonest cause of vitamin B_{12} deficiency is pernicious anaemia, but nutritional deficiency, either alone or in combination with a malabsorptive defect or increased requirements, is the commonest cause of folate deficiency.

Pernicious anaemia

This occurs in adults, usually over the age of 40, with a maximum incidence at about 60. There is a female to male ratio of 1·6 to 1 and the disease is of autoimmune origin with resultant atrophy of the mucosa of the body and fundus of the stomach, but not the antrum. In consequence there is reduced secretion of intrinsic factor and acid by the gastric parietal cells and of pepsin by the peptic cells. There may be evidence of other autoimmune diseases such as thyroid disease or Addison's disease and there is also an increased incidence of diabetes. A family history of autoimmune disease is often present.

Childhood pernicious anaemia does exist but is rare and is usually due to a congenital lack of intrinsic factor with normal gastric secretion of hydrochloric acid, but in some instances it is of the adult autoimmune type.

Clinical features

The anaemia is usually of slow onset and progressive. It is sometimes associated with haemolysis and ineffective erythropoiesis in the bone marrow and this results in a lemon yellow tint to the skin and mucous membranes. Atrophic glossitis with a red sore tongue and angular stomatitis is common. There may be loss of weight and gastrointestinal symptoms such as diarrhoea. If the anaemia becomes severe, it may be associated with purpura due to thrombocytopenia. Subacute combined degeneration of the cord (vitamin B_{12} neuropathy) consists of a peripheral neuropathy associated with degeneration of the posterior and lateral columns of the spinal cord. Demyelination occurs, particularly in the posterior columns and the corticospinal and spinocerebellar tracts. There is subsequent breakdown of the axon cylinders. Objective findings of a peripheral neuropathy are present and tenderness of the muscles, especially in the calves, is found in the early stages. Impairment of proprioception, ataxia and a positive Romberg's sign are associated with posterior column damage and there may be evidence of an upper motor neurone lesion in the lower limbs. It is one of the few disorders in which an absent ankle jerk and extensor plantar response occur together.

Megaloblastic anaemia due to causes other than pernicious anaemia present the same clinical findings with the exception of the autoimmune features associated with pernicious anaemia. Depending on the cause, they may occur at an earlier age and subacute combined degeneration of the cord is found only in vitamin B_{12} deficiency states and not folate deficiency states.

Investigations

The anaemia is macrocytic with an MCV of over 100 fl. Neutropenia and thrombocytopenia are not uncommon and examination of the blood film reveals oval macrocytes together with hypersegmented polymorphs with 6 or more lobes. The bone marrow is hypercellular and erythropoiesis shows typical megaloblastic change in the red-cell precursors in which the maturation of the nucleus lags behind that of the cytoplasm. Giant metamyelocytes are also present and the diagnosis should not be made without them. Other features include a raised level of unconjugated serum bilirubin and a raised level of lactate dehydrogenase (LDH) due to ineffective erythropoiesis. The serum iron and serum ferritin levels are also raised prior to therapy.

Deficiency of vitamin B_{12} or folate is diagnosed by detecting a low level of one or other vitamin in the blood. In true folate deficiency the red-cell folate should also be reduced.

It is always important to try and detect the underlying cause of the anaemia. A full dietary history should be taken in every case. This is a common cause of folate deficiency but only vegans are likely to suffer from vitamin B_{12} deficiency for purely dietary reasons. Vitamin B_{12} absorption may be tested by the Schilling test, in which a radioactive dose of cobalt-labelled cyanocabalomin (^{57}Co-B_{12}) is administered by mouth and the urine collected for 24 h. A flushing dose of 1000 μg of non-radioactive vitamin B_{12} is given intramuscularly simultaneously with the oral dose. The amount of radioactivity collected in the urine is an indication of the amount absorbed. Other techniques of vitamin B_{12} absorption are available but the Schilling test is most commonly used. If malabsorption is detected, then the test should be repeated with intrinsic factor to see if it can be corrected. Folate absorption may be similarly measured using tritiated folic acid (BH PGA)—but is less commonly done. Intrinsic factor antibodies in the peripheral blood are almost pathognomonic of pernicious anaemia but they are present in only about 50% of cases. Parietal cell antibodies on the other hand are present in nearly all patients with pernicious anaemia but they are not so specific. If, in folate deficiency malabsorption is detected then jejunal biopsy and other tests for intestinal malabsorption and small intestinal disease should be performed, but many cases may be due to dietary causes or excessive demands as a result of coexisting disorders. A plan of investigation for patients suffering from megaloblastic anaemia is shown in *Fig. 6.3*.

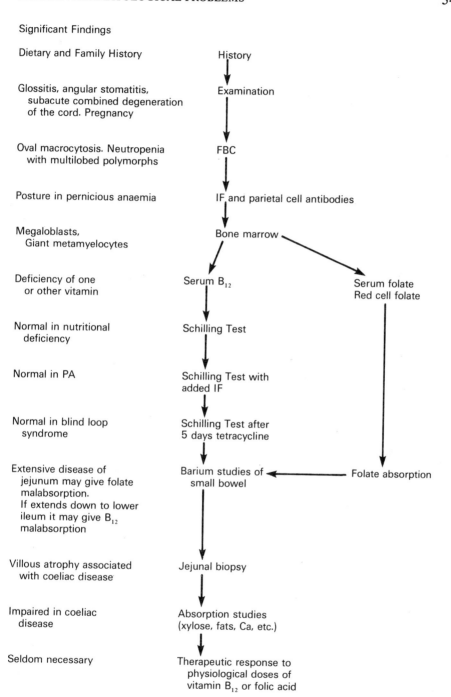

Fig. 6.3. Stepwise investigation of megaloblastic anaemia.

Management

The essence of treatment is to give the appropriate vitamin. Vitamin B_{12} is given as hydroxocobalamin 1000 μg every 2 weeks for the first month and then monthly. Monthly treatment is usually adopted but in fact one injection every 3 months is probably adequate for most patients. If pernicious anaemia or persistent malabsorption of vitamin B_{12} from any cause is responsible for the deficiency of vitamin B_{12} then life-long treatment should be instituted.

Folic acid therapy is given as folic acid tablets in a dose of 5 mg once or twice a day. The duration of therapy depends on the underlying cause. Pernicious anaemia should never be treated with folic acid alone for fear of precipitating subacute combined degeneration of the cord, but in some instances of megaloblastic anaemia it is permissible to treat with both vitamin B_{12} and folic acid until the exact nature of the anaemia is determined. Because of the chronic nature of the anaemia, blood transfusion is seldom required and should be avoided if at all possible because it may precipitate congestive cardiac failure. When anoxia makes it imperative to transfuse, then blood should be given in the form of packed red cells and very slowly. One to two units are usually sufficient. It may be advantageous to administer a simultaneous diuretic such as frusemide. Within 48 h of the commencement of therapy, the patient begins to feel better and the reticulocyte response reaches its peak at the fifth to seventh day. The haemoglobin level rises by about 1 g per week but the white cell and platelet counts return to normal within one week and the serum iron falls within 24 h to normal or subnormal levels. In every case, it is most important to determine the underlying cause of the anaemia (*see Fig.* 6.3).

Other causes of macrocytosis

Macrocytosis not due to megaloblastic change in the marrow is seen in alcoholism, liver disease, hypothyroidism, aplastic anaemia, myeloproliferative diseases and respiratory failure. The distinguishing features of the macrocytes in these disorders are that they are round rather than oval and are not associated with hypersegmented neutrophils. Alcoholism is a particularly important cause of macrocytosis and its degree is an indication of the measure of alcohol consumption by the patient. It is sometimes associated with frank megaloblastic erythropoiesis either due to a direct action of alcohol or to an associated dietary deficiency of folate.

Haemolytic anaemia

This is the result of premature destruction of red blood cells which may be intravascular when the contents of the cell are released into the circulation, or extravascular when the reticuloendothelial system particularly in the liver and spleen is responsible. The cause is either an intrinsic defect of the red cell or some extrinsic cause in the environment of the red cell, e.g. auto-antibodies. The classification of haemolytic anaemia with appropriate indication as to the cause is listed in *Table* 6.2.

Clinical features

Certain clinical features are common to all types of haemolytic anaemia and they result from the effects of increased red-cell destruction and an appropriate compensatory response within the bone marrow.

Those features which result from increased red-cell destruction include anaemia and in many cases altered red-cell morphology, e.g microsphero-cytes or fragmented red cells. There is often an increase in reticulocytes but this is a measure of increased red-cell production. Other factors indicating enhanced destruction are a raised level of unconjugated bilirubin in the serum, urobilinogen in the urine and an increased level of stercobilinogen in the stools. Haptoglobins combine with haemoglobin in the peripheral blood and are then removed by the reticulo-endothelial system so that the haptoglobin level may be reduced. Estimation of the red-cell survival time by means of chromium labelling indicates significant reduction of the normal red-cell life span.

Features associated with the compensatory increase in red-cell production include an active cellular bone marrow in which the myeloid : erythroid ratio is decreased, reticulocytosis in the peripheral blood and in some instances circulating normoblasts.

The clinical effects often result in mild jaundice, pigment gallstones and splenomegaly. Occasionally aplastic crises occur in which the bone marrow suddenly ceases to produce red cells, often in association with an infection, possibly viral. This is usually only short-lived and is followed by a further compensatory increase in bone marrow production which is reflected by a renewed reticulocytosis in the peripheral blood. Folate deficiency is a common accompaniment owing to the great demand for DNA synthesis in this situation.

Autoimmune haemolytic anaemia (AIHA)

This may be idiopathic or secondary to other diseases (*see Table* 6.2). Antibodies to red cells circulate in the peripheral blood and give rise to a positive direct antiglobulin (DAG) or Coombs test; they are described as 'warm' or 'cold' according to whether they react better at 37 °C or 4 °C respectively.

A. Warm type

Clinical features

The clinical features are those of haemolytic anaemia in general but the patient may be severely ill and run a high intermittent pyrexia. The spleen is

Table 6.2. Haemolytic anaemias

Immune	Non-immune	Intrinsic abnormalities

1. Autoimmune
  a. Warm autoantibodies
    Idiopathic
    Chronic lymphatic leukaemia
    Lymphomas
    Liver disease
    Collagen disease
  b. Cold autoantibodies
    Lymphomas
    Infections
    Infectious mononucleosis
    Atypical pneumonia
    Mycoplasma
 	
2. Drug-induced
  a. Immune:
    Penicillin, cephaloridine, phenacetin, quinidine, quinine, PAS, isoniazid, rifampicin, sulphonylureas, sulphonamides, melphalan, insulin, insecticides
 	
  b. Autoimmune
    Methyldopa, levodopa, mefenamic acid, hydantoins, methysergide, chlorpromazine
 	
3. Isoimmune
  Haemolytic disease of the newborn
  Blood transfusion reaction
	1. Infections
	  Malaria
	  Toxoplasmosis
	  Clostridium welchii
	  Infectious hepatitis
	
	2. Chemicals
	  Phenacetin, Salazopyrin, paracetamol, sulphonamides, PAS, sulphones, potassium, sodium chlorate, vitamin K analogues
	  Lead
	
	3. Mechanical
	  Cardiac surgery
	  Patch repairs
	  Aortic valve replacement
	  Mitral valve replacement
	
	4. Microangiopathic haemolytic anaemia
	  Carcinomatosis
	  Systemic lupus erythematosus
	  Polyarteritis nodosa
	  Renal cortical necrosis
	  Acute glomerular nephritis
	  Eclampsia
	  Septicaemia, e.g. meningococcal
		1. Hereditary
		  a. Membrane defects
		    Congenital microspherocytosis
		    Hereditary elliptocytosis
		  b. Red-cell enzyme defects
		    Glucose-6-phosphate dehydrogenase (G6PD) deficiency
		    Pyruvate kinase (PK) deficiency
		  c. Haemoglobinopathies
		    Thalassaemia
		    Sickle-cell disease, etc.
		
		2. Acquired
		  a. Membrane defects
		    Paroxysmal nocturnal haemoglobinuria

PAS = para-aminosalicylic acid.

often palpable and the disease tends to run a fluctuating course with remissions and relapses. Underlying causes must be looked for and they include drugs such as methyldopa or diseases such as lymphoma, chronic lymphatic leukaemia and collagen diseases (*see Table* 6.2).

Investigations

Spherocytes are usually present in the peripheral blood but they are less numerous than in hereditary spherocytosis. The other findings are those of any haemolytic anaemia but the direct Coombs test is positive due to a coating of the red cell with IgG, IgG plus complement, IgA or occasionally IgM. In a few cases, the autoantibody is directed against one of the Rhesus antigens, e.g. anti-C.

Management

The most important aspect is to look for an underlying cause and remove it if possible. Immunosuppressants are indicated and prednisolone in a dose of 60 mg or more per day is given for up to 3 weeks. If the patient fails to respond, other immunosuppressants such as azathioprine 50 mg b.d. may be tried but splenectomy is usually necessary in such cases. Some authors recommend studies with chromium-labelled red cells and surface counting over the spleen prior to splenectomy as an indication of the likely success of the operation but the correlation of such studies with clinical results is not good and the attending physician is frequently forced to undertake splenectomy in any case as a last resort.

B. Cold type

Clinical features

In patients with circulating cold antibodies, chronic haemolytic anaemia is made worse by the cold and there is a history of onset of Raynaud's phenomenon with extremities affected by the cold. Many are secondary to infections such as infectious mononucleosis or *Mycoplasma pneumoniae* and some are secondary to lymphomas (*see Table* 6.2).

Investigations

Spherocytosis is less marked than in the warm type but there is marked agglutination of red cells in the cold. Thus a blood film made at room temperature will reveal the agglutination but one made at 37 °C will not. The direct Coombs test is positive but only for complement (C_3). There is a high level of monoclonal IgM kappa specific to the antigen 'I' in the primary type of cold haemagglutinin disease (CHAD) and in those cases secondary to lymphoma; in those cases secondary to infection, the antibody is usually polyclonal and may be either anti 'I' or anti 'i'.

Management

The patient should be kept warm and the underlying cause removed if possible. Chlorambucil in a dose of 5–10 mg daily and monitored according to the blood counts may be of value in some cases. Splenectomy is not indicated.

Haemolytic anaemia due to drugs

There are two main types:

1. Autoimmune haemolytic anaemia produced by drugs such as methyldopa (*see Table* 6.2). The cause of the autoantibody formation is unknown but the clinical features are identical to those of warm type autoimmune haemolytic anaemia. The Coombs test may remain positive for many months after the drug is discontinued.

2. Immune haemolytic anaemia in which the drugs act as a hapten. The drug is attached to the red-cell membrane and antibody against the drug–membrane complex is formed, e.g. penicillin. Alternatively, the drug acts as an 'innocent bystander', i.e. antibodies are directed against the drug and this results in the fixation of complement to the red-cell membrane which in turn results in destruction of the red cell. Drugs which may cause this include quinidine, digoxin, sulphur drugs and chlorpropamide.

In every case, withdrawal of the drug results in resolution of the haemolysis within 1 or 2 weeks.

Isoimmune haemolytic anaemia

Haemolytic disease of the newborn

In this and other isoimmune haemolytic anaemias, the red cells of the patient are attacked by antibody produced by another individual. Eighty-five per cent of people have red cells which contain the Rhesus (Rh) antigen D, and such people are said to be Rhesus positive. An Rh negative woman may give rise to Rh positive children if the father of those children is himself Rh positive, since the factor is inherited as a mendelian dominant. The mother, however, becomes sensitized by the Rh positive substance in the fetal red cells and maternal agglutinins are produced. These may penetrate the placental barrier and result in haemolysis of fetal erythrocytes. Very occasionally another antigen other than anti-D is responsible.

Clinical features

The haemolytic anaemia present in the baby is usually severe and there may be enlargement of both liver and spleen with some oedema. Since the fetal liver is immature, it is unable to conjugate large amounts of bilirubin, resulting in high levels of unconjugated bilirubin in the blood. The jaundice appears about 24 h after birth and becomes gradually more severe and eventually leads to kernicterus (pigment deposition in the basal ganglia when the serum bilirubin rises above 250 μmol/l). In severe cases, the mortality is 70–80 per cent without treatment and if the condition is very severe the child may be born dead (hydrops fetalis). In mild cases, spontaneous recovery occurs.

Investigations

A full blood count will indicate that the patient has anaemia with severe haemolysis. The direct Coombs test is positive and the serum bilirubin level measured in cord blood is raised above 60 mmol/l or above 300 mmol/l in infant blood.

Management

Exchange transfusion should be given to severely affected infants and it should be given immediately. The normal exchange transfusion is 500 ml, repeated if necessary. In mild cases, simple transfusion is sufficient and in some instances no treatment at all is required. The mother of an affected child should receive 100 μg anti-D immunoglobin intramuscularly within 72 h of delivery. This will destroy the infant cells which have leaked into the mother's circulation, prevent the development of Rhesus antibodies and minimize the risk for subsequent children.

Regular checks for rhesus antibodies should be made every month throughout pregnancy. If amniocentesis during pregnancy indicates severe fetal haemolysis, then intrauterine transfusions may be administered after 27 weeks. If the infant is more than 35 weeks premature, delivery should be considered. Rh D negative women should never be given Rh positive blood if they are of child bearing age or less.

Blood transfusion reactions

ABO incompatible blood transfusions result in severe intravascular haemolysis due to the production of IgM antibodies.

Clinical features

The symptoms begin after only a few millilitres of blood have been transfused and if the transfusion is discontinued at this point, the effects may be relatively mild. If however, the transfusion is allowed to continue, severe reactions result. The patient becomes restless and nauseated, with vomiting, precordial or lumbar pain and a high fever with shivering. The skin is cold and clammy and the pulse and respiration rates both increase. The blood pressure eventually falls with the onset of severe shock. As a result of intravascular haemolysis, haemoglobinuria is present unless anuria is superimposed because of the onset of tubular necrosis. It may be some hours before the patient becomes jaundiced. In some cases, the symptoms become progressively severe with shock, uraemia and death, but most recover after about 24–48 h.

Management

The transfusion should be discontinued at once and 100 mg of hydrocortisone given intravenously. Measures for the treatment of shock should be instituted with intravenous dextran or plasma together with diuretics. If it is important to continue the blood transfusion, blood that is known to be compatible must be given. Acute renal failure is managed in the usual way including peritoneal or haemodialysis if indicated. In order to prevent such reactions the first 50–100 ml of any blood transfusion should be given slowly under careful observation and when reactions do occur, every effort must be made to determine the cause with the aid of the blood transfusion laboratory.

Haemolytic anaemia due to infective or toxic causes

Various infections, notably *Clostridium welchii*, haemolytic streptococci and staphylococci may produce haemolytic anaemia. Malaria is an important protozoal infection which may have a similar effect and falciparum malaria may give rise to blackwater fever with severe intravascular haemolysis and haemoglobinuria. Toxins include arsenic, lead, sulphonamides and potassium chlorate. The picture is one of intravascular haemolysis and the management is that of the underlying cause.

Microangiopathic haemolytic anaemia

In a variety of conditions such as thrombotic thrombocytopenic purpura, the haemolytic uraemic syndrome, some cases of adenocarcinoma, arterio-venous malformations, vasculitis and malignant hypertension, fragmented red cells (schistocytes) may be found in the peripheral blood in association with other features of haemolytic anaemia; it is thought that fibrin strands present in the arteriolar circulation are responsible.

Clinical features

There are features of the underlying disorder together with evidence of haemolysis and fragmented red cells in the peripheral blood. Other consequences of the arteriolar fibrin strands may also be evident, e.g. in thrombotic thrombocytopenic purpura there is thrombocytopenia and thrombotic lesions affecting the cerebral circulation and in the haemolytic uraemic syndrome impaired renal function is a predominant finding.

Investigations

The peripheral blood shows all the features of haemolytic anaemia and in some cases evidence of disseminated intravascular coagulation (DIC) with raised fibrin degradation products (FDPs), lowered fibrinogen levels and thrombocytopenia (*see* p. 375). Coombs test is negative but owing to the fragmentation of the red cells there is evidence of intravascular haemolysis with haemoglobinuria, haemoglobinaemia and possibly haemosiderinuria.

Management

The underlying process must be sought and eliminated. Heparin has been advocated as a means of preventing the underlying DIC in many cases, but there is now less enthusiasm for this type of therapy. More recently, plasma or whole blood exchange using a cell separator has been used with apparent success (possibly as a result of correcting blood levels of prostacyclin) in the haemolytic uraemic syndrome and thrombotic thrombocytopenic purpura.

Hereditary spherocytosis

In this condition, although the marrow produces normal red cells, in the circulating blood they become spherical instead of biconcave in shape. As a result, the cells are unduly fragile and are unable to pass through the splenic microcirculation without being destroyed. The reason for these changes is unknown. The disease is inherited in a dominant fashion with variable penetration and there is an equal sex incidence.

Clinical features

The anaemia may first be recognized at any age. It tends to fluctuate in severity, is usually associated with splenomegaly and frequently with pigment gallstones. The general features of haemolytic anaemia are usually to be found, together with microspherocytes in the peripheral blood. 'Aplastic crises' are a recognized feature of the disease and result in a sudden worsening of the anaemia. They are usually precipitated by infection and may be associated with rigors, fever and vomiting.

Investigations

Findings in the peripheral blood are those of any haemolytic anaemia but microspherocytosis is a prominent feature. These cells are smaller in diameter than normal but well filled with haemoglobin and deeply stained. Osmotic fragility is increased and there is increased autohaemolysis, i.e. when the cells are incubated in their own plasma for 48 h and the degree of haemolysis is increased but it is corrected by the addition of glucose. The direct antiglobin (DAG) test is negative.

Management

Splenectomy is curative in that it corrects the anaemia although the circulating microspherocytes are still present in the peripheral blood. The operation should not be carried out in early childhood if it can be avoided, because it makes the child more susceptible to infections, particularly pneumococcal. Any folate deficiency should be corrected by oral supplements before surgery.

Hereditary elliptocytosis

This is a similar clinical situation to hereditary spherocytosis except that the red cells take on an elliptical shape and splenectomy is required relatively rarely.

Red cell enzyme deficiencies

Glucose-6-phosphate dehydrogenases (G6PD) deficiency is one of several red cell enzyme deficiencies which may be inherited. There is impaired reduction of glutathione which results in haemolytic anaemia on oxidant stress, e.g. by certain drugs, such as antimalarials and analgesics. The disease is sex-linked, affecting males with the female as the carrier. It is found mainly in West Africa, the Mediterranean, South-East Asia and the Middle East. Management consists mainly of avoiding offending agents.

Aplastic anaemia

This is an anaemia characterized by pancytopenia in the peripheral blood and aplasia of the bone marrow. The disease may be primary or secondary to a number of known causes (*see Table* 6.1). The primary types are either congenital (Fanconi anaemia) or idiopathic acquired. It is a matter of debate whether the underlying defect is primarily a reduction in stem cells or an alteration in the microenvironment of the marrow but many patients can be successfully treated by an infusion of new stem cells as in bone-marrow transplantation. It has been suggested that in some cases suppressor T-lymphocytes bring about an autoimmune suppression of stem cells.

Clinical features
The condition occurs at any age and the clinical features are those associated with low blood counts, i.e. recurrent infections due to neutropenia, bleeding from thrombocytopenia, and anaemia. Lymphadenopathy is not a feature of the disease, nor is splenomegaly.

Investigations
Pancytopenia is invariably present. The anaemia is normochromic and normocytic unless there is associated bleeding when it may be hypochromic. In severe cases the neutrophil counts and platelet counts are below $1.5 \times 10^9/l$ and $10 \times 10^9/l$ respectively. A bone marrow aspirate usually produces a dry tap and a trephine biopsy shows the marrow spaces to be virtually empty although these findings may be patchy. As a result of the reduction in the other cell types, there is sometimes a preponderance of

lymphocytes and plasma cells in the remaining cellular elements. Clearance of radioactive iron from the blood is decreased, but this investigation is not usually necessary to make the diagnosis.

Management

Treatment consists in treating infections and haemorrhage, and transfusing blood as required. If infection is a severe problem, reversed barrier nursing is necessary together with intravenous antibiotics and occasionally granulocyte transfusions. At an early stage a decision should be made concerning bone marrow transplantation. This is reserved for severe cases with low neutrophil and platelet counts under the age of 45 with a suitable donor. Those cases consequent upon infective hepatitis fall into this category since the prognosis without bone marrow transplantation is virtually hopeless. If transplantation is contemplated, then transfusion of blood or blood products should be kept to a minimum and if possible avoided altogether until the patient is referred to a transplant unit. For less severe cases, non-androgenic steroids in the form of oxymetholone in a dose of 150–200 mg daily are usually tried. Controlled trials have not confirmed their effectiveness but most haematologists agree that occasional patients do well on this form of therapy. Some respond to high dose prednisolone therapy, e.g. 2 g daily and others appear to have responded to antithymocyte-globulin which suppresses killer T-cells. An underlying cause must be sought and eliminated in every case.

Conclusion

Aplastic anaemia is a relatively rare condition. About 25% of patients recover from this disorder but with bone marrow transplantation the prognosis has been improved considerably.

Pure red cell aplasia

This is another rare condition in which only the red cells are affected. In about 50% of cases it is associated with an autoimmune disease such as SLE or thymoma or lymphoma. There is also a congenital form known as Blackfan–Diamond syndrome.

Management

Immunosuppression may be of help and some of the congenital forms respond to androgen therapy. Treatment of the underlying disorders is of paramount importance.

Anaemia of chronic disorders

Various chronic conditions such as infections or malignancies may give rise to an anaemia of chronic disorders. The common causes are listed in *Table 6.1*.

Clinical features

Anaemia is mild and is of the normocytic, normochromic type; occasionally slight hypochromia is present. Iron stores in the bone marrow are adequate and the serum ferritin levels are normal. The serum iron is low but the total iron binding capacity is lowered rather than raised as in iron deficiency. These findings seem to be due to the fact that the reticuloendothelial system fails to release iron into the plasma. Red-cell survival is slightly reduced and in some anaemias, particularly that due to renal failure, erythropoietin production is also reduced, resulting in diminished red cell formation.

Investigation

It is important to confirm the diagnosis by measurement of serum ferritin, serum iron and total iron binding capacity and to detect the underlying cause. Some cases may be complicated by associated deficiencies of iron or folate.

Management

Blood transfusions may occasionally be required. Prednisolone in doses of 10–15 mg/day will occasionally result in release of iron from the reticulo-endothelial system with consequent improvement in the anaemia.

Conclusion

The anaemia of chronic disorders is often easily diagnosed since the underlying pathology is very evident, but in some instances this is not so and in all such cases, every effort should be made to establish the cause.

6.4 MYELOPROLIFERATIVE DISORDERS

These are a group of disorders resulting from an aberration of stem cell proliferation in the bone marrow. The stem cell disorder seems to lie somewhere between hyperplasia and neoplasia and the resulting diseases include polycythaemia rubra vera, myelofibrosis, primary thrombocythaemia and chronic granulocytic leukaemia. The last condition will be considered separately later. The general features of myeloproliferative disorders consist of a generalized proliferation of the cellular elements of the bone marrow, usually involving more than one cell line. Frequently, there is an increase in bone marrow reticulin which may proceed to collagen deposition in the more severe cases. Sometimes, cases intermediate between two of these clinical syndromes are encountered and it is for this reason that the concept of myeloproliferative disorders is so valuable.

Polycythaemia rubra vera

Polycythaemia is said to be present when the haemoglobin, red-cell count and PCV are above the upper limit of normal. Polycythaemia rubra vera is a disorder of the stem cell and is often associated with an increase in neutrophils and platelets. It must be distinguished from secondary polycythaemia due to an increase in erythropoietin which stimulates red-cell production selectively, usually without concurrent increased production of other cell lines (*Table* 6.3). Relative or 'stress' polycythaemia is an apparent polycythaemia due to a reduction in plasma volume; it tends to occur in middle-aged men and is associated with cardiovascular problems. It is much more common than polycythaemia rubra vera.

Table 6.3. Secondary polycythaemia

Anoxaemia	Renal lesions	Neoplasm	Hepatic lesions
Chronic lung lesions	Cysts	Fibroids of uterus	Hepatoma
Cardiac shunts	Renal artery stenosis	Cerebellar angioma	Cirrhosis
Intrathoracic AV shunts	Hypernephroma		
Abnormal haemoglobins	Pyelonephritis		

Clinical features

Young adults are occasionally affected but it is mainly a disease of the over-40s. Symptoms consist of headaches, dyspnoea on exertion, pruritus and occasionally night sweats. Haemorrhagic or thrombotic episodes may occur in almost any site and gout is a common accompaniment due to an increased level of uric acid in the blood.

On examination, the patient is plethoric with conjunctival injection and engorgement of the retinal veins on fundoscopy. Splenomegaly is present in 60–70% of patients and in about half the liver is also palpable. Hypertension is a feature in 25% of cases.

Investigations

There is an increase in the haemoglobin, red-cell count and haematocrit. More than 50% have a neutrophil leucocytosis and in a similar percentage there is a raised platelet count also. The neutrophil alkaline phosphatase score (NAP) is normal or increased and the bone marrow is hypercellular, often with an increase in megakaryocytes. The urate level is sometimes elevated. A definitive diagnosis is made by measurement of the red cell volume using ^{51}Cr labelled red cells and stress polycythaemia concluded by measurement of the plasma volume using ^{125}I albumin. Any cause of secondary polycythaemia should be excluded, this may necessitate an estimation of arterial oxygen saturation, intravenous pyelography to exclude a renal lesion and haemoglobin electrophoresis to exclude an abnormal haemoglobin with increased affinity for oxygen. Erythropoietin assay is not usually necessary but may be helpful in distinguishing secondary poly-cythaemia (where it is raised) from polycythaemia rubra vera (where it is not).

Management

In polycythaemia rubra vera the aim of the treatment is to keep the PCV around 45%. This may be done by venesection if the platelet count is less than $500 \times 10^9/l$ but otherwise the treatment should consist of chemotherapy with busulphan in a dose of 2–4 mg/day as required or, alternatively, radioactive therapy by means of an intravenous injection of radioactive phosphorus (^{32}P). This last is an excellent form of therapy and is probably the method of choice for severe cases. Allopurinol in doses of 300 mg daily is indicated if the urate level is high.

Conclusion

Median survival in polycythaemia rubra vera is only about 13 years. Thrombotic or haemorrhagic episodes are common and about 30% of patients progress to myelosclerosis and 15% to acute leukaemia, probably as a result of the natural history of the disease rather than therapy.

Myelosclerosis (myelofibrosis)

This disorder is due to proliferation of the stem cells with an increase in one or more cell lines and an associated reactive fibrosis in the bone marrow.

Clinical features

As in other myeloproliferative disorders, the older age groups are affected and the symptoms are those of anaemia together with a hypermetabolic state which gives rise to anorexia, weight loss and night sweats. Bone pain or joint symptoms due to gout occasionally occur and some patients suffer from haemorrhagic episodes. The spleen is usually grossly enlarged and there is frequently associated enlargement of the liver.

Investigations

Examination of the peripheral blood reveals anaemia with an increase in the white cells or platelets although they may become reduced at a later stage of the disease. The NAP score is elevated and the blood film reveals a leuco-erythroblastic picture with characteristic 'tear drop' red cells. Bone marrow aspiration produces a dry tap but bone marrow trephine biopsy shows a hypercellular marrow with an increase in reticulin or collagen with thickening of the bony trebeculae in some patients; megakaryocytes are frequently increased. Serum folate levels are often reduced and as in polycythaemia rubra vera, the urate level may be increased. Sclerotic changes on bone radiography are rare.

Management

This consists of blood transfusions as required and folic acid supplements in a dose of 5–10 mg/day if deficiency has been demonstrated. Small doses of an alkylating agent such as busulphan 2–4 mg are of benefit if there is marked splenomegaly with hypermetabolic signs. Allopurinol 300 mg daily is indicated in those patients with high urate levels. Splenectomy is advised only where massive splenomegaly results in an extremely high blood transfusion requirement or severe pressure symptoms in the abdomen; specialist advice is advised before this procedure is undertaken.

Conclusion

The median survival is only 3–4 years, although some patients live much longer. The cause of death is usually haemorrhage or infection; a small minority develop acute leukaemia or other complications such as portal hypertension.

Essential thrombocythaemia

This is a disorder in which the predominating feature is a platelet count of over $1000 \times 10^9/l$ with relatively little change in the neutrophil or red cell count.

Clinical features

In addition to the raised platelet count there may be features suggestive of polycythaemia rubra vera or myelosclerosis but these are relatively minor. The spleen is enlarged in the initial stages but splenic atrophy may subsequently occur. Bone marrow examination confirms an increase in megakaryocytes, some of which may be abnormal.

Management

Therapy is by ^{32}P or alkylating agents such as busulphan, 2–4 mg per day.

Conclusion

This is a rare disorder which is often only a preliminary to the development of frank polycythaemia rubra vera or myelosclerosis.

6.5 DISORDERS OF WHITE CELLS

Agranulocytosis

If the total neutrophil count drops below $1 \cdot 0 \times 10^9/l$ serious infections may result and below $0 \cdot 5 \times 10^9/l$ they are almost inevitable. Agranulocytosis may be a manifestation of some other disorder (e.g. acute myeloid leukaemia) but drugs as a cause should always be excluded. They may act by suppressing the bone marrow or by acting as an 'innocent bystander' (*see* Drug-induced haemolytic anaemia, p. 346).

Clinical features

Recurrent infections with fever, malaise and weight loss occur. Oral ulceration is common and infections in the skin and perianal area may be particularly troublesome; the infections are usually bacterial but viral fungal and protozoal infections also occur. Cyclical neutropenia is a rare condition in which periodic agranulocytosis occurs at intervals of weeks or months with no obvious underlying disease.

Management

The underlying cause must be looked for and offending drugs should be removed. Hypersplenism may require splenectomy but is not usually performed unless the neutropenia is actually giving rise to recurrent infections. Treatment with appropriate antibiotics, antiviral or antifungal agents should be instituted vigorously but the use of these agents prophylactically is still controversial. Corticosteroid therapy may be beneficial if there is an autoimmune disease associated with the neutropenia as in Felty's syndrome but they should be used with caution since they may themselves increase the risk of infection.

If the granulocytes fall below $0.5 \times 10^9/l$ and if the patient has an infection and is running a high fever which fails to respond to antibiotics granulocyte transfusion should be given in a special unit equipped with a cell separator.

Infectious mononucleosis (glandular fever)

This disease is thought to be due to the Epstein–Barr (EB) virus. Antibodies to the virus are present in the blood of many people who have never had the clinical manifestations of glandular fever but who presumably have had a subclinical infection. Those particularly at risk are young people between the ages of 15 and 30, especially if they live in institutions such as nurses homes or boarding schools.

Clinical features

Some patients are asymptomatic but most complain of tiredness associated with generalized aches and pains, headache, fever with enlargement and tenderness of superficial lymph nodes. The spleen may be palpable below the costal margin. Some patients develop a maculopapular rash during the first 10 days but this is often quite transient. At least 50% of patients complain of a sore throat and a small percentage (5%) develop jaundice. Rarely haemorrhagic complications may ensue as a result of thrombocytopenia or DIC.

Investigations

There is a leucocytosis in the peripheral blood with a total white count of between $10–20 \times 10^9/1$, 60–80% of which are atypical lymphocytes, the so-called 'glandular fever' cells. These are thought to be T-cells reacting against B-lymphocytes that have been infected with the EB virus. After the first week of illness the Paul Bunnell test becomes positive and is an indication of the development of heterophil antibodies to sheep red cells. Absorption studies are required to distinguish these antibodies from similar ones present in serum sickness. The Monospot test is usually used as a screening procedure. A rising titre of EB virus antibody can be detected but is not necessary for diagnosis. IgM anti 'i' autoimmune haemolytic anaemia with a positive Coombs test and autoimmune thrombocytopenia are occasional complications. It must be remembered that patients with infectious mononucleosis occasionally develop a false positive Wassermann reaction.

Management

Most require only symptomatic treatment. Antibiotics are of no avail unless there is secondary infection of the fauces or tonsils but ampicillin should never be used since it causes a generalized drug rash in 90% of patients for reasons which are not fully understood. Corticosteroid therapy is not indicated unless there are autoimmune complications. Hepatitis is frequent and patients should avoid alcohol for 3 months.

Conclusion

Most patients recover after about a month but in some instances the disease drags on for weeks or months with intermittent episodes of malaise and general debility. Recovery, however, is the rule.

6.6   MALIGNANT BLOOD DISEASES

Almost all malignant blood diseases should be treated in special centres. The possible exceptions are chronic myeloid leukaemia and chronic lymphocytic leukaemia, but even these should be referred to special centres if the best results are to be achieved. They will, therefore, be discussed only briefly with the exception of the chronic leukaemias.

Acute leukaemia

About 50% of all leukaemias are of the acute variety. The common form in children is acute lymphoblastic leukaemia (ALL), while the common form in adults is acute myeloid leukaemia (AML), although both diseases may be seen in all age groups. The main clinical features are due to anaemia, thrombocytopenia and neutropenia and the diagnosis is based on the finding of large numbers of immature cells, mainly lymphoblasts or myeloblasts respectively in the peripheral blood and bone marrow. The management involves highly specialised techniques which include reverse barrier nursing, the use of intensive chemotherapy and, in some instances, bone marrow transplantation. These procedures result in long term survival and possibly cure in around 50% of children with acute lymphoblastic leukaemia, and in a smaller percentage of adults with acute myeloid leukaemia.

Chronic myeloid leukaemia

The peak incidence is in the middle aged although it can affect people of all ages. The hallmark of the disease is the Philadelphia (Ph') chromosome i.e. chromosome number 22 which is abnormal and may be found in all cell lines in the bone marrow (granulocytic, erythroid and megakaryocytic).

Clinical features

In the initial or chronic phase of the disease, the diagnosis is occasionally made accidentally on routine examination, but features of anaemia and a hypermetabolic state are usually present. These include pallor of the skin and mucous membranes, shortage of breath on exertion, tachycardia, fever, weight loss and night sweats. The spleen is enlarged and often markedly so and is sometimes associated with pain over the splenic area. High uric acid levels resulting in gout and a raised peripheral white cell count resulting in hyperviscosity may give rise to visual disturbances, drowsiness, disorientation and occasionally priapism. If the platelet count becomes reduced it may result in bruising and bleeding such as epistaxes. In at least 70% of cases the disease terminates in an acute phase (metamorphosis or blast cell crisis), when the picture becomes similar to that of acute myeloid leukaemia in 80% of cases and acute lymphoblastic leukaemia in the remaining 20%. The onset of this phase should be suspected when the disease becomes refractory to treatment that has previously been successful. It usually occurs after 3 or 4 years, but some patients live very much longer before the acute phase develops.

Investigations

The white cell count is markedly raised with a preponderance of cells of the granulocytic series in all stages of development but blast cells are few. The platelets may be increased in number in the early stages and there is some degree of normocytic anaemia in most patients. Other features in the peripheral blood include a low NAP score and basophilia. The bone marrow is hypercellular with a corresponding increase in granulocytic cells in all stages of maturation. Bone marrow should be sent to a cytogenetics laboratory for chromosome analysis in order to detect the Ph' chromosome.

Management

In the chronic phase, the disease is responsive to a number of drugs which include busulphan, thioguanine or 6-mercaptopurine, hydroxyurea and dibromomannitol. The usual drug used is busulphan in a dose of 4 mg daily until the white cell count is reduced to near normal levels; it should then be given sufficiently often to keep the white cell count at or about normal levels, i.e. $10 \times 10^9/l$. Alternatively, it may be combined in a dose of 2 mg daily with thioguanine 80 mg daily. Whichever regime is used, it is usual to give allopurinol 300 mg daily in an attempt to control hyperuricaemia. On such regimes the blood picture usually returns to normal and the spleen regresses but the bone marrow always remains rather hypergranular and the Ph' chromosome does not disappear from the affected cell lines.

The onset of the acute phase is an extremely serious development which almost always heralds death within a few weeks or months. In an attempt to avoid this outcome bone marrow transplantation has been undertaken in the chronic phase if the patient has a suitable donor and is under the age of 45. Such procedures and the management of the acute phase are best undertaken in special centres.

Conclusion

The natural history of this disease is always fatal although a few do live 10 years or more before developing the acute phase. The only real hope, however, of long-term survival is allogenic bone marrow transplantation undertaken in the chronic phase in remission.

Chronic lymphocytic leukaemia

This may occur in middle age, but is more commonly seen in the elderly and is more common in males than females. It results from an abnormal proliferation of lymphocytes (usually B cells but occasionally T cells) affecting the blood, bone marrow, lymph nodes, liver and spleen.

Clinical features

About one-fifth of patients are symptom-free and the diagnosis is made on a routine blood count; in others, there is symptomless lymphadenopathy and splenomegaly. Neutropenia and reduced immunoglobulin levels result in increased susceptibility to infection, such as herpes zoster, and exaggerated reactions to vaccination. Lymphoid tissue anywhere in the body may be involved including tonsillar tissue; involvement of the salivary glands is known as Mikulicz's syndrome. In some patients skin infiltration is present and in those patients with T-cell leukaemia, widespread reddening of the skin (*l'homme rouge*) is frequently present.

Investigations

The diagnosis is based on a lymphocyte count in the peripheral blood in excess of $5 \times 10^9/l$ in association with bone-marrow infiltration with mature lymphocytes of 30% or more. Anaemia and thrombocytopenia are only present in the later stages of the disease and generally signify a bad prognosis. Some patients develop autoimmune haemolytic anaemia with a positive Coombs test, or thrombocytopenia. Immunoglobin levels should be monitored but these seldom return to normal with therapy.

Management

The disease has been staged by Rai and his colleagues, as shown in *Table* 6.4. In stage 0, it is customary not to treat the patient unless there is evidence of progression, and it is probably justifiable to observe asymptomatic patients in stages 1 and 2 for some months to see if the disease is progressive before treatment is begun. Most patients respond to an alkylating agent such as chlorambucil in a dose of 5 or 10 mg daily, given intermittently, or cyclophosphamide 50 mg daily given intermittently. The

Table 6.4 Classification of chronic lymphatic leukaemia (Rai et al.)

Stage		
	0	Absolute lymphocytosis ($5 \times 10^9/l$)
	I	Lymphocytosis plus lymphadenopathy
	II	Lymphocytosis and splenomegaly and lymphadenopathy
	III	Lymphocytosis plus anaemia (not autoimmune haemolytic) plus splenomegaly or lymphadenopathy
	IV	Lymphocytosis plus thrombocytopenia (not autoimmune) plus splenomegaly or lymphadenopathy

usual procedure is to give the drug for periods of 2 weeks with a rest of 2 weeks between courses. Once a satisfactory response has been achieved the duration of each course of therapy and the dose may have to be tailored to the minimum dose required for control of the disease and can be discontinued altogether if complete remission is achieved.

Corticosteroids are of value if there is bone marrow failure presenting as anaemia or thrombocytopenia. In such patients 2 weeks of prednisolone in a dose of 50–60 mg daily preceding alkylating agents may be beneficial. Corticosteroids are indicated if there is evidence of autoimmune haemolytic anaemia or thrombocytopenia.

Total body irradiation has been used in some centres, particularly in the USA, with beneficial results and occasionally good results can be achieved by splenic irradiation. More commonly, radiotherapy is used to reduce large masses of lymph nodes causing pressure effects. Splenectomy is only undertaken in those patients with autoimmune haemolytic anaemia who do not respond to corticosteroid therapy or when the spleen is so large as to be causing severe intra-abdominal pressure and possibly hypersplenism.

Care should be taken to control recurrent infections by the administration of immunoglobulins in the form of plasma infusions or intramuscular or intravenous preparations of gammaglobulin at 2–4 weekly intervals. Other supportive therapy includes transfusions with red cells or platelets but granulocytes are seldom necessary.

Conclusion

Chronic lymphatic leukaemia is a more serious disease in many patients than is commonly supposed. The average survival is less than 5 years although some elderly patients with relatively benign disease may live much longer. Some unusual variants of chronic lymphatic leukaemia do exist. They include hairy-cell leukaemia, prolymphocytic leukaemia and T-cell leukaemia but these are best treated in special centres since their management presents particular problems.

Paraproteinaemias

Immunoglobulins consist of two light chains (kappa, k or lambda, l) and two heavy chains known as gamma (γ) alpha (α) or mu (μ) according to whether it is an IgM, IgA or IgM immunoglobulin respectively.

The types of paraproteinaemia and some of the salient features are shown in *Table* 6.5. They may be defined as those disorders manifested by a monoclonal protein in the serum or urine or both, which is an apparently

Table 6.5. Paraproteinaemia

	Possible paraprotein type
Malignant	
Myeloma	Light chain IgG IgA
Macroglobulinaemia of Waldenström	IgM
Cold haemagglutinin disease (CHAD)	IgMk
Lymphocytic lymphoma	IgG IgM
Chronic lymphocytic leukaemia	IgG IgM
Amyloidosis	Lambda (l) light chains
Heavy chain disease	α γ μ heavy chains
Benign	
Monoclonal gamma paraprotein	IgG IgA IgM

non-functioning immunoglobulin in whole or in part. The monoclonal nature of the paraprotein is usually determined by the presence of a sharp band on protein electrophoresis and the fact that there is only a single type of light chain present. The exception to this rule is heavy chain disease.

Multiple myeloma

It is rare to find this disease in patients under the age of 40. It is a neoplastic disorder characterized by a monoclonal paraprotein in the serum or urine, lytic bone lesions and malignant myeloma cells in the bone marrow.

Clinical features

The clinical features are produced either by tumour growth or by the paraprotein itself. Those due to tumour growth consist of bone pain, recurrent infections due to low levels of normal immunoglobulins in the peripheral blood, anaemia, thrombocytopenia and neutropenia. Tumour growth is also associated with increased osteoclastic activity resulting in hypercalcaemia and lytic bone lesions.

The paraprotein may result in a tendency to bleed due to interference with coagulation factors and platelet function. Increased levels of paraprotein may result in hyperviscosity leading to the hyperviscosity syndrome with mental confusion, fundal haemorrhages and visual failure, purpura and heart failure. About 5% of the patients develop amyloidosis with macroglossia or the carpal tunnel syndrome, or very occasionally diarrhoea. Other features of amyloidosis may include cardiomyopathy or peripheral neuropathy. This is as a result of light chain activity. A more common consequence of Bence Jones proteinuria is renal damage. Renal failure, together with infection and paraprotein escape from therapy, accounts for the majority of deaths.

Investigations

A paraprotein may be detected in the blood or urine of almost all patients. The frequency with which a particular type of immunoglobulin is involved is in proportion to the amount of immunoglobulin normally present in the serum, that is to say, IgG is the commonest followed by IgA and IgM. IgD and IgE are rare causes. Normal immunoglobulin levels are depressed. Bence Jones proteinuria is present in over 60% of patients. The bone marrow shows an increase in myeloma cells, usually over 10% and often over 30%, and radiological skeletal survey shows osteolytic lesions in more than 50% of patients.

The peripheral blood often shows anaemia of normochromic type but may occasionally be macrocytic due to folate deficiency. Thrombocytopenia and neutropenia are less common but the ESR is always elevated with the exception of some cases of Bence Jones myeloma, in which the paraprotein consists entirely of Bence Jones protein with no immunoglobulin abnormality. In some patients plasma cells may be found in the peripheral blood (plasma-cell leukaemia).

It is important to carry out a full biochemical profile with particular reference to blood urea and serum calcium levels and in some patients serum albumin level may be reduced.

Management

All patients should be rehydrated and asked to drink at least 3 litres of fluid a day. If hypercalcaemia is present, it may respond to rehydration or specific chemotherapy (*see below*). Some patients require corticosteroid therapy, e.g. hydrocortisone 200 or 300 mg daily, intravenous or oral phosphates, calcitonin or phosphonates.

Chemotherapy, in the form of melphalan 10 mg daily together with prednisolone 40 mg daily for 4–7 days and repeated every 3–4 weeks, should be given. The exact amount of treatment depends on the degree of depression of normal bone marrow elements which usually follows the administration of melphalan. Cyclophosphamide seems to be an equally satisfactory drug and may also be given in association with prednisolone. Allopurinol is indicated if the urate level is raised. Chemotherapy is less well tolerated in the presence of renal failure.

Those patients who fail to show a reduction in the paraprotein level in response to therapy of at least 50%, or who relapse after an initial response should be treated with Adriamycin in a dose of 50 mg intravenously and BCNU in a dose of 100 mg intravenously. If there is a satisfactory response to therapy it should be continued for at least a year after the paraprotein level reaches a plateau (i.e. remains at a steady level for at least 6 months). Plasmaphoresis is usually reserved for patients with severe hyperviscosity symptoms or intractable bleeding due to the paraprotein. Other forms of therapy that are required from time to time include neurosurgery, for the relief of spinal cord compression as a result of a wedge collapse of a vertebra, and X-ray therapy as an adjunct in such patients for palliative relief of bone pain.

Conclusion
Median survival is only about 3 years. Poor prognostic features are renal failure, anaemia and impaired physical activity.

Waldenström's macroglobulinaemia

This is a rare disease occurring in the older age groups and more commonly in men than women. It is characterized by a raised level of IgM paraprotein in the peripheral blood and infiltration of the bone marrow by lymphocytes and plasma cells. Bence Jones proteinuria and lytic lesions in the bones are rare.

Clinical features
The main features are those of the hyperviscosity syndrome which is a consequence of the high IgM level in the peripheral blood. The optic fundi show engorged retinal veins, exudates, haemorrhages and papilloedema. The patient complains of fatigue, weight loss, visual disturbances and confusion, together with central nervous system symptoms and signs, haemorrhages and heart failure. Raynaud's phenomenon is rare and usually indicates the presence of a cryoglobulin. Splenomegaly and lymphadeno-pathy may be detected.

Investigations
A normocytic, normochromic anaemia is common, often with a lympho-cytosis. The bone marrow shows a corresponding infiltration with

lymphocytes and plasma cells. The ESR is elevated due to the presence of a monoclonal macroglobulin (IgM) in the serum.

Management

The hyperviscosity syndrome can be successfully treated by plasmaphoresis using a cell separator. Some patients can be maintained by this procedure once every 2–4 weeks without any further therapy but most require additional therapy in the form of an alkylating agent, such as chlorambucil 5 mg/day or cyclophosphamide 50 mg/day given intermittently for 2-weekly periods with 2 weeks rest in between courses. Blood transfusions and antibiotics may be required for anaemia or infections, respectively.

Benign monoclonal gammopathy

If a paraprotein is found in low concentration in the peripheral blood in a patient who is symptom-free and with no evidence of bone marrow involvement or Bence Jones proteinuria and no lytic lesions on radiography of the bones then a benign monoclonal gammopathy is said to exist (*Table* 6.6). The concentration of paraprotein should not be more than

Table 6.6. Features of benign monoclonal gammopathy

	Benign	*Malignant*
Paraprotein level	< 10 g/l	$<$ or > 10 g/l
Bony lesion	—	+
Bence Jones protein	—	±
Progression	—	±
Plasma cells in bone marrow	$< 4\%$	$> 10\%$
Normal immunoglobulin levels	Normal	Reduced

10 g/l and there should be no evidence of an increase in this level when it is monitored during the coming months or years. It is particularly important not to overlook the possibility of a solitary plasmacytoma since this may be associated with similar findings. Both plasmacytoma and benign monoclonal gammopathy may progress to multiple myeloma in due course although in some instances it takes many years. A solitary plasmacytoma should be treated by radiotherapy either before or after surgical excision but no other treatment is required and no treatment is required for monoclonal gammopathy unless there is evidence of progression to multiple myeloma.

6.7   MALIGNANT LYMPHOMAS

These are neoplastic disorders in which there is enlargement of lymph nodes, spleen and other structures and in which biopsy shows characteristic replacement of normal lymphoid tissue by abnormal cells. They are divided into Hodgkin's disease, characterized by the presence of Reed–Sternberg cells in the biopsy, and non-Hodgkin's lymphoma in which the lymphoid tissue is replaced by abnormal lymphocytes or histiocytes.

Hodgkin's disease

This disease occurs in both sexes with one incidence peak in adolescence and early adult life and a second in middle age. It has been suggested that the first peak is due to a virus and that the second is a truly malignant disease but a viral aetiology has never been convincingly demonstrated at any age.

Clinical features

There is an enlargement of one or more groups of superficial lymph nodes, the disease often beginning in the neck. The nodes gradually enlarge and may reach a size of several centimetres in diameter before the patient seeks help. There is subsequent spread to other lymph nodes and possibly the spleen and eventually the disease may spread outside lymphoid tissue to involve any organ in the body. Involvement of the skin is rare and tends to be a late complication. Alcohol-induced pain is an occasional presenting complaint but is by no means specific. Systemic symptoms, when present, consist of fever, with a temperature of 38 °C or more (intermittent pyrexia is known as Pel–Ebstein fever), weight loss of more than 10% during the previous 6 months, and night sweats. Pruritus in the absence of other systemic symptoms is not very significant.

Investigations

Examination of the peripheral blood may show mild normocytic, normochromic anaemia, leucocytosis and eosinophilia, and the ESR is elevated. The bone marrow aspirate is involved only in about 10% of cases. Liver function tests, if abnormal, suggest spread to the liver; the alkaline phosphatase level is a particularly good indicator. Immunoglobulin levels are not depressed until the late stages of the disease, although cellular immunity may be impaired earlier on. Bone involvement with hypophosphataemia is uncommon. The definitive diagnosis is made by gland biopsy. Clinical staging is essential (*Table* 6.7) and this may necessitate a staging laparotomy in those patients who present clinically as stages 1 or 2. Other investigations used in the staging process include chest radiography, computer tomography, bone marrow trephine biopsy and liver biopsy. Scanning techniques with isotope or ultrasound may also have a role to play. The absence or presence of systemic symptoms should be noted and a designation, either A or B, applied respectively to the clinical stage.

Management

The principles of management are relatively simple but the patients are best treated at special centres. It is customary to employ radiotherapy for stage 1

Table 6.7. Clinical stages of lymphoma

Stage 1	One group of glands involved
Stage 2	More than one group of glands involved but on the same side of the diaphragm
Stage 3	Glands involved on both sides of the diaphragm, including splenic disease
Stage 4	Spread of the disease outside lymph nodes, e.g. bone marrow, liver
	A—absence, and B—presence of systemic symptoms
	Pathological staging takes into account histological information in addition to initial biopsy, e.g. at laparotomy.

and 2 disease and chemotherapy for stages 3 and 4. In certain selected groups both therapies may be required but in such patients there is an increased risk of the subsequent development of acute leukaemia. The standard form of chemotherapy consists of pulses of four drugs used in combination; mustine or cyclophosphamide, vincristine or vinblastine, procarbazine and prednisolone.

Conclusions

The prognosis for patients suffering from this disease has been revolutionized in the last decade. Five-year survival rates vary between 85 and 50%, depending on the stage of the disease, the precise histological picture, and the presence or absence of systemic symptoms on presentation.

Non-Hodgkin's lymphoma

The non-Hodgkin's lymphomas are usually of B-cell origin and may sometimes be accompanied by monoclonal gammopathy. In some patients the tumour is of T-cell origin and in these there is a high incidence of mediastinal and skin lesions. Clinical manifestations are more varied than in Hodgkin's disease. There is a close relationship with acute lymphoblastic and chronic lymphatic leukaemia but the term is usually reserved for those patients without leukaemia manifestations. At least six histological classifications have been produced in recent years but the main feature of them all is to separate those histologies which indicate a poor prognosis from those which indicate a good one.

Clinical features and investigations

The disease may occur at any age but is commonest in middle life. Other clinical features are similar to those found in Hodgkin's disease and staging investigations required are also the same as those for Hodgkin's disease. There is, however, one important difference in that laparotomy is carried out only where special indications exist since these diseases tend to be more disseminated as a result of haematogenous spread. Immunological investigations are more commonly abnormal than in Hodgkin's disease.

Management

This should be undertaken in special centres. Stage 1 and 2 disease is treated by radiotherapy as in Hodgkin's disease and is sometimes followed by adjuvant chemotherapy. Chemotherapy is the treatment of choice for advanced disease (stage 3 and 4) but adjuvant radiotherapy may be valuable for bulk disease. The chemotherapy used depends on the histology of the tumour. Good prognosis histology usually responds well to chlorambucil or a combination of cyclophosphamide, vincristine and prednisolone but poor prognosis histology requires drug regimes containing Adriamycin. This drug is often used in combination with cyclophosphamide, vincristine and prednisolone, but may be used with vincristine and prednisolone saving cyclophosphamide for subsequent regimes should relapse occur. Supportive therapy with antibiotics and transfusion of blood and blood products as required is necessary.

Conclusion

As in Hodgkin's disease, considerable progress has been made in recent years in the management of these disorders and 'cures' can be achieved in all groups, but unlike Hodgkin's disease, the prognosis is related more to histology than staging of the disease.

6.8 DEFECTS IN HAEMAOSTASIS

The haemostatic mechanism involves capillary contraction followed by adhesion of platelets to the damaged endothelial wall and subsequent platelet aggregation with the formation of a platelet plug. The blood coagulation mechanism then gives rise to the formation of fibrin at the side of the platelet plug with red cells to form a thrombus. Fibrin is produced either by activation of the intrinsic or the extrinsic coagulation system. Injury to endothelial cells results in the activation of coagulation factors in the intrinsic pathway sequentially (*Fig.* 6.4). Tissue damage, on the other hand, results in the activation of the intrinsic pathway. Both systems unite in the final common pathway in which activated factor X, platelet factor III, calcium and factor V all act together to convert prothrombin to thrombin. Thrombin then converts fibrinogen into fibrin. It is unlikely that, following an injury, both systems usually operate and therefore a defect in either pathway will result in abnormal haemostasis (*Fig.* 6.4).

Fibrin deposition is limited by the fibrinolytic mechanism. This operates by release of plasminogen activator from damaged tissues and this in turn converts plasmin. Plasmin then breaks down fibrin to form fibrin degradation products (*Fig.* 6.4). Capillary defects, deficiency in numbers or function of platelets, or an abnormality in the coagulation system may all be responsible for haemostatic defects.

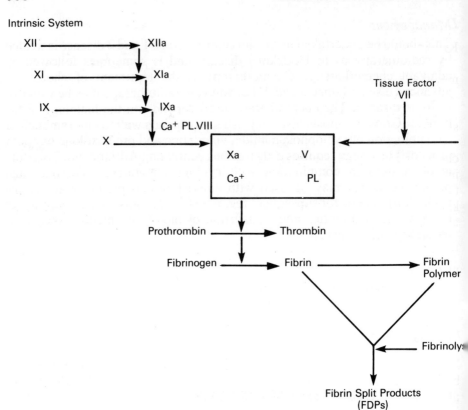

PL = Phospholipid; Ca⁺ = Calcium ions;
XII = Coagulation Factor XII;
XIIa = Activated Coagulation Factor XII.

Fig. 6.4. Coagulation cascade.

Investigation of bleeding disorders

Bleeding time	—	Platelet capillary defect
Platelet count	—	Thrombocytopenia
Prothrombin time	—	Defects of extrinsic coagulation pathway
Activated partial thromboplastin time	—	Defects in intrinsic coagulation pathway
Euglobulin clot lysis time	—	Fibrinolysis
Platelet function studies	—	Only required in presence of prolonged bleeding time and normal platelet count
Factor assay	—	Required if defect appears to be in intrinsic or extrinsic coagulation pathway

Defects of capillary endothelium

Known causes include:

1. Infections which give rise to toxic damage to the endothelium, e.g. meningococcal septicaemia.

2. Scurvy as a result of defective intercellular substance.

3. Senility because of poor supporting tissues to the vascular endothelium; steroid therapy may give rise to purpura for similar reasons.

4. The Henoch–Schönlein syndrome. Immune complex deposition occurs but the primary cause is often undetected although it may be an infection, or certain allergens. There is a leucocytoclastic vasculitis affecting the skin, particularly the skin over the legs and buttocks, the small intestine, kidneys and joints giving rise to painful arthropathy, severe abdominal pain and haematuria.

There is little effective treatment.

5. Simple easy bruising tends to occur in young women and is associated with no detectable abnormality.

6. Hereditary haemorrhagic telangiectasia is transmitted as an autosomal dominant which results in localized pinpoint swellings consisting of collections of non-contractile capillaries. These lesions are situated in the mucous membrane of the nose, mouth, tongue, lips and fingertips, and there are sometimes associated arteriovenous malformations in other organs of the body. The lesions become more progressive as the patient increases in age but seldom present a serious clinical problem before the age of 20. Epistaxes and intestinal haemorrhage result in iron-deficiency anaemia for which oral iron and blood transfusions may be required. There is no really effective therapy apart from this, although cauterization of the offending lesions has sometimes been performed.

Platelet abnormalities

Immune thrombocytopenia (ITP)

This is usually idiopathic but underlying diseases should be excluded, e.g. chronic lymphocytic leukaemia, Hodgkin's disease, autoimmune haemolytic anaemia and SLE. IgG antibodies sensitize the platelets to destruction by the spleen, but in some instances platelets are destroyed in other parts of the reticuloendothelial system, e.g. the liver.

Clinical features

The patient complains of an insidious onset of spontaneous or easy bruising, which may be associated with a tendency to bleed from mucosal surfaces, but central nervous system bleeding is rare. There is evidence of bruising and petechial haemorrhages are common but the spleen is usually impalpable and the presence of splenomegaly should give rise to considerable caution about the diagnosis.

Investigations

The platelet count is reduced while the bone marrow shows an increase in megakaryocytes, reflecting both an increased production of platelets by the bone marrow and an increased destruction in the peripheral blood. IgG platelet antibodies are present in the peripheral blood in most instances.

Management

In acute ITP spontaneous recovery is common, but it is seen only in a minority of cases with chronic ITP. Eighty per cent of such patients, however, respond to prednisolone in a dose of 60 mg daily given for a period of 3 weeks. Those patients who do not respond, or who relapse when steroid therapy is reduced, may require splenectomy. About 80 per cent of patients subjected to splenectomy have a satisfactory response. In those in whom steroids and splenectomy both fail, other immunosuppressive agents such as vincristine 1–2 mg intravenously at weekly intervals or azathioprine 50–100 mg/day may be used. Platelet transfusions are not indicated since they are rapidly destroyed in the same way as autologous platelets but they may be beneficial in life-threatening situations.

Drug-induced thrombocytopenia

Over 100 drugs have been implicated in drug-induced thrombocytopenia (*Table* 6.8). In most cases the drug combines with a plasma protein which then gives rise to an antibody and the production of immune complexes. These are adsorbed on to the platelets which are destroyed as 'innocent bystanders' (*see* Drug-induced haemolytic anaemia, p. 346).

Some drugs may depress the bone marrow with reduced megakaryocyte production, e.g. gold.

Investigations

As in ITP, thrombocytopenia is associated with abundant megakaryocytes in the bone marrow if the process causing thrombocytopenia is an immune one and with reduced megakaryocytes if it is due to bone-marrow depression.

Management

Every effort should be made to detect the offending drug (*see Table* 6.8). Withdrawal of the drug results in recovery within a few days. Platelet transfusions are not indicated unless there is life-threatening haemorrhage.

Symptomatic thrombocytopenia

Many malignant blood diseases such as leukaemia may be associated with symptomatic thrombocytopenia, but the primary condition is usually

Table 6.8. Platelet abnormalities

Thrombocytopenia	Thrombocytopathy

Drugs
Immune
    Quinidine
    Quinine
    Rifampicin
    Stipaphen, etc.
Marrow depressant
    Analgesic
    Antibiotics, etc.
    Diuretics
    Antithyroid drugs
 	
Idiopathic acute autoimmune
    Acute
    Chronic
 	
Symptomatic of other diseases
Immune
    Lymphoid malignancies
Marrow infiltrations
    Leukaemia
    Lymphoma
    Carcinoma
	Drugs
	    Analgesics (aspirin, indomethacin)
	
	Inherited
	    Glanzmann's disease, etc.
	
	Symptomatic
	    Uraemia
	    Myeloproliferative

obvious. Any condition resulting in significant splenomegaly may result in hypersplenism with splenic pooling of platelets; such patients usually respond well to splenectomy, but it should be remembered that few of them actually suffer from bleeding. Massive blood transfusions result in thrombocytopenia if stored blood is used, since such blood contains few platelets. It may be associated with bleeding which can be prevented by giving fresh blood or platelet concentrates.

Platelet function abnormalities

Rarely platelet numbers are normal but the bleeding time is prolonged and platelet function tests of adhesion and aggregation show typical inherited abnormalities, e.g. Glanzmann's disease and platelet storage pool disease. Acquired abnormalities due to drugs such as aspirin are common. The synthesis of thromboxane A2 which is a powerful platelet aggregating substance is inhibited. This action of aspirin has been utilized in the treatment of patients with certain thrombotic disorders such as transient ischaemic attacks (TIA). Trials have also been carried out in ischaemic heart disease but the results are inconclusive. Other antiplatelet compounds include sulphinpyrazone and dipyridamole.

Clinical features are similar to those of thrombocytopenia and are described above.

Bone marrow examination shows normal numbers of megakaryocytes and platelet antibodies are absent. Platelet function tests show characteristic abnormalities of adhesion and aggregation depending on the aetiology.

Management

A careful history should be taken and removal of offending drugs results in recovery in a few days. In patients suffering from inherited abnormalities platelet transfusions should be given to cover bleeding episodes or surgical intervention. It may be necessary to give packed red cells should the patient be anaemic as a result of bleeding.

Abnormalities of coagulation

Inherited deficiencies of any of the coagulation factors may occur but the commonest ones are Factor VIII (haemophilia A), Factor IX (haemophilia B or Christmas disease) and von Willebrand's disease, and even these are uncommon.

Haemophilia A

This occurs with a frequency of about 7 per 1 000 000. It is inherited in a sex-linked recessive manner and is due to a deficiency or absence of the coagulant part of the Factor VIII molecule (VIIIC).

Clinical features

Only boys are affected and bleeding begins after circumcision or when the infant begins to move around. Haemarthroses and musculoskeletal bleeds are common; other forms of bleeding occur less commonly but cerebral haemorrhage is rare. The severity of the condition relates to the level of Factor VIII present in the blood which is constant and only those patients with a Factor VIII level of less than 1% are considered to be severe.

Investigations

Both the activated partial thromboplastin time (APTT) and the prothrombin time (PT) are prolonged, indicating a defect in the intrinsic pathway of the coagulation system. This is associated with a prolonged whole blood clotting time and a low level of factor VIIIC on assay; the bleeding time is normal.

Management

Management should be undertaken in special centres where the principles of treatment include Factor VIII replacement therapy and physiotherapy to affected joints, together with orthopaedic advice as required. Regular dental care is essential in order to prevent the need for extraction. Many patients now administer their own Factor VIII therapy at home and some have prophylactic Factor VIII injections, but large doses of factor VIII seem to be responsible for the high incidence of hepatitis which occurs in these patients.

Conclusion

The life expectancy has much improved in recent years with increasing usage of Factor VIII concentrates, but with a high incidence of hepatitis some patients may go on to develop cirrhosis. However, the commonest cause of death is cerebral haemorrhage, particularly in the older age groups.

Christmas disease (Factor IX deficiency)

This condition is clinically almost identical to haemophilia A but it is much less common. The APTT and whole blood clotting time is as in haemophilia A, but the Factor VIII level is normal. Instead there is deficiency of Factor IX. The principles of management are the same as for haemophilia A.

Von Willebrand's disease

This is inherited as an autosomal dominant and affects males and females equally. It is due to a deficiency of Factor VIII-related antigen (VIII RAg) which is the other and larger part of the Factor VIII molecule and is synthesized by vascular endothelial cells. Deficiency of VIII RAg results in low VIIIC level with which VIII RAg complexes and impaired platelet adhesion to subendothelial connective tissue.

Clinical features

Unlike haemophilia, there is a tendency to bleed from mucous membranes, the gastrointestinal tract and superficial cuts and bruises, but haemarthroses are rare.

Investigations

The bleeding time is prolonged because of impaired platelet function. There is a low level of both Factor VIIIC and Factor VIII RAg and platelet aggregation with ristocetin and platelet adhesion to glass beads is impaired.

Management

Cryoprecipitate is a protein fraction of blood containing not only VIIIC but also VIII RAg and is the treatment of choice.

Conclusion

All patients with inherited coagulation disorders should be treated in special medical centres since their management requires both special laboratory and clinical expertise.

Acquired coagulation defects

Acquired coagulation defects may arise from defective synthesis of coagulation factors, disseminated intravascular coagulation or the presence of inhibitors.

Defective synthesis of coagulation factors

Vitamin K is required for the synthesis of Factors II (prothrombin), VII, IX and X. Vitamin K_1 is found in fat-soluble foods and bile salts are necessary for its absorption. Deficiency may be found in patients with coeliac disease and conditions in which an excess of bile salts is lost from the body, e.g. high intestinal fistula and disease of the lower ileum. This is because bile salts participate in an enterohepatic circulation which involves their reabsorption from the lower ileum. Haemorrhagic disease of the newborn reflects the inability to the liver to synthesize coagulation factors together with low stores of vitamin K_1. The condition is more marked in premature infants.

Defective synthesis may also occur as a result of severe liver disease and the defects may be divided into two: those dependent on vitamin K and the remainder. Obstructive jaundice with lack of bile salts in the intestine causes defective absorption of vitamin K but hepatocellular disease involves a defect in the synthesis of other clotting factors including Factor V. Fibrinogen levels are reduced only in the most severe cases and in the late stages of the disease. This may be due to the fact that fibrinogen is produced not only by the Kupffer cells of the liver but also by the extrahepatic reticulo-endothelial system. On the other hand, patients with obstructive jaundice tend to have an increase in plasma fibrinogen levels and this is also seen in some tumours of the liver, either primary or secondary. The increased levels in obstructive jaundice are thought to be due to associated infection whereas those due to deposits in the liver probably occur as a result of a non-specific response to tumours anywhere in the body. A similar increase is seen for example in patients with active Hodgkin's disease.

Clinical features and investigations

The clinical features are those of any coagulation defect. On investigation the prothrombin time is prolonged and factor assays will indicate low levels of appropriate clotting factors.

Management

Prophylactic vitamin K_1 should be given to newborn babies in a dose of 1 mg intramuscularly and 5 mg orally daily for adults. If the patient is actually bleeding, it should be given in a dose of 1 mg intramuscularly every 6 h to infants and 10 mg subcutaneously daily to adults. Fresh frozen plasma which contains the appropriate coagulation factors may also be administered. If the bleeding has been severe, then a blood transfusion may be required.

Disseminated intravascular coagulation (DIC)

This condition may occur in a wide range of diseases. The precise mechanisms are uncertain, but it results from one of two factors: the release of thromboplastin-like substances into the blood or the activation of the intrinsic coagulation mechanism. 'Triggers' include thromboplastins from inflamed necrotic or neoplastic cells, the toxins of venomous animals, bacterial endotoxin, immune complexes, particular agents and lipids. The result is a widespread occlusion of small vessels by fibrin thrombi with the consumption of coagulation factors and platelets which in turn leads to a bleeding diathesis. Variable numbers of fragmented red cells may be seen in the blood film, but the three cardinal features of the condition are lowered serum fibrinogen levels, raised fibrin degradation products (FDPs) in the blood and thrombocytopenia. The FDPs appear in high concentration as a result of increased fibrinolysis consequent upon excessive fibrin deposition.

The common causes are complications of pregnancy such as abruptio placentae, septic abortion, eclampsia and a retained dead fetus. It may also occur as a result of operations on the lungs, prostate or neoplastic tissue, or it may complicate cardiac arrest, burns and the crush syndrome. Other precipitating causes are overwhelming general infections by viruses or bacteria, and the subacute variety is sometimes seen as a complication of neoplasms of prostate, breast, lung, gastrointestinal tract, cervix and pancreas, and some forms of leukaemia. The haemolytic uraemic syndrome in childhood or adults is an example of the condition in which the microthrombi are localized to renal vessels. Renal failure is accompanied by haemolysis and red-cell fragmentation but the aetiology is unknown.

Clinical features

These may be protean as a result of the tendency to small vessel occlusion in the brain, pancreas, heart, lung, kidneys and almost any other site in the body. The most characteristic feature, however, is a tendency to haemorrhage from various mucosal surfaces and cutaneous bruising. Venepuncture wounds or any other wounds are often sites of blood loss and symptoms of the underlying disease may be apparent.

Investigations

The cardinal investigations are coagulation profile together with a platelet count, FDPs and euglobulin clot lysis time. If there is an associated haemolytic element (microangiopathic haemolytic anaemia) examination of the blood film will show fragmented red cells.

Management

The principles of treatment are removal of the cause and control of the disseminated intravascular coagulation by treatment of the underlying disease. The use of heparin to prevent further microthrombi has now been largely abandoned but platelet concentrates or transfusions of plasma or fresh blood to provide coagulation factors may be beneficial.

FOR FURTHER READING

Bloom A. L. and Thomas D. (ed.) (1981) *Haemostasis and Thrombosis.* Edinburgh, Churchill Livingstone.

Hardisty R. M. and Weatherall D. J. (ed.) (1982) *Blood and its Disorders,* 2nd ed. Oxford, Blackwell Scientific Publications.

Hoffbrand A. V. and Lewis S. M. (1981) *Postgraduate Haematology,* 2nd ed. London, Heinemann.

Hoffbrand A. V. and Pettit J. E. (1984) *Essential Haematology,* 2nd ed. Oxford, Blackwell Scientific Publications.

Israels M. G. and Delamore I. W. (ed.) (1976) *Haematological Aspects of Systemic Disease.* Philadelphia, Saunders.

Thompson R. B. (1977) *Disorders of the Blood.* Edinburgh, Churchill Livingstone.

Thompson R. B. (1979) *A Short Textbook of Haematology,* 5th ed. London, Pitman.

Williams W. J. et al. (ed.) (1983) *Haematology,* 3rd ed. New York, McGraw-Hill.

7 Common Disorders of the Kidneys and Urinary Tract

R. G. Henderson

7.1 INTRODUCTION

This section is intended for those who have not worked in a specialist renal unit and so have no 'feel' for managing patients with some form of kidney disease. There will be no problem if there is a local expert available but where there is none the unfortunate doctor is forced either to soldier on alone, relying on advice culled from textbooks, often feeling very insecure as a result, or else having to refer the patient to a Specialist Centre.

Hopefully the advice offered here will allow an inexperienced doctor to cope better with some of the problems that can occur.

The choice of topics has been made either because the condition is common or because, in the author's experience, it is less than expertly managed by most doctors. Thus the frequency dysuria syndrome is clearly justified because it affects up to 50% of women at some stage of their life. Similarly, in hospital practice an elevated blood urea is a fairly frequent event which seems to suggest a diagnosis of renal failure to most doctors even though the biochemical abnormality may reflect nothing more than dehydration resulting from inappropriate fluid therapy. Experience suggests that many doctors have a hazy understanding of this latter subject so that it has been included in a very simplified way which should help to avoid disasters. Similarly the relationship between drugs and kidney is one which most doctors have some vague knowledge of yet this is rarely enough to be translated into sound practice, so the topic is reviewed here. Finally the major syndromes of acute and chronic renal failure and the nephrotic syndrome are dealt with, recognizing the fact that they are relatively uncommon. The approach adopted is in no way comprehensive as with other textbooks but rather is pragmatic so that an inexperienced practitioner should be able to start off patient management with some degree of confidence that the patient will not get into serious trouble. Following along these lines the indications for referral to a renal unit are given.

Aspects of the patient's history and clinical findings, particularly where they are relevant to the diagnosis, are included in the individual topics and will not be discussed further. However, it is worth making a few points about the laboratory and radiological investigations which are used in the management of patients with renal disease.

Biochemistry

Laboratory results are often the basis for diagnosing renal failure, particularly an elevated blood urea. However, it is influenced by factors other than the glomerular filtration rate (GFR) (*Table* 7.1), so that it is often impossible to predict renal function from a simple measurement of blood urea. The plasma creatinine is a much more reliable guide so that in general a level of 170 mmol/l or more in males or 150 mmol/l or more in females is indicative of a reduced GFR. Note, however, that GFR is markedly reduced before the plasma creatinine concentration becomes significantly elevated. It is in fact possible, by applying a mathematical formula, to convert the plasma creatinine directly into a measure of GFR in an individual, but in practice this is rarely necessary and the reciprocal of the plasma creatinine will suffice (*see below*). Measurement of creatinine clearance which involves estimation of the level in both blood and urine together with a collection of a 24 h urine sample (with the inaccuracies that are likely to occur) is only necessary where there is some form of progressive muscular disease, the patient is postoperative, obese, oedematous, or there are rapid changes in GFR before an equilibrium has been established.

Table 7.1. Common causes of high and low blood urea

Elevated blood urea	Depressed blood urea
1. Reduced glomerular filtration rate	1. Reduced protein intake
2. Hypercatabolism	2. Liver failure
3. Gastrointestinal bleeding	
4. Drugs, e.g. corticosteroids	

Because of the inaccuracies in interpretation of blood urea plasma creatinine is used when following the progress of a patient's renal disease. Since the relationship between plasma creatinine and glomerular filtration rate is curvilinear the reciprocal of plasma creatinine is used since this has a straight-line relationship to GFR. However, even the plasma creatinine itself provides some indication of change although in moderate renal failure a greater than 30% change is necessary to indicate a change in GFR and even in advanced renal failure changes of the order of 18% are necessary before it is significant. The indications for other biochemical tests are dealt with in the relevant sections except to note here the importance of urine testing. It is interesting how often inspection of the notes of a patient with renal failure reveals previous attendances when an abnormal urinary sediment has been documented by the nursing staff. Indeed in the majority of hospitals urine testing is performed routinely by the nursing staff yet is ignored by medical colleagues. Embarrassment and occasionally fatalities will be avoided if one gets into the habit of always insisting on seeing the results of urine tests of any new patients seen either as an inpatient or outpatient.

Radiology

Although isotopic studies have an important role to play in the management of patients with renal disease they will not be considered further here since a full range is only available in specialist centres.

In general intravenous urography employing the use of a high dose of contrast medium and nephrotomography provides a great deal of extremely useful information. It may be employed even in those with very poor renal function (GFR ≤ 3 ml/min). From the films it will be possible to tell whether the patient has one or two functioning kidneys, their size, whether there is evidence of obstruction and if so its site, whether there is irregularity of kidney outline or abnormalities of the pelvicalyceal system suggestive of conditions such as analgesic nephropathy, tuberculosis or reflux nephropathy. The density of the nephrogram should not be relied upon as an index of renal function. Where GFR is poor so that the pelvicalyceal system has not become visible at 2 h the patient should have a 24 h film taken since this may reveal an unsuspected obstruction.

In general there are few problems with the investigation and in particular 'allergic' type reactions are extremely uncommon. Specific problems that require action are: (1) Chronic renal failure or myeloma where dehydration may lead to problems. (2) Diabetes mellitus, particularly where there is renal impairment since intravenous urography may result in accelerated deterioration in kidney function and is best avoided unless there is a strong indication.

With the improved quality of ultrasonic scanning and a greater experience in its use it has become possible to diagnose obstruction by this technique rather than having to resort to urography. Investigations will provide information on the size, and to some extent the shape, of the kidneys together with any gross abnormalities of the pelvicalyceal system or the presence of stones. However, unlike the urogram it will not indicate whether or not an individual kidney is functioning.

7.2 DYSURIA, FREQUENCY SYNDROME OR URETHRAL SYNDROME

Episodes of dysuria predominantly affecting women occur extremely commonly so that somewhere between one-third and one-half will have suffered from at least one episode at some stage during life. While not serious the symptoms are responsible for a great deal of misery and unless a sound diagnostic approach is used, management will be unsatisfactory.

Clinical features

Patients suffer from episodes of dysuria, frequency, urgency and strangury lasting anything between 24 hours and a week. The patient is usually afebrile and although suprapubic pain may occur loin pain is uncommon. Physical examination is unhelpful and the vital investigation is an MSU taken during an attack since it is only by doing this that one may establish whether a patient falls into the first or second group as shown in *Fig.* 7.1.

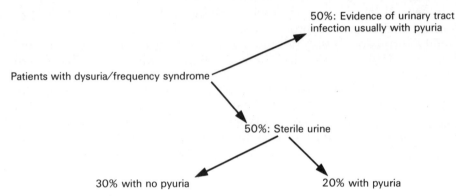

Fig. 7.1.

Table 7.2. Drugs used in dysuria

Drugs	Daily dose for long-term use
Trimethoprim	100 mg nocte
Nitrofurantoin	50 mg nocte
Ampicillin	250 mg nocte
Methenamine hippurate	1 g b.d.

Management

PATIENTS WITH EVIDENCE OF URINARY TRACT INFECTION

Where infection is present it should be treated with an appropriate antibiotic such as trimethoprim administered in the normal dosage (i.e. 200 mg b.d.) for not more than 3 days. The likelihood of recurrent attacks may be diminished by advising:

1. High fluid intake (including before retiring at night) to produce 2 litres of urine/24 h.

2. Frequent (every 3 h during the day) and complete bladder emptying.

3. Bladder emptying within ½ hour of sexual intercourse if this seems to be an aetiological factor.

Where these measures are ineffectual an intravenous urogram should be performed to exclude anatomical abnormalities or renal calculi (perhaps suggested by persistent proteus infection) which require urological advice. In the absence of these, low-dose antibiotics or urinary antiseptics may be necessary to keep the urine sterile (*Table* 7.2).

PATIENTS WITHOUT EVIDENCE OF URINARY TRACT INFECTION

This group is less satisfactory to manage. In those with sterile pyuria:

1. Exclude tuberculosis by sending three early morning urine specimens to the laboratory. If this is confirmed, treatment with ethambutol 15 mg/day as a single dose with rifampicin 600 mg and isoniazid 300 mg should be given. Once sensitivities are available it should be possible to stop the ethambutol and treat with rifampicin and isoniazid only. An intravenous urogram should be performed at the start of therapy and repeated 6 months later to exclude tuberculous stenosis of the ureters or bladder.

2. Consider gonococcal or chlamydial infection. This is best excluded by referral to a genitourinary clinic.

3. Where there is no evidence of infection re-check the history to make sure that analgesic nephropathy has not been overlooked.

In the remainder a cause for irritation should be sought and the patient should be advised:

1. To avoid nylon tights and nylon briefs.

2. To avoid using vaginal deodorants, perfumed soaps, etc.

If symptoms persist a gynaecological cause should be sought and if there is none, urethral dilatation should be considered since this sometimes improves symptoms.

7.3 ACUTE PYELONEPHRITIS

Like the urethral syndrome this is a condition predominantly affecting females during child-bearing years, yet is very much less common. Where a patient suffers from recurrent attacks there is usually an anatomical abnormality or some other explanation such as a calculus or hydronephrosis, predisposing to infection.

Clinical features

This is an acute illness with high fever, loin and suprapubic pain, dysuria and frequency; malaise and vomiting are common. The urine is often discoloured and smelly. A careful history may reveal certain relevant points:

1. Where there is a previous history of loin pain during micturition spreading from the suprapubic region up to one or both loins then this suggests reflux nephropathy.

2. There may be a history of pain starting in the loin and radiating down to the testicle or groin associated with haematuria or grit or gravel indicating stone disease.

3. Loin pain may be non-specific, occurring at periods of high fluid intake and associated with urinary sediment, suggesting a diagnosis of hydronephrosis.

4. Progressively worse loin pain associated with malaise and weight loss may indicate a renal tumour. It may also be possible to elicit symptoms which suggest abnormal bladder function which can predispose to infection,

calculus formation and reflux. Enquiry should be made about the initiation of micturition, strength of stream and terminal dribbling together with the capacity to pass a significant amount of urine after micturition thereby suggesting either ureteric reflux or a bladder diverticulum.

Examination often reveals a toxic and unwell patient but specific features are usually absent. Occasionally there may be an enlarged kidney resulting from a tumour or hydronephrosis or, alternatively, there may be evidence of lower urinary tract obstruction with a palpable bladder.

Investigations

1. Urine culture should be set up before antibiotic therapy is started but emergency microscopy is unnecessary. Dipslides, if available, are perfectly adequate.

2. Full blood count and ESR. Leucocytosis and raised ESR favour infection rather than calculi.

3. Blood cultures. These may be positive.

4. Urea and electrolytes, plasma creatinine. Evidence of some degree of renal impairment is common.

5. Liver function tests. These may be abnormal in septicaemia thereby falsely implicating the biliary tract.

6. Straight radiograph of the abdomen. Renal calculi may be visible.

7. Ultrasound of abdomen may demonstrate obstruction.

Management

The diagnosis depends on demonstrating infected urine but often treatment is warranted before results are available. Since similar symptoms, signs and laboratory findings may be seen in cholecystitis, appendicitis, salpingitis, acute glomerulonephritis, hydronephrosis, renal calculi, etc. the diagnosis should be questioned in those with no urinary tract symptoms. The possibility of urinary obstruction due to calculi, necrotic papillae or neoplasia should be borne in mind and may be excluded by ultrasound examination.

Once a urine specimen and blood for culture have gone to the laboratory the patient may be started on treatment, with the choice of antibiotics depending on the local prevalence of resistance. In the UK ampicillin is now unsuitable and intramuscular gentamicin or a cephalosporin should be used. After 24–48 h when bacterial sensitivities are available therapy can be changed to an oral agent such as trimethoprim, ampicillin, a cephalosporin amoxycillin or Augmentin. Nalidixic acid and nitrofurantoin are best avoided. A high fluid intake is important, often initially by intravenous infusion because of nausea and vomiting. Care is necessary in those with evidence of renal impairment and a reduced urine output. Where urinary obstruction is demonstrated a urological opinion should be sought.

An intravenous urogram is warranted after the acute attack has settled in males after the first attack or in females who have had multiple episodes.

Acute pyelonephritis occurring during pregnancy poses a particular problem. It occurs most commonly in those with an asymptomatic urinary infection and is particularly liable in those who are multigravidae and from lower social classes. The likelihood of its development will be reduced by screening all pregnant women regularly to ensure that there is no evidence of urinary infection and where it exists treating it with ampicillin or nitrofurantoin. Tetracycline should be definitely avoided under these circumstances. Where acute pyelonephritis develops the patient will need treatment along the lines given above taking care to choose those antibiotics which are least likely to cause problems.

Indwelling catheters
In these circumstances the urine will inevitably be infected and antibiotic therapy should be reserved for systemic illness such as fever and loin pain. The start of treatment should coincide with a change of catheter in the following ways: 100 ml 0·02% chlorhexidine is instilled into the bladder and left for ½ hour with the catheter clamped. After emptying the bladder the catheter is changed and antibiotic treatment should be given for 5 days. There is no case for long-term antibiotic therapy since this will result in colonization with resistant organisms. The urine may be kept socially acceptable by bladder washouts performed anything from daily to weekly depending on the state of the urine. Normal saline is as good as anything for this purpose.

Antibiotic prophylaxis against bacterial endocarditis
Antibiotics in the form of ampicillin 500 mg and gentamicin 80 mg (assuming a 70 kg patient) should be given with the premedication and continued for 24 h to those undergoing any urological procedure who are at risk from bacterial endocarditis.

7.4   ACUTE RENAL FAILURE

Some knowledge of the causes of acute renal failure is necessary if management is to be logical.
    1. Prerenal (functional renal failure), e.g. dehydration.
    2. Renal
       a. Acute tubular necrosis
       (or vasomotor nephropathy)
       Haemorrhage ⎫
       Burns   ⎪
       Septicaemia ⎬ Potentially
       Hypotension ⎪ reversible.
       Dehydration ⎭
       etc.

  b. Intrinsic renal disease, e.g. glomerulonephritis
  c. Drugs, e.g. cephaloridine
  d. Toxins, e.g. carbon tetrachloride, ethylene glycol
  e. Vascular insufficiency.
 3. Postrenal obstruction.
  a. In the kidneys, e.g. uric acid or sulphonamide crystals or myeloma.
  b. Ureters, e.g. by retroperitoneal fibrosis, calculi, tumour, etc.
  c. Bladder, e.g. by benign prostatic hypertrophy or tumour.

Clinical features

The patient may be ill because of conditions which may predispose to the development of acute tubular necrosis, e.g. hypotension, resulting from a bleeding peptic ulcer. It is important that this is recognized since, if it is uncorrected, it may result in acute renal failure, making management more difficult.

 Less commonly, acute renal failure may be seen in a previously fit individual who becomes oliguric perhaps because of acute glomerulo-nephritis or ingestion of a toxin. The history often provides clues if the above list is remembered. In general examination is unhelpful but evidence of dehydration (*see Table* 7.14) should be sought carefully. In general, blood pressure is normal in acute tubular necrosis but raised in condition such as poststreptococcal glomerulonephritis.

Table 7.3. Differentiation between prerenal failure and acute tubular necrosis

	Prerenal	Acute tubular necrosis
Urine: plasma osmolality (mOsmol/kg)	>1·1	0·9–1·05
Urine: plasma creatinine	>15	>15
Urine: plasma urea	>10	>10
Response to fluid loading plus diuretic	Diuresis	None

Management

PRERENAL FAILURE OR ACUTE TUBULAR NECROSIS?

This question often arises when a patient presents. The biochemical tests in *Table* 7.3 may help to distinguish between the two, but they are time-consuming and may not always provide a definite answer. If the history is less than 48 h the situation may be resolved by assessing the effects of diuretic therapy after fluid loading. This is performed as follows: a central venous pressure line is inserted and normal saline is infused until the CVP reads +5–8 cm of water. The infusion is then stopped and the patient is given frusemide 40 mg intravenously or 200 ml of 20% mannitol. If there is no diuresis acute tubular necrosis has occurred.

MANAGEMENT OF ESTABLISHED RENAL FAILURE

Exclude obstruction by ultrasound examination; if this is present surgical advice should be sought. Where uric acid or sulphonamide are thought to be responsible the urine should be alkalinized with bicarbonate and fluid intake should be at least 2 litres/24 h.

If there is no reversible cause, management is aimed at *keeping the patient alive until the kidneys recover;* there is nothing that can be done to speed up this process.

1. Water and sodium balance.
   24-hour intake of water and sodium should be restricted as follows:
   Water: 500 ml + volume equal to previous 24 h urinary output.
                + volume equal to any other loss (e.g. vomit).
                + allowance of 100 ml/1 °C if patient is pyrexial.
   Sodium: Restricted to replacement of loss in urine (and any other loss, such as vomit or diarrhoea). In severely oliguric patient sodium intake may have to be as little as 10–20 mmol/24 h.

If replacement is correct the patient's weight will remain constant or will fall slightly because of muscle breakdown (*see* p. 398).

Frusemide may increase urine output thus making fluid balance easier, but will do nothing to hasten recovery of the kidney.

2. Rising blood urea

The rate of rise of the blood urea may be reduced by restricting protein intake to approximately 0·5 g/kg body weight, provided that calorie intake is also satisfactory. It must be remembered that the sodium content of food will usually have to be restricted. Where a patient is hypercatabolic because of major injury (e.g. burns or the crush syndrome), protein breakdown will be inevitable and uninfluenced by protein restriction so that a low protein diet in these circumstances will only result in negative nitrogen balance. The use of androgens to retard catabolism has fallen into disuse with availability of dialysis; it is of no benefit in those who are hypercatabolic. Intravenous feeding may be necessary in some patients but restriction of fluid intake will often be the limiting factor. It is important not to equate the volume of nutrient with that of water since 1 litre of 20% Intralipid only contains 750 ml of water and 1 litre of Aminoplex 14 940 ml of water.

3. Potassium balance

Hyperkalaemia is common, particularly in those who are hypercatabolic, where it affects both the heart and the skeletal muscle leading to asystole and weakness respectively. The ultimate effect is a ventricular arrest so that treatment is essential as follows:

    a. Protect the heart with a slow intravenous injection of 10 ml 10% calcium gluconate.

    b. Lower the plasma potassium with an intravenous injection of 100 ml 50% glucose plus 20 units of soluble insulin. The effect lasts for about 4 h.

c. Give a potassium binding resin, such as calcium resonium 15 g q.d.s. given orally or rectally. In the latter case it may be necessary to wash out the resin after a few hours to prevent it from solidifying and causing rectal ulceration.

4. Risk of infection

The incidence is increased so that bladder catheterization, even though it may facilitate measurement of output, should be avoided and intravenous infusion kept to a minimum. Regular cultures of urine, blood and any skin lesions, etc. should be made and if there is evidence of infection prompt treatment with an appropriate antibiotic should be undertaken, modifying the dose as necessary.

5. Documentation

The measurements indicated in *Table* 7.4 should be made and are best recorded in a flow chart.

Table 7.4. Useful indices to monitor acute renal failure

Observation	Frequency	Comments
Fluid balance	Daily	Often inaccurate
Weight	Daily	Accurate, simple
Urea and electrolytes	Daily	
Haematocrit	Daily	Guide to blood volume
Na^+ content of urine + any other losses, e.g. vomit	Daily	Essential for assessing Na^+ requirements
Plasma proteins	Weekly	Indication of nutritional status

The period of oliguria compatible with recovery of kidney function may be as long as 12 weeks and despite conservative measurements the patient's condition may deteriorate. Dialysis may be necessary if:

a. The clinical condition deteriorates.

b. There is pulmonary oedema.

c. Hyperkalaemia is not controlled by the measures outlined (particularly likely in hypercatabolic patients).

In non-specialist units peritoneal dialysis may be performed but this should not be undertaken by the inexperienced but rather the patient should be transferred to a specialist centre.

Recovery

This is heralded by a polyuric phase where the patient passes large volumes of urine containing increased amounts of sodium and potassium. Unless these are replaced the patient may become dehydrated leading to a further episode of acute tubular necrosis. The urine contains little in the way of urea and creatinine so that the blood levels of these will continue to rise for the first few days of a diuretic phase.

At some stage it is necessary to establish whether tubular function has returned. This is done by weighing the patient and measuring his urea and electrolytes. Fluid intake is then restricted to see if the urine volume falls. If this does not happen replacement is continued and a further assessment is made in a few days.

7.5   CHRONIC RENAL FAILURE

The pathophysiology of chronic renal failure is different from that in acute renal failure in that there is a progressive loss of nephrons leaving a functionally normal nephron population which is subjected to an increased osmotic load. Urine output is maintained and because of the chronicity remarkable adaptation occurs so that the patient often presents late.

The common causes shown in *Table* 7.5 are largely of academic interest since in the majority there is no effective treatment. Where the patient

Table 7.5. Common causes of chronic renal failure

Causes	Incidence
Glomerulonephritis	50–60%
Interstitial nephropathy (including pyelonephritis, analgesic nephropathy, uric acid nephropathy, etc)	20–30%
Polycystic disease of kidneys	10%
Others	10%

presents with very advanced disease it may be difficult or impossible to make a diagnosis but it may be gleaned from a careful history. Pyelonephritis is likely in those who in childhood have suffered from persistent enuresis, intermittent fever, dysuria, loin pain, or episodes of non-specific ill health. A past history of acute glomerulonephritis may be elicited so that the patient may recall an illness characterized by swelling of the face and ankles which led to a long period of absence from school. The loin pain as described on p. 381 may point to stone disease, hydronephrosis, or reflux nephropathy. Similarly a history suggesting abnormal bladder dysfunction is important. Enquiry should be made into all systems since the renal involvement may be part of a multisystem disease such as diabetes mellitus, multiple myeloma, amyloid or tuberculosis. The family history is important since the patient may suffer from polycystic disease, renal tubular acidosis leading to renal calculi, Alport's syndrome, etc. A drug history should also be taken since not only are certain agents directly nephrotoxic while others, in certain individuals, cause an acute interstitial nephropathy. Analgesic abuse should be sought in every patient presenting with chronic renal failure. It is often useless to ask the patient directly if he or she has been taking analgesics since this may lead to a denial, but rather enquiry should be made whether the patient has suffered from any chronic pain for which they have bought medicines from the chemist. The length of time that 100 tablets lasts the patient usually gives a guide to intake. Unlike other conditions which cause chronic renal failure the outlook in analgesic nephropathy is less gloomy since if the patient can be persuaded to stop the habit then renal function may stabilize or even improve. Finally, occupation history may point to exposure to nephrotoxins such as lead, dry cleaning fluids, etc. There is increasing evidence to suggest that hydrocarbons may be associated with an increased incidence of glomerulonephritis.

Clinical features

The patient may be known to have chronic renal disease for which he is under regular medical review. Polyuria and nocturia become complicated by tiredness and lethargy as the disease progresses. Symptoms may arise from complications such as anaemia, hypertension and renal osteodystrophy.

The patient may present for the first time with advanced renal failure and under these circumstances it may be difficult to be certain whether the problem is one of acute or chronic renal failure. *Table* 7.6 outlines the important distinguishing features.

Table 7.6. Important distinguishing features between acute and chronic renal failure

	Acute renal failure	*Chronic renal failure*
Urine volume	Reduced (often 400 ml/24 h)	Normal but history of nocturia and polyuria
Symptoms in relation to biochemical abnormality	Early	Late
Haemoglobin	May be normal	Normochromic, normocytic anaemia
Kidney size on X-ray	Normal or increased	May be decreased (<10 cm in length)
Hand X-ray	Normal	May have subperiosteal erosions

Physical examination is very often unhelpful in establishing the diagnosis but enlarged kidneys may suggest hydronephrosis, polycystic disease of the kidneys or tumour and an enlarged bladder may point to outflow obstruction. There may be evidence of multisystem disease pointing to diabetes mellitus or disseminated lupus erythematosus. Finally, the presence of peripheral neuropathy, renal osteodystrophy, etc. should be sought.

Management

Exclude reversible causes of chronic renal failure; in practice renal function may stabilize or improve if obstruction is relieved, analgesic abuse stopped,

Table 7.7. Potentially reversible causes of chronic renal failure

Causes of renal failure	Reversible/irreversible	Diagnosis
Glomerulonephritis	Virtually all irreversible	Renal histology
Pyelonephritis	Irreversible	IVU Micturating cystogram
Analgesic nephropathy	Partially reversible	History of analgesics IVU
Polycystic disease	Irreversible	Family history IVU
Disseminated lupus erythematosus (DLE)	May respond to steroids	Renal histology ANF, DNA
Polyarteritis nodosa (PAN)	May respond to steroids	Renal histology Renal arteriography
Obstruction	May reverse when obstruction relieved	Ultrasound
Myeloma	Irreversible	Protein strip Bence Jones protein in urine Bone marrow

or disseminated lupus erythematosus and polyarteritis nodosa are treated (*Table* 7.7).

If there is no reversible cause, management is aimed at:
1. Preserving renal function for as long as possible.
2. Preventing or treating complications of uraemia.

Deteriorating GFR will inevitably occur because of the underlying renal disease; the object is therefore to prevent the rate of decline from being accelerated by:

1. Dehydration
2. Hypertension ⎬ Water and sodium balance
3. Heart failure
4. Urinary tract infection
5. Drugs, such as tetracycline, cephaloridine

WATER AND SODIUM BALANCE

Chronic renal failure is associated with both an inability to excrete a large sodium load (so that oedema, hypertension, and heart failure ensue) or to conserve sodium even in the face of additional losses from diarrhoea or vomiting so that dehydration occurs. Either state needs correction until the patient is oedema-free without postural hypotension (*see* p. 396). Most patients tend to retain sodium so that their dietary intake is restricted to a no-added salt diet (50 mmol/24 h) or if necessary a low sodium intake (20 mmol/24 h). Frusemide (up to a maximum of 1 g/day, without potassium supplements) may be necessary in some patients, who despite sodium restriction, remain oedematous. Hypertension is treated initially with a beta-blocker to which a vasodilator such as hydralazine or prazosin is added. No change in dose is necessary. Instead of a beta-blocker, captopril may be used in combination with a loop diuretic to induce sodium depletion. The patient should attend as a day case for the first 25 mg dose since profound hypotension may occur. The dose may be increased to a maximum of 150 mg/day since at levels greater than this side effects, particularly loss

Table 7.8. Useful parameters in follow-up of patients with chronic renal failure

Observations	Interval	Comments
Weight	Each clinic visit	Good guide to fluid balance
Urea and electrolytes	Each clinic visit	
Plasma creatinine	Each clinic visit	
Full blood count	Each clinic visit	
Calcium phosphate	Each clinic visit	Follow progress of renal
Alkaline phosphatase		osteodystrophy
MSU	Each clinic visit	Exclude infection
24-hour urinary protein	3/12–6/12	Important in relation to protein intake
Plasma proteins	3/12–6/12	Nutritional status
Chest X-ray	6/12	Heart size and lung fields
Radiological skeletal survey	12/12	Assess renal osteodystrophy

of taste and skin rashes, are likely to occur. A large dose of diuretics, e.g. frusemide 80 mg b.d., is often necessary for the captopril to exert its hypotensive action. If despite diuretic therapy and sodium restriction the hypertension persists a vasodilator should be added.

URINARY TRACT INFECTIONS

Urinary tract infections are treated as previously discussed avoiding nephrotoxic drugs, although it must be admitted that as a cause for deterioration in renal function they are extremely uncommon.

Prevent or Minimize Uraemic Complications. The idea is to prevent or minimize uraemic complications in the following systems. Appropriate monitoring is outlined in *Table* 7.8.

Haemopoietic system. Anaemia is inevitable. Haematinics should only be given if there is evidence of deficiency. Transfusion is best avoided since its effect is only transient.

Cardiovascular system. Heart failure and hypertension have been discussed. Pericarditis usually settles spontaneously and only if tamponade develops is aspiration necessary. Indomethacin provides symptomatic relief if pain is severe.

Gastrointestinal system. Nausea and vomiting are common and are related to the blood urea. A low protein diet will prevent or diminish these symptoms and until recently its use would not have been advocated until the blood urea was 30 mmol/l or greater. However, there is recent evidence to suggest that the use of a low protein diet may also do something to prevent deterioration in renal function and it may well be that it will be advocated much earlier in the disease. Protein intake should be increased in those with proteinuria by an equivalent number of grams as the 24 h urinary protein loss. Peptic ulceration is more common and may be treated with cimetidine. Uraemia colitis tends to be a terminal event only.

Endocrine system. Most hormone levels are depressed but in practice infertility in women and impotence in men are the main problems. Bromocriptine may be of benefit in those with high prolactin levels, but its use may be complicated by hypotension.

Calcium metabolism. Phosphate retention is common and should be treated with phosphate binding agents such as Alu-Cap 1–3 taken ¼ h before each meal. Hyperparathyroidism may be treated with 1 α-hydroxycholecalciferol 0·5–2 μg/day with weekly checks of the plasma calcium in those who are normocalcaemic, but parathyroidectomy is necessary in those with hypercalcaemia. Osteomalacia responds poorly to treatment with 1 α-hydroxycholecalciferol and vitamin D may be more effective. Since therapy is likely to be complicated by hypercalcaemia, expert advice should be sought.

Pruritus. This is difficult to control but may respond to chlorpheniramine (4 mg q.d.s.) or cyproheptadine (4 mg q.d.s.). It may improve following parathyroidectomy.

Neurological system. Peripheral neuropathy may occur and worsen despite dialysis treatment. It improves following a successful renal transplantation. Coma and convulsions occur with high levels of blood urea. In general the following points should be borne in mind.

1. It is better to seek expert advice from a regional centre early, since it will be easier for them to decide whether the patient is ultimately suitable for dialysis treatment if the patient is seen relatively fit and well. In addition, shared management can be achieved providing the opportunity to learn.

2. The possibility of dialysis treatment should not be discussed with the patient before referral to a specialist unit; refusal is much more difficult under these circumstances.

3. Intravenous infusions should not be put into the forearms since valuable vascular access sites may be permanently destroyed. The dorsum of the hands should be used.

7.6 NEPHROTIC SYNDROME

This syndrome, which is characterized by proteinuria, hypoalbuminaemia and oedema, may result from:

1. Some form of glomerulonephritis.
2. A multisystem disease such as diabetes mellitus or disseminated lupus erythematosus (DLE).
3. Immune complex disease arising from infection such as malaria, syphilis, SBE, etc.
4. Drug therapy, e.g. penicillamine.

Clinical features

Apart from ankle oedema there is nothing specific in the history except in those patients with a multisystem disease, such as DLE or amyloid. Frothy urine correlates with proteinuria.

Physical findings

The physical findings are those of oedema in the absence of heart or liver disease. There is significant proteinuria on ward testing. The differential diagnosis includes:
1. Congestive cardiac failure.
2. Constrictive pericarditis.
3. Liver disease.
4. Protein-losing enteropathy.

Management

Specific treatment will depend on an accurate diagnosis, often from renal histology. Biopsy probably should be undertaken where there are facilities for light and electron microscopy and immunofluorescence. However, some causes may be diagnosed by simple tests without resorting to biopsy and these should be excluded first (*Table* 7.9).

Although there are accepted dosage schedules for corticosteroid administration in minimal change glomerulonephritis and DLE it is probably better to transfer the patient to the care of the relevant specialist.

Symptomatic treatment:

This therapy is aimed at reducing oedema and is applicable to all patients with the nephrotic syndrome.

1. Diuretic therapy to increase the excretion of sodium and water. Frusemide in an initial dose of 40 mg/day should be taken with the aim of producing a weight loss of 0·4 kg/day. If this has not been achieved with 160 mg of Lasix, spironolactone 50 mg b.d. may be added.

2. It is traditional to prescribe a high protein diet for patients with the nephrotic syndrome. The basis for this is suspect and patients are often overwhelmed by the amount they are expected to eat, so that it is probably necessary only to give 70–80 g of protein/24 h for an adult to prevent a negative nitrogen balance.

3. Sodium restriction in the form of not adding salt at the table and avoiding salty foods such as bacon, packet soups, sausages, etc.

4. Protein infusion; there is a small group of patients in whom diuretic

Table 7.9. Causes of nephrotic syndrome which may not require biopsy confirmation

Causes of nephrotic syndrome	Diagnostic features	Specific treatment
Minimal change glomerulonephritis	Selective proteinuria in children (but often not in adults) (IgG/transferrin clearance ratio)	Corticosteroids
Disseminated lupus erythematosus (DLE)	ANF, DNA binding	Corticosteroids ± azathioprine
Diabetes mellitus	History of diabetes retinopathy common	None
Amyloidosis	History of underlying condition (e.g. rheumatoid arthritis). Rectal biopsy	Remove source of suppuration if possible
Drugs, e.g. penicillamine, troxidone	Drug history	Discontinue drug

therapy does not provoke a diuresis or does so at the expense of the circulating blood volume rather than the oedema fluid. Infusion of 2–4 bottles of plasma protein fraction (preferably salt-poor) is often all that is needed to initiate a diuresis which once started will continue despite the fact that the plasma albumin falls progressively once the infusion has been stopped.

The aim of therapy is to render the patient oedema-free, institute specific treatment if applicable and to follow the renal function over the long term, instituting therapy for chronic renal failure should this become necessary. Suggested routine investigations are shown in *Table* 7.10.

Complications

Infection was a common cause of death in the preantibiotic era. There is a loss of immunoglobulins in the urine and the oedema fluid makes an ideal culture medium. A high index of suspicion is important.

There is a thrombotic tendency—spontaneous venous thrombosis is common in the nephrotic syndrome, particularly in those with amyloidosis. Where the renal veins are affected there may be:

1. Worsening of the nephrotic syndrome.
2. Acute renal failure.
3. Hypovolaemia—the most dramatic form is seen in children where there is sudden loss of blood volume leading to hypotension and shock. If not treated with plasma protein infusion, death may ensue. In adults diuretic therapy may result in fluid loss from the blood compartment and this

Table 7.10. Routine investigations in the nephrotic syndrome

Observation	Interval	Remarks
Weight	Daily if inpatient or each clinic visit	Guide to fluid balance
Urea and electrolytes	2 × weekly or each clinic visit	
Plasma creatinine		
Haematocrit	2 × weekly or each clinic visit	Guide to changes in blood volume
Plasma proteins	Weekly or each clinic visit	Guide to nutritional status
24 h urinary protein	2–3 monthly	Guide to either natural history or response to treatment

may be detected by a progressive rise in haematocrit and blood urea. Again plasma protein infusion will help to correct this.

7.7   DRUGS AND THE KIDNEY

Renal damage due to drugs

Many drugs may be responsible, solely or in part, for renal damage which may manifest itself as asymptomatic proteinuria, the nephrotic syndrome, acute or chronic renal failure. The mechanisms whereby renal disease may occur are outlined in *Table* 7.11 but the list is not comprehensive since it is always being expanded. It is important for a clinician to remember all the drugs which may be responsible for renal problems and the best safeguard is a high index of suspicion. Where proteinuria or renal failure develops unexpectedly the drug therapy should be examined. Renal toxicity may be elicited by consulting the *Extra Pharmacopoeia* (*Martindale*) or by telephoning the manufacturer.

Prescribing in renal failure

Extra care is required when prescribing for a patient with renal failure. The following questions need answering:

1. Is the drug excreted by the kidneys?
2. If it is, then is its use likely to be accompanied by side-effects?
3. In the treatment of urinary tract infection in a patient with renal failure does the antibiotic get into the urine in a high enough concentration?

Table 7.11. Mechanisms of drug-induced renal damage

Mechanism of renal injury	Examples of drugs	Comments
1. Hypercatabolism, elevated blood urea	All tetracyclines *except* doxycycline	No direct effect on kidneys but elevated blood urea may lead to vomiting and dehydration
2. Prerenal failure	Diuretics, laxatives	
3. Obstructive uropathy	Uric acid, sulphonamides	Crystalluria in tubules
	Methysergide, methyldopa	Retroperitoneal fibrosis
	Anticoagulants	Retroperitoneal haemorrhage
4. Glomerular damage *a.* Lupus syndrome	Procainamide, hydralazine, INAH	Present with proteinuria
b. Membranous glomerulonephritis	penicillamine, gold, troxidone	Present with proteinuria
5. Interstitial nephropathy *a.* Hypersensitivity reaction with fever	Penicillins, frusemide, thiazides	Renal biopsy is necessary to confirm the diagnosis
b. Potassium depletion	Diuretics, laxatives	
c. Hypercalcaemia	Vitamin D and its analogues	
6. Proximal tubular damage	Aminoglycosides, polymixins, cephaloridine, amphotericin	Disadvantages of toxicity often outwayed by benefits of treating infection
7. Papillary necrosis	Analgesic combinations	The actual drugs which can cause this remain uncertain

Table 7.12. Creatinine clearance as a guide to severity of renal functional impairment

Severity of impairment	Creatinine clearance (ml/min)
Mild	>30
Moderate	10–20
Severe	<10

If a drug is renally excreted, problems are more likely the worse the renal function, which in practice is assessed by measurements of creatinine clearance (*Table* 7.12).

If dosage modification is necessary this may be achieved by:
1. Using the usual maintenance dose but giving the drug less frequently.
2. Reducing the dose while maintaining the dosage interval.
3. Reducing the dose and increasing the dosage interval.

Most hospitals have guidelines for the use of antibiotics in patients with renal failure and it is sensible to consult the microbiology department before prescribing. If no local advice is available the drug manufacturer should be consulted. Toxicity should be avoided if blood concentrations are measured where this is possible (e.g. gentamicin or vancomycin).

Do not be put off prescribing a drug such as gentamicin because of its nephrotoxicity. It is true that the plasma creatinine may increase slightly but will often be offset when treating a septicaemia caused by a gentamicin-sensitive organism. *Table* 7.13 outlines the more common problems seen in prescribing for patient with renal failure; the list is not complete and it is important to check before prescribing rather than assume that there will not be problems.

7.8 SIMPLIFIED INTRAVENOUS THERAPY AND SOME DISTURBANCES OF ELECTROLYTE AND ACID–BASE BALANCE

In general it is difficult to have electrolyte problems with oral fluids but this is easily achieved with intravenous therapy so that hyponatraemia is often due to the unthinking use of 5% dextrose solution. Careful assessment of the patient's needs and accurate replacement is the key to avoiding problems. It is possible to manage the majority of patients using a combination of 5% dextrose and normal saline solutions to which potassium chloride is appropriately added providing that one remembers:

1 g NaCl = 17 mmol of Na^+ and Cl^-, so that 1 litre normal saline contains 150 mmol Na^+ and Cl^-.

Similarly 1 g KCl = 13 mmol of K^+ and Cl^-, so that a 10 ml ampoule containing 1·5 g KCl will have 20 mmol of K^+ and Cl^-.

When a regimen of intravenous therapy is planned the following questions should be considered:

1. At the start is there any evidence of overhydration or dehydration (*Table* 7.14)?

If there is then this should be corrected first.

The treatment of overhydration is as follows:

a. Restrict sodium intake.

b. If plasma sodium falls below 115 mmol/l restrict water intake to less than 1 litre/24 h.

c. If necessary give a diuretic to increase urinary water and sodium loss.

d. Continue treatment till the patient is oedema-free.

The treatment of dehydration is as follows:

a. In clinical practice this is almost always a mixed deficiency of sodium and water and should be replaced with saline. Use normal saline unless

Table 7.13. Problems in prescribing for patients with renal failure

Drug	Modification	Comments
Antibiotics		
Cephalosporins	Avoid cephaloridine. Others safe but dosage interval may need to be increased	Toxicity of cephaloridine increases if given with frusemide
Aminoglycosides, e.g. gentamicin	Reduce dose and/or increase interval	Nephrotoxicity plus ototoxicity, blood levels essential
Tetracycline	Avoid all except doxycycline	Cause elevation of blood urea
Ethambutol Rifampicin Isoniazid	Modify in moderate and severe renal failure	
Penicillins	Safe	Possible toxicity with long-term use
Trimethoprim	Safe	
Metronidazole	Safe	
Carbenicillin	Dosage interval increased	
Vancomycin	Dosage interval increased markedly	
Nitrofurantoin Nalidixic acid	Avoid in moderate and severe renal failure	Inadequate urine concentration
Diuretics		
Thiazides	Do not use in moderate and severe renal failure	No natriuresis if GFR 20 ml/min
Loop diuretics		Effective to GFR 3 ml/min
Aldosterone/triamterene	Avoid in moderate and severe renal failure	Cause K^+ retention
Other drugs		
Digoxin	Dose interval increased	Measure digoxin levels
Allopurinol	Reduce dose to 100 mg daily in severe renal failure	
Hypotensives	No dose change	Renal function may deteriorate temporarily when treatment started

Table 7.14. Indicators of state of hydration

Dehydration	Overhydration
Weight loss	Weight gain
Postural hypotension	Peripheral oedema
Skin turgor ↓ *	Pulmonary oedema
Intraocular pressure ↓	
Haematocrit ↑	Haematocrit ↓

*Skin overlying the cheek is the best site for assessment. A dry tongue is a poor sign of dehydration and is more commonly caused by mouth breathing

the plasma sodium is below 115 or greater than 150 mmol/l when twice normal or ½ normal saline respectively should be used.

b. Assess patient's replacement needs from loss in weight (if this is known) so that if this is 2 kg then 2 litres of saline should be given.

c. Fluid should be replaced over 24–48 h. The patient should be examined frequently for signs of pulmonary oedema and in the elderly, where risk of heart failure is greatest, central venous pressure monitoring is recommended.

d. Continue intravenous fluids until postural hypotension is abolished and the jugular venous pressure is approximately +4 cm.

2. Once the patient is in balance what sort of fluid and how much should be given to maintain the status quo?

In an average-sized adult this may be achieved safely with a daily intake of 1·5 litres consisting of 1 litre of 5% dextrose and 500 ml of normal saline with the addition of 15 mmol of potassium chloride to each 500 ml.

3. If there are additional fluid losses (e.g. diarrhoea, vomiting, fistula drainage) how should these be replaced?

These fluid losses all have a high sodium content and in a patient with normal renal function should be replaced with an equal volume of normal saline since the kidneys will perform any fine adjustments which are necessary. Where there is moderate or severe renal impairment it is better to analyse the sodium and potassium concentration of the fluid and replace it exactly using a combination of 5% dextrose and normal saline to which potassium chloride is added since under these circumstances the kidney will be unable to adjust electrolyte concentration.

It is particularly important to correct hypokalaemia since this may give rise to:

a. Cardiac dysrhythmias in the presence of digoxin.

b. Weakness of skeletal muscles.

c. Impaired renal tubular function leading to polyuria.

d. Intracellular acidosis and extracellular alkalosis.

These abnormalities will persist until the potassium is replaced. This is best done orally using either effervescent potassium chloride tablets

(12 mmol of potassium per tablet) or Slow K tablets (8 mmol of potassium per tablet), but if oral therapy is not possible then an intravenous infusion of potassium chloride added to dextrose or saline infused at a maximum rate of 20 mmol in 4 h should be used.

If a patient is maintained on a correct intake of water and electrolytes then the following will be observed:

a. The weight will remain steady or if muscle wasting occurs it will fall slightly (0·3 kg/day).

b. Plasma sodium and potassium concentrations remain within the normal range.

c. The haematocrit is unchanged.

d. Oedema or postural hypotension will not develop.

Hypernatraemia

This is likely in two situations:

1. Inadequate water intake in an unconscious or semiconscious patient. This is usually the result of a tube feed high in sodium and containing inadequate water in a patient who is unable to protest. Use of a more dilute feed will overcome this problem.

2. Diabetes insipidus. Patients present with polyuria, unlike those with psychogenic polydypsia (usually psychologically disturbed females) in whom thirst is the predominant feature. The diagnosis should be obvious in those who have suffered a head injury or have a brain tumour, but will be more difficult where there are no such clues.

Table 7.15. Diagnosis of diabetes insipidus

Body weight	Urine for osmolality	Plasma for osmolality
Before water deprivation		
and at 4 h	0-1 h	½ h
6 h		
7 h	6–7 h	6½ h
8 h	7–8 h	7½ h
Values at the end of the test	Normals	Diabetes insipidus
Plasma osmolality	<300 mOsmol/kg	>300 mOsmol/kg
Urine osmolality	>600 mOsmol/kg	<600 mOsmol/kg
Urine flow rate	<0·5 ml/min	Little change (often >2 ml/min)

After excluding impaired GFR (by measuring creatinine clearance) and a tubular abnormality (due to hypokalaemia, hypercalcaemia, or drug therapy with lithium, amphotericin, etc.) the diagnosis is confirmed by performing a water deprivation test. The protocol is given in *Table* 7.15 and the test is continued for 8 h or until 3% of the body weight is lost, whichever is the sooner. A patient should not be given prior warning so that he is not afforded the opportunity of drinking excessively in anticipation. The criteria necessary to make the diagnosis are shown in *Table* 7.15 and where failure to concentrate the urine has been shown, then nephrogenic diabetes insipidus may be distinguished from a posterior pituitary lesion by the intramuscular injection of 2 μg of DDAVP. Urine is collected ½ hourly for a further 2 h and in the former there will be no change in urine osmolality and body weight will continue to fall whereas in the latter the urine will become concentrated. Management of diabetes insipidus will not be considered further here. Nephrogenic forms are usually congenital but may occur with acquired tubular lesions such as papillary necrosis. Treatment is unsatisfactory but it is important to ensure that the patient does not become dehydrated.

Hyponatraemia

Where this is not due to the injudicious infusion of 5% dextrose then this occurs in:

1. Secondary hyperaldosteronism which is probably the commonest cause of hyponatraemia in clinical practice. It may be due to:
   a. Congestive cardiac failure
   b. Renal failure
   c. Nephrotic syndrome
   d. Cirrhosis.

It is imperative to appreciate that in an oedematous patient the total body sodium must be increased even though the plasma sodium concentration is often low. Under these circumstances, any attempt to treat hyponatraemia with a saline infusion is likely to have dire consequences.

2. Salt-losing nephropathy. This is seen most often in interstitial nephropathy, such as chronic pyelonephritis, and manifests itself with postural hypotension, weight loss and deterioration in renal function. Intravenous saline may be necessary followed by slow sodium tablets in some patients.

3. Addison's disease and pituitary failure which require the appropriate endocrine investigations and subsequent replacement if necessary.

4. The syndrome of inappropriate ADH secretion. Patients suffer from weakness, lethargy, mental confusion and convulsions. The diagnosis should only be considered if points 1–3 above have been excluded, and is confirmed by demonstrating urine osmolality which is greater than that of plasma. Treatment consists of restricting fluid intake to less than a litre a day. Where the plasma sodium is less than 115 mOsmol/l infusion of twice normal saline may be necessary.

Metabolic acidosis

This may be apparent clinically with sighing respiration or may be detected by a low plasma bicarbonate and confirmed by blood gas analysis. The common causes are:

1. Aspirin ingestion
2. Diabetic ketoacidosis
3. Lactic acidosis
4. Renal failure.

The management of the first three will not be considered here except to stress that where acidosis is treated with intravenous bicarbonate it will result in hypokalaemia (as potassium is driven back in to the cells) which if uncorrected can result in death. Acidosis in renal failure where it becomes symptomatic is an indication for dialysis treatment but other than this no action is warranted.

Metabolic alkalosis

The only cause which will be considered here is loss of gastric juices whether by vomiting or aspiration. This is corrected by replacement with normal saline but it is important to correct the potassium deficiency at the same time.

FURTHER READING

General

Black, Sir Douglas and Jones N. F. (1979) *Renal Disease,* 4th ed. Oxford, Blackwell Scientific Publications.
Earley L. E. and Gottschalk C. W. (ed.) (1979) *Struss and Welt's Diseases of the Kidney,* 3rd ed. Boston, Little Brown.

Chapter 7.2

Whitworth J. A. (1982) Urinary tract infection and reflux nephropathy in adults. *Med. Int.* **24,** 1096–1100.
Asscher A. W. (1977) Therapy of urinary tract infection. *Br. Med. J.* **1,** 1332–1335.

Chapter 7.4

Evans D. B. (1978) Acute renal failure. *Br. J. Hosp. Med.* **19,** 597–604.
Clarkson A. R. (1980) Acute renal failure. *Medicine* **25,** 1279–1284.
Adu D. (1982) Acute renal failure. *Med. Int.* **23,** 1079–1085.

Chapter 7.5

Meyers A. M. (1982) Conservative management of chronic renal failure. *Med. Int.* **23,** 1086–1088.

Chapter 7.6

Parfrey P. S. (1982) The nephrotic syndrome. *Br. J. Hosp. Med.* **27,** 155–162.

Chapter 7.7

Cove-Smith R. (1982) Drugs and the kidney. *Med. Int.* **24,** 1124–1138.
Bennett W. M., Muther R. S. and Parker R. A. (1980) Drug therapy in renal failure—dosing guidelines for adults. *Ann. Intern. Med.* **93,** 62–89, 286–325.

Chapter 7.8

Eastham R. D. (1983) *A Guide to Water, Electrolyte and Acid-base Metabolism.* Bristol, Wright.

8 Common Endocrinological Problems

R. D. Hill

8.1 INTRODUCTION

Disorders of the endocrine system are often slow in onset and run a prolonged course. They are often life-long disorders which bring long-term complications. Early diagnosis and treatment are essential. A delay in diagnosis may prolong unnecessary suffering and produce permanent irreversible structural changes (e.g. in diabetes mellitus and myxoedema).

The importance of *a good history* with selected direct questioning cannot be over-emphasized. This must be followed by *a careful clinical examination* and *investigation* to confirm the diagnostic suspicions aroused during history taking. Only a high index of suspicion that endocrine disease may be present will result in early diagnosis and prevent missed or delayed diagnosis. Much information can be obtained by asking simple direct questions regarding the patient's appetite, weight and micturition.

Obesity with an apparently 'normal' appetite is a common problem in clinical practice. The presence of polyuria, polydipsia, pruritus vulvae, balanitis or other infection should suggest diabetes mellitus to the physician yet the diagnosis is so often missed because the relevant questions are not asked. The presence of obesity might also suggest the polycystic ovary syndrome, but this is very rare and hypothyroidism is much more likely to be the cause if an endocrine abnormality is present. Rarely, Cushing's syndrome causes difficulty, particularly if the patient is hypertensive and hirsute. Mainly truncal obesity and the presence of a 'buffalo hump' would support the diagnosis. However, most patients have obesity due to inappropriate calorie intake rather than endocrine abnormality. A simple steroid suppression test will differentiate between simple obesity and Cushing's syndrome. If dexamethasone 2 mg orally is given at 10.00 p.m. and a plasma cortisol measured at 9.00 a.m. the following morning then Cushing's syndrome can be excluded if the plasma cortisol is less than 60 nmol/l (2·17 μg%).

Weight loss accompanied by a normal or increased appetite should suggest a diagnosis of hyperthyroidism. However, in the elderly the weight loss may be insignificant and fatigue may be the main complaint. Weight loss with polyuria which at first may be seen as nocturia (only discovered if the relevant question is asked) should suggest diabetes mellitus. Weight loss with a poor appetite, lethargy, fatigue, pigmentation and a low blood pressure should also suggest the possibility of Addison's disease. However, this is a rare disorder. Because of its rarity the diagnosis is usually initially missed. If you do not consider a diagnosis, you cannot make it.

Increased frequency of micturition associated with increased volume of urine voided (polyuria) and thirst (polydipsia) should suggest the possibility of diabetes. If glycosuria is absent then hypercalcaemia or chronic renal failure must be considered.

The classic clinical picture and appearance of acromegaly represents a 'spot diagnosis'. Hypopituitarism is rare and may be more difficult to 'spot'. However, this diagnosis is important since hypoglycaemia leading to coma and death may result from a delayed or missed diagnosis. Full treatment of these and other rare endocrine conditions, particularly those related to delayed puberty, virilism, hirsutism and amenorrhoea are beyond the scope of this book.

Diabetes mellitus, thyroid disease and hypercalcaemia constitute the most common endocrine abnormalities seen by the general physician in both primary and secondary health care.

8.2 DIABETES MELLITUS

Diabetes mellitus is not a single entity but is a group of diseases characterized by an increased blood glucose concentration and an inappropriately low secretion of insulin. A patient is said to have diabetes when the fasting blood glucose is 7 mmol/l or more and the blood glucose taken 2 hours after a meal is 10 mmol/l or more. A full glucose tolerance test is rarely if ever needed in normal clinical practice and at the most a modified (2 point) glucose tolerance test is all that is necessary in cases of doubt. Here a fasting blood glucose is measured and a glucose load of 75 g is given by mouth. The blood glucose is measured 2 hours later and if the fasting blood glucose is greater than 7 mmol/l and the 2-hour blood glucose is 10 mmol/l or more than the diagnosis is established.

Types of diabetes mellitus
Insulin-dependent diabetes mellitus (IDD)
This was formerly known as juvenile-onset or ketosis-prone diabetes. Recently it has been called type I diabetes. In the absence of insulin therapy these patients develop ketoacidosis. Usually the disorder is of acute onset and occurs in the younger age group. However, there is now good evidence to suggest that the disease process leading up to insulin-dependent diabetes may be present for many months or even years before clinical presentation. In addition, insulin-dependent diabetes with typical acute onset and ketoacidosis can occur at any age.

In this group there is an interaction between genetic factors (e.g. the dual axis of susceptibility indicated by the presence of certain histocompatibility factors) and environmental agents.

Non-insulin-dependent diabetes mellitus (NIDD)

This was formerly known as maturity-onset diabetes and more recently as type II diabetes. These patients do not become ketoacidotic in the absence of insulin therapy and are usually controlled by a diet with or without the addition of an oral hypoglycaemic agent. However, insulin therapy may be necessary to achieve good control of the blood glucose.

Insulin-dependent diabetes and non-insulin-dependent diabetes are not mutually exclusive. Occasionally an apparently non-insulin-dependent diabetic will become ketoacidotic and will then require insulin therapy. Rarely an apparently insulin-dependent diabetic will remit and then become easily controlled on a diet with or without an oral hypoglycaemic agent.

Non-insulin-dependent diabetics typically occur in the older age group (maturity onset) but can occur in the young (maturity-onset diabetes) in the young or 'MODY' syndrome).

Secondary diabetes—this may be defined as diabetes secondary to:
1. Pancreatic disease (pancreatitis, surgery).
2. Hormonal abnormalities (e.g. Cushing's syndrome).
3. Drugs (e.g. thiazides and cortisone).

Clinical features of diabetes mellitus

In 20% of cases patients have been ill for more than 6 weeks before the diagnosis is made. Only a high index of suspicion and simple urine testing can reduce the time from presentation to diagnosis.

Insulin-dependent diabetes mellitus

The clinical presentation of IDD may be summarized as follows:
1. Polyuria (with nocturnal enuresis in children) leading to dehydration.
2. Polydipsia.
3. Weight loss with a failure to thrive in children.
4. Ketoacidotic precoma leading, if untreated, to coma (*see later*).
5. Recurrent infections of the skin or genital tract are not usually presenting features of insulin-dependent diabetes although they may be the factor which precipitates ketoacidosis.

Non-insulin-dependent diabetes

The clinical presentation of NIDD may be summarized as follows:

1. Polyuria.
2. Polydipsia.
3. Weight loss.
4. Fatigue.
5. Infection.
    a. Skin—often severe and extensive.

    b. Vulvovaginitis, pruritus vulvae, balanitis.

    c. Dental and other ENT infections.

6. Changes in visual acuity.

7. Peripheral vascular disease.

8. Neuropathic symptoms.

9. Glycosuria found on routine testing at insurance medical examinations or discovered during coincidental illness.

10. An abnormal taste in the mouth.

11. Hyperglycaemic non-ketoacidotic precoma or coma (often precipitated in an unknown diabetic by an intercurrent illness).

It is sometimes suggested that non-insulin-dependent diabetes which is easily controlled with a diet or a diet plus oral hypoglycaemic agents is a 'mild' disease. The term 'mild' should not be used to describe any disease which may eventually lead to blindness and/or severe peripheral vascular disease and amputation.

The routine management of the diabetic in the non-emergency situation

Having found glycosuria it is important to test for ketonuria. If ketones are present the question should be asked 'How ill is the patient'? If the patient is ill, dehydrated and ketoacidotic, then admission should be sought. If ketones are present, but the patient is not ill, dehydrated, or ketoacidotic then the decision should be made as to whether the patient requires admission for the initiation of insulin therapy or whether this can be done in the home. This will of course depend on local specialist advice and local diabetic support service availability. It has been shown that those patients who are stabilized on insulin at home gain control of the blood sugar more quickly and return to work more quickly than those who are admitted to hospital (*Fig.* 8.1). The cost of managing the patient at home is a fraction of that following admission to hospital. If the patient is managed at home then this is best done with the help of a nurse specializing in diabetes who, in partnership, with the doctor can give dietary advice and educate the patient in insulin therapy. Whatever the course of action it is important that at some time in the early part of the illness the patient should be seen by a specialist in diabetes.

If ketones are absent, again the question should be asked 'How ill is the patient'? If the patient is ill and dehydrated then obviously admission is necessary. If ill but not sufficiently dehydrated to require intravenous therapy then the patient may be managed in the home. Again it would be reasonable to arrange for the patient to be seen by a specialist in diabetes.

In children extreme caution should be exercised. On finding glycosuria the advice of the local paediatric department or diabetic specialist (if he looks after children in the area) should be sought. The rapidity with which children may become severely ill cannot be over-emphasized. An early

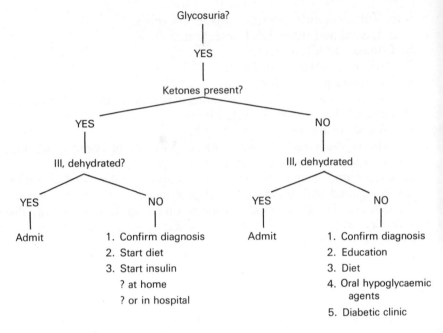

Fig. 8.1. Routine management of the diabetic patient.

diagnosis may mean that a child can be stabilized at home with the help of a diabetic specialist nurse. The child is then saved from the trauma of admission to hospital and intravenous therapy.

In all cases the diagnosis must be established beyond doubt by determining the blood glucose level.

Initial investigation of the diabetic

In addition to the blood glucose estimation the haemoglobin Ai (HbAi), electrolytes, urea, serum creatinine, liver function tests and chest radiograph should be undertaken. After stabilization blood lipids should be measured.

Initiation of treatment

Diet

Our ability to change a patient's lifelong eating habits is limited. Studies have shown compliance with dietary advice to be poor. The advice should therefore be simple and with attainable objectives.

General principles

1. Take a limited dietary history and attempt to modify the existing diet rather than change the whole pattern of eating.

2. Aim for an energy intake to maintain body weight within the accepted limits for the patient's height, age and sex.

3. Remember, that to lose 1 lb (0·5 kg) in weight per week it is necessary to eat 500 calories less per day than that energy requirement to maintain a steady body weight.

4. Do not restrict carbohydrate intake excessively since very low carbohydrate diets impair carbohydrate tolerance and high carbohydrate diets tend to improve it. Aim to give 50–55% of the energy intake as carbohydrate.

5. Advise that most simple carbohydrates such as monosaccharides and disaccharides should be removed from the diet. Replace these with complex carbohydrate foods with a high fibre content. These are more slowly digested, absorbed and tend to reduce the total calorie intake per day.

6. Advise a low cholesterol, low animal fat diet rich in polyunsaturates. Although there is no proof that such a dietary change will be effective in reducing the high incidence of coronary artery disease and peripheral vascular disease in diabetics, epidemiological studies do show that in populations taking such a diet, the incidence of these disorders is low (*see* Further Reading, Co-operation Record Book, diet section).

Oral hypoglycaemic agents

Non-insulin-dependent diabetics who fail to achieve satisfactory blood glucose levels and HbAi concentrations on diet alone should be considered for treatment with an oral hypoglycaemic agent. These should not be used until a period of dieting has been tried (2–3 months). Adherence to the diet can be assessed by measuring the patient's weight. A fall in weight to or the maintenance of a normal weight suggests good compliance. In obesity, failure to lose weight may mean either poor compliance or that too many calories have been given in the diet.

Oral hypoglycaemic agents fall into two groups, the sulphonylureas and the biguanides.

SULPHONYLUREAS

Sulphonylureas act by stimulating the pancreas to produce insulin. They probably also increase the number of insulin receptors and have some effect on platelet adherence. The relevance of the latter to vascular disease is as yet unknown. Many sulphonylureas are commercially available and a list is shown in *Table* 8.1. When prescribing sulphonylureas the following points are worth noting.

1. Sulphonylureas should not generally be given to the obese since this usually results in a further weight increase.

2. Chlorpropamide is a long-acting drug and may cause prolonged severe hypoglycaemia in the elderly. It also causes fluid retention and may precipitate heart failure. It is advisable not to give chlorpropamide to patients over the age of 60 years.

Table 8.1. Oral hypoglycaemic agents

Sulphonylureas and related drugs

Tolbutamide	(Pramidex, Rastinon)
Chlorpropamide	(Diabinese, Melitase)
Glibenclamide	(Daonil, Euglucon)
Acetohexamide	(Dimelor)
Glibornuride	(Glutril)
Gliclazide	(Diamicron)
Glipizide	(Glibenese, Minodiab)
Gliquidone	(Glurenorm)
Glymidine	(Gondafon)
Tolazamide	(Tolanase)

Biguanides

Metformin	(Glucophage)

3. Tolbutamide is a short-acting drug which has to be taken twice or three times a day. Patients often forget to take the second or third dose but dangerous hypoglycaemia is unlikely and fluid retention is not a problem.

4. Gliquidone is a short-acting compound which has to be taken three times a day. However, its action is not affected by renal failure and it may therefore be useful in this situation. However, it is expensive.

5. It is important to get to know one oral hypoglycaemic agent and use it safely and effectively. Glibenclamide is a useful drug which is effective and safe. With a starting dose of 2·5 mg/day it should be increased at 4-day intervals by 2·5 mg increments to a maximum dose of 10 mg b.d. or until a satisfactory blood glucose is achieved. It is unlikely that a further increase in dose will bring any benefit.

6. Fortunately the side-effects of sulphonylurea therapy are infrequent and not severe. Facial flushing sometimes occurs after taking alcohol, particularly in patients on chlorpropamide. This may be distressing for the patient but is not dangerous. Other side-effects are listed below.

Gastrointestinal—anorexia, nausea, vomiting, epigastric discomfort and diarrhoea.

Neurological—weakness, paraesthesiae.

Skin—photosensitivity, reactions, other rashes.

Other—jaundice, eosinophilia, fever.

There is a great deal of cross-reaction between one sulphonylurea and another. A reaction shown to one compound will almost certainly be produced by another.

If normoglycaemia or at least a satisfactory blood glucose is not achieved with good dietary compliance and the addition of a sulphonylurea, then the addition of a biguanide or conversion to insulin therapy must be considered.

BIGUANIDES

Biguanides reduce blood glucose concentration by stimulating anaerobic glucose metabolism with the production of lactic acid. Both insulin and sulphonylureas not only lower the blood glucose concentration but also reduce the concentration of lactate towards those concentrations found in the non-diabetic. Biguanides increase the concentration of lactate. In the presence of renal or hepatic dysfunction or in a situation of high lactate production (e.g. severe hypotension in myocardial infarction), lactate levels may rise sufficiently to produce a severe lactic acidosis. Coma in lactic acidosis has a mortality of 50%. Before prescribing a biguanide the doctor must consider all these factors. Phenformin should not be prescribed because of this danger. Metformin should only be used in selected cases. These are usually obese subjects failing to obtain satisfactory blood glucose values on diet or who gain weight on sulphonylureas. They must have normal renal or hepatic function. The dose of metformin (hydrochloride) is 500 mg every 8 h or 850 mg every 12 h. Biguanides produce the gastrointestinal side effects of nausea, vomiting and diarrhoea.

Treatment with insulin

INDICATIONS FOR TREATMENT WITH INSULIN

1. Ketoacidotic hyperglycaemic precoma or coma.
2. Non-ketoacidotic hyperglycaemia precoma or coma.
3. Insulin-dependent diabetes mellitus.
4. Non-insulin-dependent diabetes mellitus with poor control despite adherence to diet and maximum dose of oral hypoglycaemic agents.

The treatment of precoma and coma will be dealt with separately (*see below*, p. 419.

In the non-diabetic the islet cells of the pancreas maintain a steady background concentration of insulin with burst of activity increasing insulin concentrations when carbohydrate is taken or when catecholamine or cortisol secretion increases. This maintains normoglycaemia in the range of 3–6 mmol/l. This can be achieved in the diabetic by using the artificial pancreas and be very closely approximated to by using continuous intravenous or subcutaneous infusion of insulin. However, these techniques are of limited value and are used for special circumstances only. They are not routinely used and are not within the scope of this chapter. In the practical everyday management of the diabetic the nearest one can come to this state of affairs is by giving a long-acting insulin to maintain a background concentration of insulin together with multiple injections of a short-acting insulin. This technique has its limitations since most diabetics are not prepared to give themselves more than two injections of insulin per day.

When faced with the problem of starting a patient on insulin, the doctor is confronted by a bewildering number of decisions. There are a large number of insulins (*Table* 8.2) some of which are purified and some highly purified,

Table 8.2. List of insulins available

The strength of insulin to be dispensed must be stated in the prescription (i.e. U-20, U-40, U-80 or U-100, indicating the number of units per ml).

Short-acting insulin preparations

Purified (pH 3·2)   *Highly purified* (Neutral)

Pork/bovine mixture   *Bovine origin*

Soluble insulin BP   Hypurin Neutral (Weddel)
Regular insulin USP   Neusulin (Wellcome)
                                                 Quicksol (Boots)

                                                 Porcine origin

                                                 Velosulin (Nordisk)
                                                 Actrapid MC* (Novo)

                                                 Human Insulin

                                                 Human Actrapid (Novo)
                                                 Humulin (Lilly)

                                                 *MC = Monocomponent

Insulins of longer duration of action suitable for use with twice-daily regime when mixed with a short-acting insulin

Purified   *Highly purified*

Bovine origin   *Bovine origin* (NPH Type)

Isophane insulin   Hypurin Isophane (Weddel)
  injection (NPH)   Neuphane (Wellcome)
                                                 Monophane (Boots)

                                                 Porcine origin (NPH Type)

                                                 Insulatard (Nordisk)

                                                 Monocomponent insulins of porcine origine

                                                 Monotard MC (Novo)
                                                 Semitard MC (Novo)

                                                 Human insulin (NPH Type)

                                                 Human protophane (Novo)
                                                 Humulin I (Lilly)
                                                 Monotard (Novo)

Ready-mixed insulins suitable for twice-daily regimes when patients cannot or find difficulty in mixing their own insulins ('biphasic insulin')

Table 8.2. List of insulins available (*cont.*)

Porcine/bovine mixture

Rapitard MC (Novo)
A mixture of crystalline bovine insulin and neutral porcine insulin. The mixture contains 25%
of a short-acting component and 75% of the longer-acting component.

Porcine mixtures
Mixtard (Nordisk) contains crystalline neutral highly purified insulins in a mixture having
30% of the insulin as a short-acting component and 70% as a long-acting component.

Initard (Nordisk)
Also a mixture of highly purified isophane and neutral insulin but having 50% as the short-
acting component and 50% as the long-acting component.

Note

1. The varying composition of mixtures in respect of the proportion of short-acting and
long-acting components.
2. Rapitard contains insulin of bovine origin and is not suitable if allergy to bovine insulin
exists.

Insulin mixtures suitable for a once-daily regime

Containing a short-acting component (30%) and a long-acting component (70%). They all
contain bovine insulin or a bovine/porcine insulin mixture.

Insulin Zinc Suspension Lente (bovine)
Hypurin Lente (Weddel) (bovine)
Lentard MC (Novo) (bovine and porcine)
Neulente (Wellcome) (bovine)
Monotard MC (Novo) (porcine)

Neutral insulin can be mixed with the above mixtures to increase the short-acting component.
However, they must not be mixed with insulins having a pH of 3.

Other insulins having long duration suitable for background insulin therapy in
combination with short-acting insulins

Bovine origin

Insulin Zinc Suspension (Crystalline) Ultralente
Ultratard MC (Novo)
Tempulin (Boots)

some of bovine origin and some of porcine origin. There are many different
insulin regimes with combinations of short-acting, intermediate acting and
long-acting insulins. The starting dose appears arbitrary and adjustment of
the dose is difficult.

As with most forms of therapy it is better to become familiar with one or
two regimes and then use them safely and effectively. For this reason only
two regimes will be described. A twice-daily regime using Actrapid and
Monotard (or soluble and isophane) and a once-daily regime using Lentard
MC (or Insulin Zinc Suspension Lente).

TWICE-DAILY INSULIN REGIME

Insulin dose:
1. Total units per day = 0·2–0·5 units/kg body weight.
2. Morning dose = two-thirds of total daily dose.
3. Evening dose = one-third of total daily dose.
4. Ratio of Actrapid (soluble) to Monotard (isophane) = 1 : 2.
5. Timing of injection—30 min before meal given subcutaneously.

Fig. 8.2 may be used as a teaching aid to show patients how the twice-daily regime works. A step-by-step explanation must be given to give the patient full understanding.

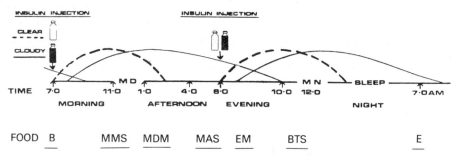

Fig. The twice-daily insulin regime in diabetes (*see text*).

1. The horizontal line represents the time course through the day divided into periods as indicated, i.e. morning, afternoon, evening and night. MD = midday, MN = midnight.

2. Below the horizontal line is indicated approximate meal times. B = breakfast, MMS = midmorning snack, MDM = midday meal, MAS = midafternoon snack, EM = evening meal, BTS = bedtime snack. Below each mealtime the appropriate number of grammes of carbohydrate taken may be written in.

3. Above the line is shown the time course and action of insulin injections. Injections of two insulins are given as a mixed dose before breakfast and before the evening meal. The more rapidly acting insulin (clear, i.e. Actrapid or soluble) is shown by the dotted line and the more prolonged acting insulin (cloudy, i.e. Monotard or isophane) is shown as the solid line.

4. To monitor the effect of insulin therapy, blood glucose (home monitoring or laboratory) or post-voided urine specimen must be taken before breakfast, before midday meal, before evening meal and before retiring to bed.

5. Rules for the adjustment of insulin (by patient):
a. Not more than 2–4 units should be added or subtracted in any one day.
b. Only one insulin should be adjusted at any one time.

c. Changes should be made gradually to allow adjustment throughout the day.

d. If a high blood glucose value or glycosuria is found in the fasting state then the evening Monotard or NPH should be increased. If a high blood glucose value or glycosuria is found before the evening meal the morning Monotard or NPH should be increased. Similarly, if glycosuria or a high blood glucose value is found before retiring to bed then the evening Actrapid or soluble should be increased.

e. If hypoglycaemia is experienced during the morning then it is the morning Actrapid that should be decreased. Similarly, if hypoglycaemia is found in the afternoon then the morning Monotard should be decreased. Hypoglycaemia during the evening is an indication for a decrease in the evening Actrapid. Hypoglycaemia during the night is an indication that the evening Monotard should be decreased.

By gradually adjusting the dose of insulin good control of the diabetes is usually possible. Fine tuning of the control and adjustments for exercise can be achieved by increasing and decreasing the carbohydrate intake at the various times indicated on the chart.

This regime is particularly suitable for all diabetics under the age of 60 and during pregnancy.

SINGLE-DOSE REGIME

1. Choice of insulin—Lentard MC or insulin zinc suspension Lente.
2. Starting dose 0·2–0·5 units/kg body weight.
3. The insulin is given subcutaneously 30 min before breakfast. The dose is increased by increments of 2–4 units/day until urine tests show no glycosuria at some time during the day. The dose is then increased with the object of making the patient free of glycosuria at all times of the day without including hypoglycaemia. This may be difficult on a single dose of insulin and it may be necessary to adjust both the quantity and timing of carbohydrate intake to avoid hypoglycaemia.

This regime is suitable for patients over the age of 60 in whom tight diabetic control is not absolutely necessary and who require less than 50 units/day.

SPECIAL SITUATIONS

1. Patients who are not able to mix their own insulins may find it useful to use a biphasic insulin which is a mixture of a rapidly acting and intermediate acting insulin. This is only a second best to the use of a twice-daily regime indicated above.

2. For patients who have difficulty in seeing the marks on the insulin syringe a 'click count' syringe (which has a ratchet mechanism making a click every time two units on the syringe are passed) may be useful. Similarly, for those patients who have difficulty in measuring their

insulin intake, a fixed-dose insulin syringe may be used. However, the adjustment must be constantly checked as this tends to work loose and a variable dose is then given by the patient.

INSULIN SYRINGES

It is essential to use a syringe which is appropriate for the strength of insulin used. At present insulin of 20 units/ml, 40 units/ml, 80 units/ml, 100 units/ml are in use throughout the world. In the United States, Canada, New Zealand, Australia, and Great Britain U100 insulin is now in general use. It is essential to use a U100 syringe clearly marked in units of insulin when using U100 insulin.

In the UK glass syringes are still used and the British Standard for the appropriate syringe must be prescribed (BS1619/2). However, by far the best syringes are disposable syringes of the plastic type with needles attached and of low dead space (e.g. the Plastipak 1 ml syringe made by Becton and Dickinson (UK) Ltd, York House, Empire Way, Wembley, Middlesex, HA9 OPS). Although these syringes are made for once-only use a diabetic can often use one syringe for 14 injections, i.e. for one week or more. It is not necessary to re-sterilize these syringes. After injection any residual insulin should be removed from the syringe by drawing air in and out of the syringe. The cap over the needle and top should then be replaced and the syringe stored in the refrigerator until used again for the next injection. When glass syringes are used they should be stored in industrial spirit. A suitable syringe case which is spirit proof is made by Hypoguard Ltd, Dock Lane, Melton, Woodbridge, Suffolk, IP12 1PE.

NEEDLES

The best needles are those found on disposable syringes. If glass syringes are used or other disposable syringes then disposable needles 5/8 inch long, 27 or 28 gauge should be used. Disposable needles may be used several times until they become blunt. Non re-usable needles are a second best. These should be of 27 or 28 gauge 5/8 inch long. It should go without saying that needles which are re-used without sterilization should only be used by one person.

SWABBING THE SKIN

It is now considered unnecessary to swab the skin before injection.

DRAWING UP THE INSULIN

It is important to draw air into the syringe equivalent to the number of units of insulin to be given. This air should be injected into the bottle of insulin before the insulin is withdrawn into the syringe. This will enable the insulin to be withdrawn easily without creating a vacuum. Many diabetics do not appreciate this important simple fact. When drawing up 2 types of insulin into a syringe for the twice-daily routine it is important to draw up the clear insulin first and then follow this with the cloudy insulin. When using the technique it is vital to inject air into the bottles first as failure to do so may result in insulin from the syringe being sucked back into the insulin bottle by a vacuum previously created.

SITE OF INJECTION

Injection into one site repeatedly should be avoided as this produces fibrosis, fatty tumour development and irregular absorption. In children there is a tendency to do this as sites which are repeatedly injected with insulin often become painless. This should be discouraged and a rotation pattern of injection sites should be advised. It is important to remember that the rate of insulin absorption depends on the site of the injection. For instance the rate of absorption of insulin from the leg is different from that of the abdomen or the arm.

INJECTION TECHNIQUE

This can only be learnt by practical demonstration. The needle should be inserted at near a right angle to the surface of the skin. The needle must go right through the skin into the subcutaneous tissues. Failure to do this will result in an intradermal injection and ulceration. After insertion of the needle the plunger should be gently withdrawn to test for intravenous placing of the needle. If no blood is withdrawn the injection should be made.

MONITORING OF THE STANDARD OF CONTROL ACHIEVED

In order to make the most of treatment available the diabetic must learn to monitor the standard of control achieved. It is not enough for him to be symptom-free. An attempt must be made to achieve as near normoglycaemia as is possible. This may be achieved by monitoring in the home and in the laboratory.

MONITORING IN THE HOME

Monitoring the standard of control achieved in the home may be done by urine testing and/or blood glucose measurements.

Urine testing

Limitations. The concentration of glucose in the blood at which glucose appears in the urine will depend on the renal threshold for glucose (on average, around 10 mml/l or 180 mg%). This renal threshold may increase with age and in renal disease. It must always be borne in mind, particularly when the urine tests do not correlate with blood glucose estimations. Remember, if the renal threshold for glucose is 10 mmol/l then the blood glucose is twice normal before glucose appears in the urine.

METHODS

1. Diastix (Ames)
2. Urine Testing Strips (Boehringer)

3. Clinitest (Ames)

The basic rules for urine testing are set out below.

Non-insulin-dependent diabetes

1. Test urine four times a day until stable then daily but at varying times.

2. To catch the postprandial glucose peaks, ask the patient to empty the bladder before eating and then test the next specimen of urine passed after food (on average 2–3 h postprandial).

3. Test (*a*) specimen on rising (urine collected in bladder overnight); (*b*) after breakfast; (*c*) after midday meal; (*d*) after evening meal.

Insulin-dependent diabetes

1. Test urine four times a day until good control is achieved and then reduce the frequency of testing to suit individual needs and the standard of control needed. Test at least once per day but at varying times.

2. To assess blood glucose at the time of urine collection the post-voided technique must be used. Here the bladder is emptied and the urine discarded; 30 min or so later the bladder is emptied again and it is this specimen that is tested.

3. Test the urine before breakfast, before the midday meal, before the evening meal and before retiring to bed.

Home blood glucose monitoring

Measuring the blood glucose concentration at home may be done by using test strips alone or in a combination with a meter. Dextrostix (Ames) may be used with the Glucometer (Ames), the Glucochek (Medistron) and Hypocount (Hypoguard) meters. They may also be used without the aid of a meter using the colour scale on the container. They have the disadvantage that the test area must be washed and blotted dry before reading.

The Glycemie 20–800R strips made by Boehringer have the advantage in not having to be washed before reading, the blood being simply wiped off. There may be used alone or in conjunction with a meter (Glucochek II, or Reflux-Boehringer). They also have a double scale and wider range of accuracy.

SOURCES OF ERROR

1. Not enough blood on test area. Hypodermic needle is used to prick the skin instead of a suitable lancet (Monolet made by Hypoguard). The hypodermic needle produces a deep painful wound but not much blood!

2. Swabbing the skin with alcohol may damage the enzymes in the test strip. It is not necessary to swab the skin, providing the skin is socially clean, i.e. washed with soap and water.

3. Inaccurate timing.

4. With Dextrostix incorrect technique for washing off blood and blotting afterwards.

Some patients find it difficult to prick the finger to produce adequate quantities of blood. A simple finger pricking device (Autolet, Owen Munford Ltd, Medical Division, Brook Hill, Woodstock, Oxon, OX7 1TU) overcomes this difficulty.

Laboratory monitoring

From time to time (3–6 months) the patient should attend the laboratory for a blood glucose and HbAi* estimation. The blood glucose taken 2 h after a meal (the 2-hour interval blood sugar or IBS) correlates well with 24 h glucose profiles. The 2-hour period after a meal is often a convenient time for patients to attend the laboratory. By attending the laboratory in the week preceding the visit to the doctor, the result may be to hand when the patient is seen. Patients living a long way from the laboratory may have the blood glucose measured at the time of attending the diabetic clinic or the consulting room (office) of the doctor. In the latter case a simple glucose meter measurement may be made on the premises.

Desirable standards of control

'Good control' is all that we can hope for and suggested standards for this are indicated in *Table* 8.3 below. Ideal control is of course normoglycaemia 24 h of a day. At present this is impossible to maintain in most cases.

Table 8.3. Desirable standards of control

Type	Treatment	IBS	Urine glucose
NIDD	Diet	3–7 mmol/l	0%
NIDD	Diet and oral hypoglycaemic agents	3–10 mmol/l	0%
IDD	Diet and insulin	3–11 mmol/l	0–1%

However:

1. With increasing age standards of control may be relaxed.
2. During adolescence, instability is often the rule.
3. The ideal is rarely achieved.
4. Weight should be steady in the adult and near to that which is ideal for patient's age, height and sex.
5. HbAi should be less than 9%.

*Haemoglobin Ai (HbAi). The contact between glucose in the blood and haemoglobin in the red cell produces glycosylated haemoglobins (HbAi). The reaction is not enzymatically mediated. The degree of glycosylation depends on the concentration of glucose in the blood and time. As the red blood cell lives approximately 100 days, the concentration of HbAi is an indication of the average blood glucose over a period of 2–3 months. It is therefore a good method of assessing the overall standard of control achieved over this period. The concentration correlates well with daily blood glucose profiles and the outcome of diabetic pregnancy. The measurement is particularly useful when there is a discrepancy between the recorded urine tests, interval blood sugar and the HbAi. Patients can cheat for a single interval blood sugar but not for 2–3 months!

Diabetic emergencies

Hypoglycaemia

INCIDENCE

Hypoglycaemia is the commonest cause of unconsciousness in the diabetic. The incidence may well be rising as diabetologists attempt to tighten diabetic control in order to prevent long-term complications. This has particular implications in terms of the diabetic driving cars and motor cycles.

CAUSES

Hypoglycaemia occurs mainly in insulin-treated diabetics although occasionally it occurs in those on oral hypoglycaemic agents, particularly the elderly who have gone without food.

Precipitating factors usually are:
1. A late meal.
2. Unaccustomed or excessive exercise.
3. Mistakes in insulin dosage.

SIGNS AND SYMPTOMS

The signs and symptoms of hypoglycaemia are due to adrenergic discharge and neuroglycopaenia. All insulin-dependent diabetics should have a minor hypoglycaemic episode induced in order to allow them to recognize early symptoms. The onset may be slow with minor alterations in behaviour noticed only by relatives. However, it may also be rapid leading to sudden unconsciousness without warning and neuroglycopaenic fits. Often the patient experiences hunger, trembling, tingling sensations in the limbs and around the mouth and sweating. Early morning headaches may be a clue to nocturnal hypoglycaemia.

DIFFERENTIAL DIAGNOSIS

This is usually not difficult but if there is any doubt, intravenous glucose should be given. It can do no harm to the patient with hyperglycaemia but more insulin given to the patient with hypoglycaemic coma can be fatal.

PREVENTION AND TREATMENT

The most important factor in the treatment and prevention of hypoglycaemia is patient education. The frequency of hypoglycaemia may be reduced by introducing multiple daily doses of insulin, particularly the twice-daily regime. Patients must always carry glucose with them and take this when symptoms first appear. They should always take a meal before driving and should never drive immediately before a meal particularly if there is likely to be any delay. Relatives should be given a glucagon pack containing a small disposable syringe and 1 mg of glucagon which can be given intramuscularly or subcutaneously. This often has a tremendous psychological effect on a family and although it may never be used they all know that it is there as a safety net in an emergency.

Doctors should carry in their emergency kit glucagon 1 mg in a disposable pack and glucose as Dextrose solution BP 50% weight volume (Minijet system. IMS 50 ml size).

As soon as a patient recovers consciousness following an hypoglycaemic episode it is essential to feed him to prevent him lapsing back into unconsciousness.

A patient requiring hospital treatment for hypoglycaemia represents a failure in patient education and in primary health care.

Hyperglycaemia with ketoacidosis

INCIDENCE

A District General Hospital (catering for a population of 200 000) might expect to see 20–30 cases per year. A doctor in Primary Health Care looking after 2000–3000 patients might expect to see one case in 3–5 years.

MORTALITY

In good centres a mortality of 5–10% might be expected but in the average District General Hospital this may be 20–25%. The mortality amongst geriatric patients is 50%.

PATHOGENESIS

Severe insulin deficiency leads to hyperglycaemia secondary to hepatic gluconeogenesis and ketoacidosis secondary to uninhibited lipolysis and resultant hepatic ketogenesis. The intracellular acidosis thus induced causes intracellular potassium to migrate across the cell membrane to the extracellular space in order to maintain ionic equilibrium. Extracellular potassium concentrations rise and severe potassium deficiency occurs owing to the coincident osmotic diuresis. If the pH falls below 6·8 death is likely. Acidosis causes insulin resistance.

Insulin deficiency also prevents peripheral glucose uptake and stimulates muscle catabolism. Muscle catabolism results in a rise in amino acids available for the liver to use as a substrate for gluconeogenesis.

PRECIPITATING FACTORS

1. Intercurrent illness, e.g. infection, myocardial infarction, cerebro-vascular episode.
2. Surgery—trauma.
3. Failure to take insulin.
4. Delayed diagnosis in a new diabetic.
5. A decrease in the dose of insulin on the mistaken advice of a doctor when the patient is ill.

PREVENTION

The mainstay of prevention must lie in patient and primary health care doctor education. During any illness, the patient must be encouraged to take a high fluid intake and increase the dose of insulin according to home glucose monitoring. However, if vomiting occurs and i.v. replacement therapy becomes necessary, admission should be arranged without delay.

PRESENTATION

In the undiagnosed diabetic there is often a history of fatigue, weight loss, polyuria and polydipsia for some weeks or months. More severe symptoms of thirst, polyuria and vomiting may, together with symptoms of intercurrent illness, be present for a few days before the diagnosis is made. Severe leg cramps, abdominal pain and breathlessness may occur in the late stages.

SIGNS

The main physical signs are related to dehydration and acidosis. The skin is warm and dry. With increasing dehydration the skin loses its turgor and the muscles have the texture of wet cardboard. Ocular tension is lost and if dehydration proceeds, peripheral shutdown occurs with a cyanosed cold periphery, tachycardia, loss of peripheral pulses and a fall in blood pressure.

With increasing acidaemia, acidotic hyperventilation occurs (Kussmaul respiration) and the patient smells strongly of ketones.

Higher cerebral function may be normal at first but as the condition deteriorates, impairment leads from precoma confusion to deep coma. It is worthwhile noting that even in the presence of frank infection only 10% of patients have a fever and mild hypothermia may even develop.

INITIAL INVESTIGATIONS

At the bedside to confirm the diagnosis

   1. Blood glucose (Glycemie 20–800R test strips or Dextrostix with or without a meter).
   2. Urinary ketones (Ames ketostix).

Laboratory investigations

   1. Blood glucose.
   2. Plasma urea.
   3. Plasma electrolytes.
   4. Full blood picture to assess the packed cell volume.
   5. Blood pH (hydrogen iron concentration), $P\text{co}_2$ and $P\text{o}_2$.
   6. Blood ketones.
   7. MSU for microscopy and culture.
   8. Blood culture.
   9. Throat swabs.

OTHER INVESTIGATIONS

Chest radiography and ECG (patient to remain connected to monitor).

TREATMENT

This must begin as soon as the diagnosis is confirmed (or if suspected with high probability) and if possible in the home.

Rehydration. Rehydration alone will considerably improve the patient and lower the blood sugar. The peripheral circulation will be restored and urine flow re-established. If the patient is not severely ill, not grossly ketoacidotic and not vomiting, the rehydration may be possible orally. However, intravenous rehydration is usually necessary. Peripheral veins may be used but a central line allows central venous manometry to be carried out. This is useful in the severely ill patient and is particularly helpful in the elderly to eliminate the risk of fluid overload.

Types of fluids and rates of infusion
1. Isotonic (normal) saline equivalent to sodium 155 mmol/l (mEq/l).
2. Half-normal saline.
3. 5 or 10% dextrose.
Half-normal saline or dextrose should replace normal saline if the plasma sodium exceeds 155 mmol/l or when the blood glucose falls to less than 10 mmol/l.

The rate of infusion is shown in *Table* 8.4 below.

Table 8.4. Rate of infusion

Time (hours)	Time interval (hours)	Volume of solution (litres)	Sodium (mmol)
0–1	1	2	310
1–2	1	1	155
2–3	1	1	155

This is continued until the central venous pressure (CVP) is 1 cm and then to maintain the central venous pressure at around 1 cm (Sonksen).

On average 4–6 litres of fluid are *retained* in the first 48 h indicating the size of the deficit at onset.

Insulin therapy

The low-dose insulin regimes have now become accepted as standard treatment for diabetic ketoacidosis. Two regimes are in use.

1. LOW-DOSE INTRAMUSCULAR REGIME (ALBERTI)

In this regime insulin is given intramuscularly. It is therefore essential that adequate rehydration is achieved otherwise the insulin will not be absorbed.

This regime is particularly useful in centres where constant nursing is not available.

Insulin—soluble or Actrapid MC.

Route—intramuscular.

Dose—the dose used in this regime is shown in *Table* 8.5 below.

Table 8.5. Low-dose regime

Time (hours)	Dose (units of insulin)
0	20
1	6
2	6
3	6

This regime is followed until the blood glucose is between 10 and 15 mmol/l; 5 units every 2 h are then given to maintain a steady blood sugar of around 10 mmol/l. If blood glucose does not fall in 2 h it is essential to give insulin intravenously.

2. LOW-DOSE INSULIN INTRAVENOUS INFUSION (SONKSEN)

The aim of this regime is to maintain the plasma insulin at around 50 mu/l. The insulin concentration is proportional to the rate of infusion. The insulin plasma half-life is 4 min.

Insulin—soluble or Actrapid MC or equivalent.

Route—the i.v. line may be a separate peripheral line or piggybacked on to a central venous line.

Infusion technique.

a. By use of a syringe pump.

b. Using insulin mixed in the infusion solution.

Rate of infusion—4 units/h until the blood glucose is 10 mmol/l and then 1–0·5 units/h to maintain a steady blood glucose of around 7–10 mmol/l.

PRACTICAL POINTS

1. The blood glucose should be monitored at the bedside with test strips (with or without a meter). The blood glucose should be measured every 30 min and from time to time (2–4 hourly) the values should be checked in the laboratory. Beware leaving this task to inexperienced nurses. Inaccurate information is more dangerous than no information at all.

2. Sonksen advocates the use of an additive to insulin-containing solutions to prevent the insulin adhering to equipment and lowering the actual quantity of insulin infused. He advocated the addition of human serum albumin, Polygeline, plasma protein fractions or 2 ml of the patient's own blood.

3. If the blood glucose does not fall the rate of insulin infusion should be doubled.

4. Take care to watch the connections between the pump and i.v. line and that the pump does not get inadvertently switched off if electrically driven. These are the commonest causes of failure to lower the blood glucose!

Correction of electrolyte imbalance

SODIUM AND CHLORIDE

Sodium and chloride replacement is adequately taken care of by the rehydration regime indicated above.

POTASSIUM

Rehydration and insulin therapy tend to lower the plasma potassium concentration dramatically. Severe hypokalaemia may result and may be responsible for the patient's death when all appears to be going well. Potassium should therefore be given early in the rehydration process and the level of plasma potassium monitored throughout.

Replacement potassium

Route—intravenously mixed with the normal saline solution.
Dose—the dosage schedule is shown in *Table* 8.6 below.

Table 8.6. Dosage schedule for potassium

Plasma potassium concentration (mmol/l)	Dose (mmol/h)
Greater than 5	0
4–5	13
Less than 4	26
Less than 3	39

Practical points

1. Even if plasma potassium is greater than 5 initially the plasma potassium may drop dramatically in the first hour and this must be monitored.

2. ECG monitoring is sometimes helpful. 'Tented' T waves suggest hyperkalaemia and flat T waves with T wave inversion indicate hypokalaemia. However, the plasma potassium may be less than 2 mmol/l before definite ECG signs occur and this is too late!

3. Patients with ketoacidosis often have gastric atony. This can sequestrate several litres of electrolyte-rich fluid in the stomach. A nasogastric tube should therefore be passed in patients with ketoacidosis developing precoma or coma to prevent vomiting and the danger of aspiration pneumonia. This also aids the restoration of electrolyte and acid–base balance.

Correction of acid–base deficit

In most cases rehydration and insulin therapy are sufficient to correct the acid–base deficit. However, if the pH is less than 7 insulin resistance becomes a problem and at that pH life is threatened. At a pH of 7 or less bicarbonate solution should be given. Correction of the acidaemia will allow potassium to pass into the cells and produce hypokalaemia which must be corrected.

DOSE AND ROUTE

Aliquots of 50 mmol of 8·4% sodium bicarbonate solution together with 13 mmol of added potassium should be given over a 20-min period. After an equilibration period of approximately 10 min the pH should be estimated again. The process should be repeated until the pH is greater than 7.

PRACTICAL POINTS

1. As little as 50 mmol of bicarbonate will relieve distressing hyperventilation due to acidosis.

2. For every mmol of bicarbonate given 1 mmol of sodium is given. Excessive quantities of sodium given in this way will produce severe hyperosmolarity due to the hypernatraemia. Intracellular dehydration will result with prolongation of the coma. Under no circumstances should infusions containing 250–500 ml of 8·4% sodium bicarbonate solutions be set up as there is a real danger that these may run in accidentally and kill the patient.

OTHER MEASURES

1. Early use of antibiotics is indicated if infection is suspected, if a central venous line is used or the patient is catheterized. Many advocate the routine use of prophylactic antibiotics.

2. In the severely hyperosmolar patient and when the patient is unconscious heparinization should be used to prevent postcoma thrombosis and diffuse intravascular coagulation syndrome.

3. Oliguria or anuria after adequate rehydration with a central venous pressure of greater than 1 cm and a blood pressure of greater than 100 mmHg should be treated with 120 mg i.v. frusemide. If this fails the patient should be treated as having acute renal failure.

4. If hypotension (a blood pressure less than 80 mmHg systolic persists for 2 h after onset of treatment and adequate rehydration 2 units of whole blood should be given.

5. If the Po_2 is less than 11 kPa (80 mmHg) oxygen via face mask or nasal catheter should be given.

6. Precipitating factors must be treated.

Hyperglycaemia without ketoacidosis leading to precoma or coma

Of patients with severe hyperglycaemia leading to precoma and coma, 5–10% do not have significant ketoacidosis. However, if severely shocked they may have a lactic acidosis or a uraemic acidosis. These patients are usually elderly and often previously non-insulin dependent. The condition is sometimes associated with the excessive intake of sweetened drinks in an attempt to assuage thirst. Patients with hyperglycaemia without significant ketoacidosis probably have enough insulin to switch off lipolysis and ketone production but not enough circulating insulin to prevent the very high blood glucose concentration seen (often greater than 50 mmol/l).

PRESENTATION

This is similar to hyperglycaemic ketoacidosis, precoma or coma but without the signs of acidosis. Dehydration is the most significant sign and hyperosmolarity is often extreme (greater than 360 mmol/l).

PRACTICAL POINTS

Calculation of plasma osmolarity:
Plasma osmolarity = 2 (Na + K) + glucose + urea mmol/l
The concentration of sodium, potassium, glucose and urea are measured in mmol/l. The concentration of urea is less important in that it has equal distribution between intracellular and extracellular spaces and therefore does not contribute greatly to osmolar imbalance.

TREATMENT

This is essentially the same as that for hyperglycaemia with ketoacidosis. Rehydration is the most urgent need. The danger of contributing to the osmotic imbalance cannot be over-emphasized. If the plasma sodium is 150 mmol/l or more than half-normal saline or 5% dextrose should be used in place of normal saline. A central venous line is desirable.

Patients with this condition are often sensitive to small dose of insulin and treatment must be carefully monitored.

Plasma sodium and potassium values must be monitored on a 2–4 hourly basis.

Patients with severe dehydration are at risk from diffuse intravascular coagulation and postcoma venous thrombosis. Heparin should be used prophylactically with these patients unless there is a definite contraindication.

Lactic acidosis
Fortunately this rare cause of coma in diabetics is likely to become even more rare as the dangers of phenformin are recognized. However, the diagnosis must be suspected in a diabetic taking a biguanide who becomes severely acidotic, particularly if there is any intercurrent illness. The mortality in this condition is in the region of 50%. Patients are severely ill and require large quantities of bicarbonate. However, peritoneal dialysis or even haemodialysis may be necessary because of the resultant sodium

overload. Blood glucose control is not a problem and often the blood glucose is within the normal range.

Management of the diabetic pregnancy

The importance of good diabetic control during pregnancy cannot be overstated. Good diabetic and obstetric care reduces the perinatal mortality from 25·8% to 4%. Good control before and at conception may reduce the incidence of fetal abnormalities.

1. Before pregnancy. Education programme—importance of control, insulin adjustment, home blood glucose monitoring.

2. Obtain normoglycaemia and a normal HbAi before conception if possible.

3. Supervise patients during pregnancy every 2 weeks, if possible at a joint clinic with the obstetrician to reduce the number of visits the patient has to make to the hospital.

4. At each visit assess the patient's own blood glucose monitoring results and check an interval blood sugar measured in the laboratory. Every three months measure the HbAi. The blood pressure should be measured at regular intervals and the eyes inspected once per month.

5. Aim for a full term normal delivery.

6. The confinement and labour should be managed by a joint team of specialists in diabetes and obstetrics. The diabetes should be controlled during labour using an insulin pump and a low-dose insulin infusion technique, aiming to maintain a blood glucose of 8–10 mmol/l.

7. A specialist in neonatal care with special care facilities for the infant should be on hand.

The conclusion of a successful pregnancy in a diabetic is a tribute to the joint efforts of the patient, the obstetrician and the diabetologist.

Diabetes and surgery

Good metabolic control in the postoperative period has the following important effects.

1. Reduces length and severity of postoperative catabolic state.

2. Reduces the danger of infection.

3. Increases rate of wound healing.

4. Aids fight against infection should it occur.

Anaesthetists often fear hypoglycaemia during the operation. Good metabolic control can be achieved and the anaesthetist's task made much easier by adherence to simple rules as follows.

1. If possible achieve good control preoperatively (i.e. in the cold case) blood glucose values 3–7 mmol/l.

2. For the diabetic controlled by diet alone. The patient should be treated as if non-diabetic on the day of operation. However, the blood glucose must be monitored closely in the postoperative period (*see below*).

3. For the diabetic controlled on diet and oral hypoglycaemic agents the

patient should be fasted preoperatively in the usual way and not be given an oral hypoglycaemic on the day of operation. Chlorpropamide is a long-acting substance and should be stopped at least 24 h before the operation. The blood glucose should be monitored during and after the operation using a simple portable meter such as the Ames Glucometer.

4. For the insulin-dependent diabetic undergoing a minor procedure it may only be necessary to fast the patient and not give the patient insulin on the morning of operation. However, it is important to remember that a long-acting insulin taken the night before the operation (e.g. Monotard) may still be acting in the morning and not covered by carbohydrate because the patient has been fasted. A reduction of the evening Monotard dose on the night before operation will prevent this problem occurring. Simple monitoring of blood glucose values on the morning of operation will detect this danger and if present the situation can be countered by giving i.v. glucose.

After recovery from the procedure the patient must be fed and given short-acting insulin to cover the carbohydrate intake. On the day following such a procedure the patient should be able to return to the former diet and insulin regime.

5. For the insulin-dependent diabetic undergoing a major procedure two methods are available:

a. The PIG regime (potassium, insulin, glucose).

3 days preoperatively: Stabilize on twice daily or preferably thrice daily soluble or Actrapid insulin.

Day of operation: Arrange operation in a.m.; first on the list if possible. Set up infusion of 10% dextrose, 500 ml, + Actrapid insulin 10 u, + potassium chloride 1 g.

Infuse over a period of 4–5 h and repeat until oral feeding restarts, altering doses as shown in *Table* 8.7.

Table 8.7. Postoperative insulin infusion regime

Blood glucose results	Insulin dose
Up to 5 mmol/l	5 units/500 ml 10% dextrose
5–9 mmol/l	10 units/500 ml 10% dextrose
10–19 mmol/l	15 units/500 ml 10% dextrose
Greater than 20 mmol/l	20 units/500 ml 10% dextrose

When oral feeding begins: stop infusion, give thrice-daily Actrapid or Soluble Insulin subcutaneously with meals. Daily dose = preop. dose + 20% if there is infection and an additional 20% if on steroids.

b. Low-dose insulin infusion by pump. In this regime the PIG regime outlined above is used but the insulin administered separately by an infusion pump. The rate of insulin infusion is usually between 2 and 5 units/h.

For obvious reasons it is important to run in the insulin-glucose by a separate i.v. line from that used for other infusions such as saline and blood. During a surgical procedure it may be necessary to increase the rate of infusion of blood or saline. This would interfere with the rate of delivery of insulin and glucose and upset the patient's metabolic control.

Whether the PIG regime or low-dose infusion by pump is used, the blood glucose must be monitored during and after operation. Electrolytes must be measured pre- and immediately postoperatively and then as frequently as is necessary during the postoperative period.

6. Remember, the stresses of a surgical procedure and anaesthetic together with an i.v. glucose solution may cause severe hyperglycaemia even in patients formally very well controlled on diet alone or on diet and an oral hypoglycaemic agent. It follows that the blood glucose must be monitored if good metabolic control is to be achieved.

7. Postoperative period. Again normoglycaemia should be the aim. In patients on intravenous infusions of insulin this is a simple matter. Adjusting the rate of infusion is all that is necessary. In other patients becoming hyperglycaemic during the postoperative period, i.v. infusions of insulin and glucose should be introduced if the patient is on intravenous therapy. If the patient is eating normally then multiple doses of short-acting insulin should be given throughout the day, with each meal. A dose of Monotard may be given in the evening to cover insulin requirements during the night. The dose of Monotard necessary may be assessed by measuring the fasting blood glucose.

As soon as stitches are removed and wound healing is complete, the patient may be returned to the former diet and treatment regime. This may need to be modified to maintain good control.

Diabetes mellitus and intercurrent illness

In the fasting state the blood glucose is maintained by hepatic glyconeogenesis. Glyconeogenesis is enhanced by relative insulin deficiency and an increase in catecholamine, glucagon and cortisol secretion. All these factors are present during illness. It follows that even when a patient cannot eat during an illness, severe hyperglycaemia may result. During intercurrent illness insulin must not be reduced and if anything should be increased on the basis of urine testing or home blood glucose monitoring. Patients should be encouraged to adjust their own insulin in this situation. They should also be encouraged to give themselves multiple doses of a short-acting insulin such as Actrapid. If the patient is not able to take a normal diet then he should be encouraged to take fluids containing carbohydrate. For example the following contain 20 g of carbohydrate (2 standard portions):

1. A glass of milk containing 2 teaspoonsful of Ovaltine, Horlicks or Bournvita.

2. 320 ml of fresh or tinned unsweetened orange juice containing 2 teaspoonfuls of sugar.

3. Diabetic fruit squash or lemon juice containing 4 teaspoonfuls of sugar.

If the patient is vomiting or unable to take fluid then hyperglycaemia and ketoacidosis may develop rapidly and the patient should be admitted without delay.

The long-term complications of diabetes mellitus

Some years after the diagnosis of diabetes mellitus, widespread vascular and neural damage may be detected. The severity and extent of the damage is a function of time, related to the duration of the diabetes mellitus. Thus after 15–20 years, 80% of diabetics have clinically detectable retinopathy. However, other factors such as severity of the metabolic upset, a genetic predisposition and other unknown factors may also be important.

The long-term complications of diabetes fall broadly into three groups.
1. Microvascular disease.
2. Macrovascular disease.
3. Neuropathy.

Microvascular disease

Widespread arteriolar and capillary lesions can be demonstrated in the diabetic. The most important and dramatic clinical manifestations of this damage are seen in the eye and the kidney.

DIABETIC RETINOPATHY

Diabetic retinopathy is a common cause of blindness. In Western countries it is the single most common cause of blindness in the 35–65-year-old age group.

The overall prevalence of retinopathy within a diabetic population is 26%. Any patient with retinopathy has a potentially blinding disorder. The detection of retinopathy together with its prevention and treatment have become important clinical problems.

Clinical features. The detection of diabetic retinopathy is a clinical skill which can only be learnt by practising the art of medicine. The visual acuity should be measured using a Snellen's chart and the eye examined ophthalmoscopically. A good ophthalmoscope with a clean mirror and a bright light should be used. Patients should be observed in a darkened room with the pupils dilated (using 1% tropicamide).

Features of diabetic retinopathy to be observed
1. Early background retinopathy—dots and blots only.
2. Exudative background retinopathy—dots, blots and hard exudates.
3. Ischaemic background retinopathy—dots, blots, sheet haemorrhages, deep dark round haemorrhages, and retinal infarcts (cotton wool spots or soft exudates).

4. Mixtures of (2) and (3) above.

5. Pre-proliferative retinopathy. As in (3) above but more extensive, associated with large areas of capillary closure, haemorrhage, intraretinal vascular abnormalities, venous bleeding and tortuosity.

6. Proliferative retinopathy. Any of the above features (1)–(5) associated with either peripheral new vessels or disc new vessels or both. The presence of fibrous tissue indicates retinitis proliferans and if the vessels bleed a vitreous haemorrhage is produced.

7. End-stage diabetic eye disease, retinal detachment and glaucoma.

8. Any of the above conditions may cause a severe deterioration in visual acuity due to a maculopathy.

Management of diabetic retinopathy. Early detection is most important. All diabetic patients should have visual acuity measured and their eyes examined once per annum. If retinopathy is detected the patient must be followed up by a specialist in diabetes with access to expert ophthalmological opinion. These three groups of patients should be followed by an ophthalmologist, preferably in consultation with a specialist in diabetes in a joint retinal clinic:

1. Severe retinopathy requiring treatment (new vessels on the disc, peripheral new vessels and maculopathy);

2. Severe retinopathy in danger of developing a maculopathy (i.e. exudative lesions, haemorrhages or dots and blots close to the macula);

3. Severely ischaemic retinae with a danger of developing proliferative retinopathy.

Prevention and treatment. The aim must be prevention, not just cure.

It is now generally accepted that good control (most blood glucose values less than 10 mmol/l, aiming for a range of 3–7 mmol/l, and HbAi values within the normal range) is the best insurance against retinopathy. Pirart in his monumental study of 4400 patients between 1947 and 1973 has demonstrated the importance of control. The treatment of associated features such as hypertension and renal failure are of paramount importance. The possible value of agents which reduce platelet stickiness such as aspirin and Persantin have yet to be evaluated.

The prompt treatment of disc new vessels by pan photocoagulation (xenon arc or argon laser) will reduce the 5-year incidence of blindness by 60%. Because of the danger of vitreous haemorrhage from new vessels they must be regarded as an emergency requiring immediate treatment. Peripheral new vessels do not carry the same prognosis for visual loss as disc new vessels. However, they should be treated to remove the danger of vitreous haemorrhage.

Focal photocoagulation of an area producing hard exudates threatening the macula may prevent the development of maculopathy. Such treatment of established exudates at the macula do not improve visual acuity but may prevent a further deterioration. Photocoagulation for ischaemic maculopathy is of doubtful benefit.

The development of end-stage diabetic eye disease represents a failure in medical treatment. The surgical management is difficult and the results are poor. Discussion of the subject is beyond the scope of this chapter.

DIABETIC NEPHROPATHY

Changes in renal function may be observed at the time of diagnosis of the diabetes. The glomerular filtration rate in IDD may be increased by 30%. Microalbuminuria (albumin excreted in the urine at a rate which is in excess of normal as measured by radioimmunotechniques but not detectable by standard tests) is present and is also found in poorly controlled diabetics. These abnormalities can be reversed by good control.

The functional changes indicated above may be related to the eventual structural changes in diabetic nephropathy. This relationship is as yet not clear.

The development of intermittent proteinuria as detected by standard clinical techniques (e.g. Albustix—Ames) precedes established proteinuria which indicates the development of diabetic nephropathy. Of patients with established proteinuria 90% have hypertension. Only rarely do patients develop the nephrotic syndrome or the Kimmelsteil–Wilson syndrome (nephrotic syndrome, hypertension and haematuria).

With the passage of time renal function progressively deteriorates and in some patients chronic renal failure develops. The Joslin Clinic experience indicates that in IDD diagnosed before the age of 20 years, 48% will die of renal failure after an average of 22 years' duration of diabetes. This compares with only 6% of patients with diabetes diagnosed after the age of 20 years.

Prevention and treatment. Prevention must be the aim, rather than the cure.

The reversibility of early functional changes and animal experiments suggest that good control may prevent or delay the development of nephropathy. Again Pirart has demonstrated the difference between those patients who have been poorly controlled (a prevalence of nephropathy approaching 20%) compared with those patients who have been well controlled (prevalence of nephropathy less than 1–2%) over a period of 25 years.

It is unlikely that any degree of obsessional good control will affect the outcome in established chronic renal failure and the accompanying permanent structural changes. However, hypertension and coincident infection must be treated effectively.

In end-stage chronic renal failure, dialysis and transplantation must be considered. Haemodialysis has not been effective in improving the quality of life or the survival time of patients with diabetic nephropathy. Continuous ambulatory peritoneal dialysis has been more successful. Transplantation in the diabetic is less successful than in the non-diabetic. However, more recent experience suggests that early transplantation is associated with much better results.

The patient should be referred to a renal centre as soon as the diagnosis of chronic renal failure has been established. The criteria for such a referral vary widely. However, the following are suggestions:

1. Age less than 50 years.
2. No significant clinical coronary artery disease.
3. No significant clinical peripheral vascular disease.
4. Retinopathy adequately treated with a visual acuity of 6/9 or better.

Microvascular disease affects all parts of the body. The eyes and kidneys are the most dramatically affected and microvascular changes in the heart may give rise to a cardiomyopathy which, at least in the early stages, may be reversible by good control. However, the most serious danger to the heart is from macrovascular disease.

Macrovascular disease

Atherosclerosis affects both the diabetic and the non-diabetic; however, the diabetic suffers more extensive disease at an earlier age than the non-diabetic. The mortality following a coronary thrombosis is higher in the diabetic than in the non-diabetic. The consequences of peripheral vascular disease are more severe in the diabetic when compared with the non-diabetic. The combined effects of peripheral vascular disease, neuropathy and infection produce disastrous diabetic foot disease which often necessitates amputation for diabetic gangrene. Intermittent claudication and angina pectoris reduce mobility.

PREVENTION AND TREATMENT

Prevention must the the aim. Good control should be attempted since there is some evidence that the advance of macrovascular disease is retarded in patients with interval blood sugars (blood sugars taken 2 h after a meal) of less than 10 mmol/l (180 mg%).

Smoking should be vigorously discouraged.

It is not known what effect the more recent diabetic dietary advice will have on the incidence of macrovascular disease. Epidemiological studies suggest that diet may be important. Many diabetics have hypercholesterol-aemia and hyperlipidaemia. A diet with more carbohydrate and less fat together with a high fibre content and rich in polyunsaturates is unlikely to do very much harm and may well do some good. It may also help with weight reduction. The value of lipid-lowering agents is unknown.

The treatment of hypertension, particularly with peripheral vasodilating drugs (e.g. hydralazine) may be helpful in retarding the progress of macrovascular disease and in reducing the incidence of strokes and myocardial infarction. In the treatment of hypertension it should be noted that thiazide diuretics worsen carbohydrate tolerance and the blood glucose must be monitored carefully. Treatment with beta-blockers in the IDD is safe but the recovery time from hypoglycaemia may be prolonged.

The treatment of the diabetic with ischaemic heart disease, peripheral vascular disease and cerebrovascular disease does not differ from that of a non-diabetic.

Myocardial infarction carries a worse prognosis in the diabetic when compared with the non-diabetic. Myocardial infarction usually results in a severe disturbance of carbohydrate metabolism and the diabetes may become seriously out of control. On the other hand, hypoglycaemia must be avoided. If hyperglycaemia develops then the low-dose continuous intravenous infusion technique should be used to control the diabetes.

DIABETIC FOOT DISEASE

The rotting diabetic foot is an all too common and depressing feature of the diabetic ward. Prevention is better than cure. In addition to the general methods of treatment outlined earlier in this section, foot care must form part of any patient education programme.

Diabetic neuropathy

The cause of diabetic neuropathy is unknown. It is thought to be a combination of disordered neural metabolism and vascular disease. Either of these mechanisms may predominate in any given clinical situation. In typical diabetic peripheral neuropathy the metabolic component may well be the most important factor whereas a vascular incident may be the cause of a mononeuritic episode. Diabetic neuropathy affects the peripheral, cranial and autonomic divisions of the nervous system.

DIABETIC PERIPHERAL NEUROPATHY

Diminished vibration perception in the legs and absent ankle reflexes are often the first objective signs of diabetic peripheral neuropathy. However, even in the absence of objective neuropathy the patient may complain of numbness, tingling and painful sensation in the feet and legs indicating a subjective peripheral neuropathy. With advancing neuropathy and loss of pain sensation in the feet, local minor trauma becomes an important factor in the development of diabetic foot disease (*see above*). The disturbance of peripheral nerve function associated with autonomic neuropathy may result in the development of a Charcot joint.

CRANIAL NEUROPATHY

Isolated mononeuritic cranial nerve lesions are almost certainly vascular in origin and are fortunately transient with full recovery.

AUTONOMIC NEUROPATHY

The importance of autonomic neuropathy has only recently been appreciated. It may be responsible for unexplained and unexpected sudden death in diabetics, particularly when undergoing surgery or general anaesthesia. The most important manifestations of autonomic neuropathy are listed below.

Cardiovascular system. Tachycardia, postural hypotension, blood flow abnormalities in the feet.

Skin. Sweating abnormalities, particularly postgustatory sweating.

Pupillary abnormalities. Argyll Robertson pupil.

Genitourinary tract abnormalities. Bladder atony, retention of urine, impotence (however, many cases of impotence are due to psychosexual problems and not related to autonomic neuropathy).

Gastrointestinal tract. Gastric dilatation, constipation, diarrhoea.

GARLAND'S AMYOTROPHY

This syndrome is characterized by pain, wasting and weakness in the proximal muscle groups affecting usually the pelvic girdle and thighs but also seen in the pectoral girdle. The syndrome is often associated with extensor plantar responses and a raised c.s.f. protein. The condition is seen in the elderly and is resistant to treatment. Good control seems to be the most important therapeutic factor.

PREVENTION AND TREATMENT

It appears that good control reduces the incidence of diabetic neuropathy. Pirart showed that neuropathy was at least six times more common in poorly controlled diabetics than in those patients with good control over a period of 25 years. When neuropathy is established little can be done apart from maintaining good control, giving simple analgesia and protecting the feet from trauma. When pain and abnormal sensations in the feet and legs become a problem, it is worthwhile trying the effect of phenytoin 250 mg to a maximum dose of 400 mg/day or carbamazepine 100 mg b.d. to a maximum dose of 1·6 g/day. In cases resistant to treatment aspirin 300 mg/day or dipyridamole 100–200 mg t.i.d. or q.i.d. may be tried. Multivitamin preparations have also been used. The value of anything but simple analgesia and good control is uncertain. There is little point in persisting with treatment longer than one month if no benefit is seen. Time seems to be an important therapeutic factor.

Conclusions. General management of the diabetic
The objectives of following-up a diabetic regularly may be summarized as follows:
1. To achieve good control.
2. To prevent and treat short-term problems.
3. To prevent and treat long-term problems.

4. To continue education and advice.

The aim is to allow a diabetic to live as normal a life as possible within the constraints set by his disease.

Because diabetes is a chronic disorder, the diabetic must undertake a large part of his own treatment. The most important person in the health care team looking after the diabetic is the diabetic himself. The first task of the health care service must be to educate the diabetic in the art of looking after himself. No matter what efforts are made they are unlikely to affect the patient's intelligence, educational, cultural and social background. They can, however, influence his attitude towards his diabetes, motivate him and imbue him with a spirit of co-operation which will allow him to make the most of the educational facilities provided. A full education programme should be given (*see* Further Reading).

Even after an effective educational programme the diabetic cannot be expected to look after his diabetes without additional support from the health care services. The following supporting facilities must be made available.

1. Initial and continuing education.

2. Dietary advice.

3. Laboratory monitoring blood glucose and glycosylated haemoglobin).

4. Annual clinical review by competent observers to detect diabetic eye disease, changes in blood pressure and detect diabetic foot disease.

5. Help in the management of special problems such as pregnancy, retinopathy, peripheral vascular and coronary artery disease, neuropathy, diabetic foot disease and chronic renal failure.

Diabetes mellitus is a common disease and most doctors will be involved in its day-to-day management. Because of the numbers of patients involved the management of diabetes must be shared between Primary Health Care on the one hand and Secondary Health Care on the other (*see* Further Reading).

Whether routine follow-up of the diabetic is carried out in Primary Health Care or Secondary Health Care, the follow-up can be greatly assisted by the use of well-trained nurses.

Only by efficient organization of the health care service will the diabetic gain the health care he so desperately needs.

8.3 DISEASES OF THE THYROID

Introduction

Diseases of the thyroid form a common group of disorders. In a Secondary Health Care Unit with a catchment area containing 200 000 patients we might expect to see no less than 2300 patients with thyrotoxicosis under treatment at any one time. In the Primary Health Care Unit with 2300 patients a doctor might expect to see 26 patients with thyrotoxicosis under treatment at any one time. In addition there will be a similar number of patients with hypothyroidism and non-endocrine abnormalities of the gland. The prevalence of hyperthyroidism in the female is 2%. This is 5–10 times commoner than in the male.

Hyperthyroidism

Diffuse toxic goitre (Graves' disease) and multinodular toxic goitre account for 99% of all patients presenting with thyrotoxicosis. Diffuse toxic goitre is seen most frequently in the age group 20–40 years. Toxic nodular goitre is seen most frequently in the group aged 40–70 years. Symptoms and signs are due to the excess production of the thyroid hormones T3 and T4. However, the patient may also complain of pressure symptoms from the enlarged goitre or from the unsightly nature of the enlarged gland.

Clinical features

The onset of thyrotoxicosis is usually gradual but occasionally acute. Symptoms depend largely on the age of onset.

In the young, weight loss associated with a good appetite, hyperactivity, tremor, emotional lability, anxiety, sweating and heat intolerance are common symptoms.

In the older age group tachycardia, palpitations (often due to atrial fibrillation) are frequently seen and may proceed to dyspnoea and heart failure. Because of the peripheral vasodilatation the pulse may be 'collapsing' in character.

Sometimes the characteristic hyperactivity is not seen and the patient complains of lethargy and weakness. In some patients a typical myopathy occurs affecting mainly the muscles of the pelvic and pectoral girdles. The myopathy may involve the diaphragm producing dyspnoea which may be mistaken as being caused by heart failure. Rarely, symptoms suggesting myasthenia gravis and periodic paralysis may be seen.

Ocular manifestations of the disease are common. Characteristically, there is lid retraction producing the thyroid stare which may be mistaken for exophthalmos. However, prominence of the eyes may be due to exophthalmos and, in addition, exophthalmic ophthalmoplegia may produce diplopia. Pain and grittiness associated with lacrimation is sometimes seen and it is essential to exclude corneal ulceration secondary to poor closure of the eyelids over the globe. Failure to recognize this problem may result in perforation and loss of vision.

In women oligomenorrhoea or amenorrhoea is common. In men gynaecomastia is occasionally seen and in both sexes loss of libido may be a problem.

Nausea, vomiting and loose bowel actions occur in thyrotoxicosis and rarely steatorrhoea is present.

Palmar erythema and spider naevi are sometimes present and may lead to the erroneous suggestion that hepatocellular disease is present.

Thyrotoxicosis rarely affects children. When it does it tends to produce a growth spurt, agitation and behavioural disorders, associated with chorea-like movements. In pregnancy the fetal thyroid may be stimulated by maternal thyroid-stimulating immunoglobulins and produce neonatal thyrotoxicosis. Fortunately this condition settles naturally after 2–3 months as the immunoglobulins are metabolized.

Investigations

The diagnosis must be established by the demonstration of an increased concentration of T4 or, in rare cases (T3 toxicosis), of T3 in the circulation. Many modern laboratories now measure the free T4 and T3 concentrations which will give a direct indication of biological activity.

Normal values: free T4 26–39 pmol/l, 20–30 ng/l
free T3 3–12 pmol/l, 2–8 ng/l

Some laboratories are still measuring total T4 and T3.

Normal values: T4 50–150 nmol/l, 40–110 μg/l
T3 1–3 nmol/l, 0·7–2·0 μg/l

However, T4 and T3 are 99·96% protein bound to thyroid-binding globulin (TBG) and thyroid-binding pre-albumin (TBPA). The values are therefore affected by conditions which disturb protein binding and protein concentration. Some of these are listed below:

INCREASED SERUM TBG

1. Pregnancy, oestrogens and contraceptives.
2. Clofibrate and similar compounds.
3. Liver disease.
4. Myxoedema.

DECREASED SERUM TBG

1. Androgens.
2. Cortisone and similar derivatives.
3. Conditions lowering serum proteins such as protein malnutrition, malabsorption and the nephrotic syndrome.
4. Acromegaly.
5. Severe prolonged illness of any kind.

The free thyroid (T4) index (FTI) has been measured to overcome some of the problems of measuring total T4 values:

$$FTI = \frac{\text{Serum (total) T4} \times \text{T3 resin uptake (patient)}}{\text{T3 resin uptake control}}.$$

Similarly, the serum T4 TBG ratio has been used in the past but these have been superseded by free T4 and T3 measurements.

The avidity of the thyroid for iodine is an indication of its activity. By measuring the ^{131}I uptake of the gland the activity may be assessed. In some centres the ^{131}I uptake is considered an essential precurser to the therapeutic treatment with radioiodine. However, ^{131}I uptake may be normal in patients who are clinically thyrotoxic with a raised T4. This situation is particularly seen in:

1. Thyroiditis.

2. Iodine-induced thyrotoxicosis (self-administered iodine preparations often contained in seaweed extracts).

3. Self-administration of excess thyroxine (thyrotoxicosis factitia).

4. Steroid therapy.

Occasionally thyrotoxicosis is caused by a single hyperactive thyroid nodule (adenoma). This 'hot nodule' may be detected by scanning the thyroid isotopically.

Management and treatment

In managing the patient with thyrotoxicosis it is important to remember the natural history of the disease. Before treatment was available natural remissions and exacerbations of the disease were seen. With treatment relapse is frequently encountered (e.g. 50% of medically treated patients relapse) and even in patients never having had any treatment at all, hypothyroidism sometimes develops at a later date. It is important to explain this natural history to the patient and explain that life-long annual follow-up is essential. The annual follow-up need be nothing more than the measurement of a serum free T4 and thyroid-stimulating hormone (TSH– see Hypothyroidism, p. 441.

The three methods of treatment should be explained to the patient and their various advantages and disadvantages discussed. The doctor and patient must make a decision individually suited to the given patient.

MEDICAL TREATMENT

Immediate short-term treatment should be given in severely thyrotoxic patients to reduce the adverse effects of excessive quantities of T4 and T3 in the circulation. This may be done by beta-blockade. The patient should be given propranolol 40 mg t.d.s. increasing to 80–160 mg up to q.d.s. if necessary. This will reduce restlessness, anxiety, heat intolerance, tremor and tachycardia. Beta-blockade must not be stopped abruptly since a thyroid 'storm' or 'crisis' may result (see later). If failure is present the patient should be digitalized and given diuretics.

Long-term medical treatment has the advantage of being simple and effective. However, it does mean taking medication for a year or more. In addition, even after 1–1½ years' medication the relapse rate on stopping medication is in the region of 50%. If relapse occurs then again the three methods of treatment should be explained to the patient and an independent decision made as to which treatment should be given.

Induction of remission:
1. Carbimazole (Neo-Mercazole), 30–60 mg/day as a single or divided dose for 4–5 weeks, or
2. Propylthiouracil, 300–600 mg/day as a single or divided dose for 4–6 weeks.

Maintenance dose:
1. Carbimazole, 5–15 mg/day as a single or divided dose for 12–18 months, or
2. Propylthiouracil, 100–200 mg/day as a single or divided dose for 12–18 months.

PROBLEMS

Both carbimazole and propylthiouracil have similar side-effects. However, most problems arise within the first three months and there is no cross-reactivity between the two drugs. Thus if one drug is found unsuitable the other may be tried.

SIDE-EFFECTS OF CARBIMAZOLE AND PROPYLTHIOURACIL

These are uncommon but include skin rashes, arthralgia, fever, nausea and vomiting, jaundice and lymphadenopathy. Fortunately these are only transient and often may be treated with antihistamines. However, the most dangerous side-effect of carbimazole and thiouracil is a toxic neutropenia. A full blood picture should therefore be checked before the patient is started on one of these drugs (a mild leucopenia is often seen in thyrotoxicosis) and repeated at monthly intervals. The patient should be warned that if they develop a sore throat which becomes ulcerated they must report immediately for a blood count. Provided that the drug is stopped immediately the condition is reversible.

SURGICAL TREATMENT

The most important factor in deciding to advise surgery is the availability of a competent and experienced surgeon. In such hands, partial thyroidectomy is seldom followed by hypoparathyroidism or recurrent laryngeal nerve palsy. However, the relapse rate following surgery is in the region of 5–10% and 30% of patients become hypothyroid some years later. Pre- and postoperative care is important. Patients must be rendered euthyroid by medical treatment before surgery is undertaken. This will usually involve a period of medical treatment for about 8 weeks (*see* Medical treatment, *above*). The patient should be treated with iodine for 8 days prior to operation to reduce the vascularity of the gland. This is usually given in the form of Lugol's iodine or potassium iodine tablet 60 mg t.d.s.

Surgery is indicated if:
1. There is an enlarged goitre giving rise to pressure or cosmetic symptoms.
2. The patient does not wish to take prolonged medication.
3. The patient has fear of radioiodine therapy.

Treatment with radioactive iodine

This treatment is simple and effective. The patient may be reassured that there is no danger from cancer or leukaemia. In the UK radioiodine treatment is usually reserved for patients who are over child-bearing age. However, no such reservation exists in the USA. It should not be used in pregnancy.

Failure to control the thyrotoxicosis occurs in 30% of patients and late-onset hypothyroidism is common.

Carbimazole or propylthiouracil or their derivatives must be stopped at least 48 h before ^{131}I therapy otherwise the gland will not take up the radio-iodine. However, beta-blockade may be continued. Drug therapy may be re-started one week after radioiodine therapy and continued until control is achieved, usually in about 2 months. If relapse occurs a second dose of radioiodine should be given but the interval between doses should be greater than 4 months.

Radioactive iodine dosage

1. Small goitre, 3–4 mCi ^{131}I.
2. Large goitre, 6 mCi ^{131}I.

Treatment in special situations

1. Pregnancy. Surgical or medical treatment may be given during pregnancy. If medical treatment is given it is important to stop antithyroid drugs one month before delivery.

2. Thyroid crisis. Causes:

a. Surgery on an ill-prepared patient.

b. Withdrawal of beta-blockade without first rendering the patient euthyroid.

The thyroid crisis or storm is characterized by extreme tachycardia, hyperpyrexia and restlessness. Delirium may proceed into coma, collapse and death. Treatment must be prompt and effective. A suggested regime is as follows:

1. Propranolol, 1 mg i.v. given over a 1-min period. This should be repeated up to 5 mg; 20–80 mg 8-hourly may be given orally.

2. Sedation with chlorpromazine 50–100 mg i.m. 8-hourly.

3. Carbimazole 60–120 mg or propylthiouracil 600–120 mg immediately followed by carbimazole 30–60 mg/day or propylthiouracil 300–600 mg/day.

4. One hour after initiating the above therapy potassium iodide 1 mg should be given orally or as a rectal infusion. This should be continued twice daily for 2 days.

5. Dexamethasone, 2 mg 6-hourly reducing gradually when the condition is controlled.

The patient should be kept in a cool, quiet, dark room and fanning should be used to reduce the hyperpyrexia.

Hypothyroidism

Thyroid hormone deficiency produces a slowing down of the body's metabolic processes. In severe deficiency states the tissues become thickened with a mucinous material and the classic picture of myxoedema is produced. In extreme deficiency myxoedema coma may follow.

Transient hypothyroidism sometimes follows ^{131}I therapy and after partial thyroidectomy for thyrotoxicosis. It is also seen after acute thyroiditis.

Probably the commonest cause of long-term hypothyroidism is iatrogenic, following ^{131}I therapy, surgical treatment or medical treatment of hyperthyroidism, thus underlining the importance of long-term follow-up. However, hypothyroidism may also follow autoimmune disease of the thyroid producing thyrotoxicosis and thyroiditis.

Rarely, hypothyroidism is secondary to hypothalamic or pituitary disease. Carcinomatous infiltration of the gland may also produce hypothyroidism.

Thyroid agenesis or an inherited enzyme defect are important causes of cretinism and juvenile myxoedema.

Clinical features

The onset is insiduous, producing multisystem disease. The diagnosis is frequently missed. The peak age group affected is between 40 and 60 years.

Symptoms and signs are best remembered by listing as follows:

General—Mental and physical malaise, cold intolerance and weight gain.

Skin changes—Dry skin with hyperkeratosis and a yellow tinge (due to abnormal carotene metabolism). The skin is often pale and there is a malar flush tinged with cyanosis. The hair is usually dry and brittle. Alopecia may be present.

Eyes—The skin changes mentioned above together with puffiness around the eyes give the classic myxoedema. A spot diagnosis.

Periods—Menorrhagia.

Musculoskeletal change—'Aches and pains', myopathy and stiffness.

Neurological changes—Polyneuropathy, carpal tunnel syndrome, cerebellar ataxia and psychosis.

Cardiovascular change—Hypertension, angina, atrial fibrillation and pericardial infusion.

Deafness

Thyroid—This is usually small although a goitre may be present in iodine deficiency, familial goitre, and secondary to goitrogenic drugs such as the antithyroid drugs, sulphonamides and sulphonylureas.

Anaemia—This may be normochromic-normocytic, hypochromic-normocytic or macrocytic-normoblastic. Occasionally a macrocytic anaemia is seen which is megaloblastic indicating the coincidence of B_{12} deficiency anaemia (pernicious anaemia).

Investigations

The finding of a low T4 and/or T3 and a raised TSH confirms the diagnosis. A low T4 and/or T3 and a low TSH indicates hypothyroidism secondary to pituitary–hypothalamic disease. A TSH stimulation test will produce a rise in the T4 and T3 concentration in the blood indicating that hypothyroidism is secondary to pituitary or hypothalamic disease (*see* Further Reading).

Management and treatment

If the diagnosis is clear on clinical grounds, blood should be taken to confirm the diagnosis (T4 and TSH) and treatment started immediately. Patients with hypothyroidism are very sensitive to thyroxine and should be given an initial dose of L-thyroxine, 50 μg daily. The dose should be increased gradually by increments of 50 μg/day at intervals of not less than 2 weeks. The dose may be halved and the interval lengthened if the patient cannot tolerate the replacement therapy due to angina. The addition of beta-blockade may help.

The maintenance of L-thyroxine is usually between 100 and 300 μg/day as a single dose. Replacement therapy should be monitored by measuring TSH concentrations in the blood. The dose of L-thyroxine should be increased until TSH values are normal.

Patients must be told, and the message must be repeated, that replacement therapy is for life and that annual follow-up for assessment of TSH is essential. The most efficient and least labour intensive way of follow-up is by means of a computer register. Patients with thyroid disease should be entered into a computerized register together with details of the T4 and TSH values. This register may be used to send for patients for measurement of the TSH on an annual basis. The computer may be programmed to pick out abnormal results and non-attenders and doctors in both Primary and Secondary Health Care alerted.

Myxoedema coma

It is salutory to note that many of the patients developing myxoedema coma do so in hospital. The condition is precipitated by cold, infection, anaesthetics and drugs such as chlorpromazine and narcotics.

Clinical features

To the signs of myxoedema are added increasing somnolence and torpor which proceed to coma with a 50% mortality. Hypothermia (a low reading thermometer measuring rectal temperature is essential) is characteristic with a temperature falling to 24 °C in 80% of patients. (It is worthwhile noting that 18% of patients with hypothermia are myxoedematous.)

Investigations

Blood should be taken for T4 and TSH and treatment started immediately.

Management and treatment

The patient should not be actively rewarmed but should be allowed to rewarm at the ambient room temperature.

L-Thyroxine, 400–500 μg i.v. as a bolus should be given immediately. However, a similar dose via a nasogastric tube is also effective. Other resuscitative measures should be administered as necessary.

Hydrocortisone 100 mg 6-hourly i.v. is often given but there is no good evidence that it is necessary. If, however, hypopituitarism is a possibility then the patient should be given hydrocortisone.

There is no evidence that the use of T3 has any place in treatment. If recovery takes place it is usually within 24–48 h.

8.4 HYPERCALCAEMIA

Introduction

With the advent of 12-channel auto-analysers in routine District General Hospital biochemistry laboratories, hypercalcaemia has become a common chance finding. In this situation, hypercalcaemia is frequently asymptomatic and totally unrelated to the reason for doing the investigation in the first place. It therefore troubles and perplexes the physician, forcing him to decide how far he should investigate such a chance finding.

Hypercalcaemia found in hospital populations is most frequently (greater than 50%) related to malignant disease. Hypercalcaemia discovered in outpatients is most frequently (greater than 50%) asymptomatic and may be due to insignificant primary hyperparathyroidism.

Action to be taken on finding hypercalcaemia

1. Repeat the investigation. Blood must be taken without a constricting venous cuff.
2. Check the serum phosphate, bicarbonate, electrolytes and urea, hydrogen ion concentration or pH, and alkaline phosphatase.
3. Review the patient's symptoms by direct questioning.

Symptoms suggesting hypercalcaemia

Polyuria, polydipsia.
Anorexia, nausea, vomiting, constipation.
Weakness, lassitude.
Depression, poor concentration, confusion leading to coma.
Renal stone formation (45% of patients with primary hyperparathyroidism produce renal stones).
Other symptoms may suggest a cause for the hypercalcaemia.

Causes of hypercalcaemia

1. Malignant disease.
   a. Bone metastases.

    b. Myltiple myeloma.

    c. Haematological malignancy.

    d. Hypercalcaemia due to malignancy but not due to metastases, i.e. due to humoral factors produced by malignant cells. This type of hypercalcaemia is usually associated with hypophosphataemia, hypokalaemia and alkalosis.

  2. Hyperparathyroidism.

    a. Primary hyperparathyroidism. This is usually associated with hypophosphataemia, hyperchlorhydria, and acidosis.

    b. Secondary hyperparathyroidism (related to chronic renal failure or malabsorption syndrome).

  3. Sarcoid.

  4. Vitamin D intoxication (usually iatrogenic in the treatment of renal osteodystrophy or hypoparathyroidism).

  5. Thyrotoxicosis.

  6. Addison's disease.

  7. Paget's disease.

  8. Milk-alkali syndrome.

Diagnosis

The most important step is to decide whether the hypercalcaemia is significant or not. This decision can only be made by taking an adequate history with appropriate direct questioning followed by a careful clinical examination and further investigation.

If hypercalcaemia is significant and the cause is not clear then a steroid suppression test should be performed.

Steroid suppression test

  1. Serum calcium measured on a fasting subject using an uncuffed venous sample.

  2. Prednisolone, 10 mg 8-hourly, or hydrocortisone, 40 mg 8-hourly, orally, for 10 days.

  3. Serum calcium measured as in (1) above on the 8th, 9th and 10th days.

INTERPRETATION

Hypercalcaemia due to hyperparathyroidism does not suppress with steroids. On the other hand most patients with hypercalcaemia due to other causes show a gradual and progressive fall towards normality with steroids.

Treatment

In most cases where hypercalcaemia is found to be significant, the treatment is that of the cause of the hypercalcaemia. However, in asymptomatic patient with hypercalcaemia which does not suppress with steroids, the problem arises as to whether further investigation should be undertaken. It is these patients with hypercalcaemia which is probably due to chronic mild primary hyperparathyroidism that are the most perplexing. In the long term such 'mild hypercalcaemia' may produce renal damage and soft-tissue calcification. There is, however, no definite evidence on this subject. If the patient is under 60 years of age and possible long-term effects are feared then referral to a specialized centre is indicated. Primary hyperparathyroidism is treated by surgery.

Hypercalcaemia secondary to sarcoid is an indication for treatment with steroids. Prednisolone, 30 mg daily, should be given with a gradual reduction in dose over a period of months, the dose being titrated against the serum calcium.

Treatment of severe life-threatening hypercalcaemia

Severe hypercalcaemia produces polyuria and eventual dehydration which may lead to confusion and coma. This condition is most frequently seen in malignancy, primary hyperparathyroidism and vitamin D intoxication. It is important to realize that even in malignancy treatment is worthwhile since the patient may be quite well, despite the malignancy, if the hypercalcaemia is controlled.

1. Fluid replacement with normal saline and 5% dextrose.
2. Reduction of the serum calcium. This may be achieved rapidly by giving 50 mmol of buffered phosphate intravenously. This should only be done after adequate hydration which in itself will reduce the serum calcium by 1 mmol. The buffered phosphate should be given over a period of 6 h and should not be given to patients in chronic renal failure. It is important to realize that if too much phosphate is given pulmonary oedema may develop. Local leakage of buffered phosphate may cause localized calcification.
3. Prednisolone, 30 mg per day, may be given but takes 3–7 days to be effective. Mithramycin is very effective and can be used to lower the serum calcium. It should be given in a dose of 15 μg/kg body weight as a single dose in a 5% dextrose solution (1 litre) given over a period of 4–6 h. The calcium lowering effect has a varied duration from a few days to 3 weeks.
4. Peritoneal and haemodialysis is useful in patients with renal failure or fluid overload.
5. Calcitonin may be used in some patients with malignant hypercalcaemia.

FURTHER READING

Chapter 8.2

WHO (1980) Expert Committee on Diabetes Mellitus, second report, Technical report series 646. Geneva. WHO.
Medicine International (1981) Vol. 1, No. 8. Various authors.

Keen H. and Jarrett (ed.) (1982) *Complications of Diabetes Mellitus.* 2nd ed. London, Arnold.

Hill R. D. (1976) Running a diabetic clinic. *Br. J. Hosp. Med.* **16,** 218–226.

Hill R. D. (1976) Community Care Service for Diabetics in the Poole Area. *Br. Med. J.* **1,** 1137.

Co-operation Record Book for diabetic patients, free of charge from Hoechst (UK) Limited, Pharmaceutical Division, Hoechst House, Salisbury Road, Hounslow, Middlesex TW4 6JH. This booklet was designed by members of the Community Care Scheme for Diabetics in the Poole Area and is used extensively as a record book and as a means of educating the diabetic patient.

Chapter 8.3

Medicine International, 1981, Volume 1:
  Endocrine Disorders Part 1, No. 6, June 1981; Part 2, No. 7, July 1981
  Metabolic Disorders Part 1, No. 8, August 1981; Part 2, No. 9, September 1981.

Chapter 8.4

Kanis J. A. (ed.) (1979) *Hypercalcaemia, a Symposium on Aetiology and Medical Management of Hypercalcaemia,* London 28.9.79. Published by Armour Pharmaceutical CY Ltd, Hamden Park, Eastbourne, Sussex BN22 9AG (Great Britain).

9 Common Psychiatric Disorders

J. C. Little

9.1 INTRODUCTION

Attention has been particularly concentrated on those common psychiatric disorders in which the intervention of the non-psychiatric clinician is most likely to be of practical value.

Hence no attempt has been made to effect a comprehensive, but inevitably superficial, survey of all common psychiatric disorders within the compass of one chapter, a policy which would have required coverage of much of the content of child and adolescent psychiatry, mental deficiency practice, the whole range of sexual disorders and therapies, and all of the varied psychotherapeutic philosophies and techniques.

Anorexia nervosa, obsessional states and phobias, despite advances in treatment, have been omitted as insufficiently common, while common conditions for which contemporary lines of treatment are of doubtful value or downright disappointing are only dealt with briefly.

9.2 THE RELATIVE IMPRECISION OF PSYCHIATRIC DIAGNOSES AND TREATMENTS

The ideal, if not always the actuality, of clinical diagnostic practice assumes a system of defined categories each with specific pathology and treatment. Psychiatric disorders hardly present in this manner for: the personality of the individual influences the expression of the disorder; more than one syndrome may coexist with relative prominence altering over time; psychological pathology is far from clear, demonstrable physical pathology is usually absent; and most of the treatments available are not specific for particular syndromes. Tolerance of uncertainty and ambiguity are characteristic, even from medical student days, of those attracted to the practice of psychological medicine.

Psychiatric diagnostic concepts can be likened to cloud formations: recognizable cumulus, cirrus, nimbus and stratus formations do exist, even though each shape never repeats identically. We frequently observe more than one type of cloud in the sky, are hard put at times to judge which is dominant, and note that as time passes the patterns change. In some skies the cloud shapes are so indeterminate, fleeting and changeable that we cannot classify at all.

447

9.3   THE AFFECTIVE DISORDERS (Disorders of Mood)

The affective disorders comprise those states in which anxiety or depression of inappropriate intensity dominate subjective awareness. They arise exogenously in over-reaction to psychological stress or endogenously as expressions of specific changes in brain chemistry.

There is long-standing disputation within psychiatry between those who hold that, as anxiety and depression commonly coexist, 'affective disorder' is an adequate diagnostic category, and those who maintain that the concept is too broad and requires further division. In so far as treatment response is the key consideration there are grounds for splitting affective disorder at least into the further clinical categories of anxiety state, depressive neurosis and endogenous depression.

Anxiety state—with an introduction to psychotherapy

Anxiety state presents:

1. As a subjectively distressing psychological state of fear, either attached to some focus of anxiety or 'free floating'.

2. As a state of over-arousal of the sympathetic nervous system, at once both subjective and objective.

3. Commonly as a mixture of both mental and somatic distress.

Pathological and normal anxiety

Whatever the patient is anxious about, the true cause of the anxiety lies elsewhere. Detection of the hidden cause and its acceptance by the patient are essential components of the treatment. Anxiety, however intense, is not pathological when the subject knows its cause. The racing car driver before the flag drops and the soldier before battle experience intense anxiety but are in no sense neurotic for both know why.

Selection for treatment

Psychotherapy is time-consuming and the non-psychiatrist should concentrate on those patients likely to benefit most. At the one extreme the acute situational anxiety response arising in a person of sound personality is likely to resolve spontaneously, especially if the provocative situation is itself transient. At the other extreme the chronically anxious personality, in need perhaps of psychological support through crises, is unlikely to benefit from any but the most skilled and protracted therapy. In plain words, time should not be wasted on those who are going to get better anyway, and the non-specialist should not bite off more than he can chew.

The patient most likely to benefit from psychotherapy has an acute anxiety state of recent origin but of uncertain cause, and although possibly constitutionally inclined to anxiety has nevertheless coped reasonably well in the past. Psychological nous is more important than higher intelligence. A quite unsophisticated relative or friend may offer surprisingly valuable insights into the psychopathology. Freud claimed only to report what every nursemaid knows.

The physical examination and iatrogenic neurosis

Anxiety-provoked physical symptoms induce a natural enough fear of physical disease, a fear which inflames the initial anxiety and sets in motion the vicious circle of symptoms → fear → more symptoms → more fear, as exemplified by the interaction of tachycardia and fear of heart disease.

The first step in psychological management is a comprehensive medical history and examination. Unsuspected physical disease may be found and treated as appropriate, but most commonly no significant physical disorder is detected. At this juncture a very common mistake is often made: the patient is sent on his way with the assurance that nothing is the matter. Inevitably new fears emerge of harbouring serious, early, obscure or undetectable illness as causes of the continuing symptoms. The expressed opinion that nothing physical is the matter *must* be followed by an acceptable explanation of the symptoms. The most potent iatrogenic anxiety-provoking programme of all involves referral for investigations round a carousel of specialist departments with little outcome other than growing uncertainty for patient and doctor. Six months on this roundabout can establish a neurosis even in the psychologically robust. A more effective technique for the induction of psychiatric breakdown could hardly be devised. The patient's best friend is the doctor who concludes that there is obviously no hidden physical disorder common enough or serious enough to warrant further unnerving examinations. Specialists may be driven on to protect their reputation for thoroughness when it is in the patient's interests to call a halt.

The clinician with laboratory back-up will exclude such diagnoses as thyrotoxicosis or the rare phaeochromocytoma, and positive features will establish the presence of pathological anxiety, one of the commonest disorders encountered in medical practice.

Sensitizing experiences

Unwinding the spiral of mounting anxiety is the key to success in treatment, and of all the means available the induction of confidence and understanding in the patient are paramount. A reasoned and comprehensible explanation to the patient of how and why the anxiety has occurred of itself reduces anxiety, but first the clinician must determine why in this particular patient the precipitating events to which others would make a normal adjustment have induced maladaptation. A keen awareness of historical time sequences is vital for it is surprising how frequently a neurotic reaction is confidently attributed to events which commenced following its onset. In particular, one is searching for earlier disturbing emotional experience. The immediate precipitant may appear quite trivial until it is linked with a deeply disturbing earlier experience which left an oversensitivity to any similar experience in the future.

Organizing time for the new psychiatric patient

Before the patient is ready to understand the underlying emotional causes of the illness, considerable medical time has already been expended. How much time should be devoted to the psychotherapy of one patient by a doctor involved with so many other demands? The answer depends very much on the doctor's hierarchy of priorities. Initial reluctance to become involved is understandable, for once pulled in by the intellectual challenge and emotional appeal it is neither easy nor desirable to opt out again.

There is some truth in the claim that the psychiatrist is now the only medical practitioner to attempt a comprehensive history. The first interview with a psychiatric patient requires a full three-quarters of an hour, at the end of which the practitioner should have a fair idea of what is wrong and what is required of him. The patient is comforted in that for the first time a professional has sat down, listened, and seems to know what he is about.

The brief interview and hastily written prescription is a travesty. The patient returns shortly and the superficial medical response is repeated. In time, the increasingly irritated doctor and increasingly frustrated patient come to dislike each other and no progress has been made. The short time available at first contact is best spent arranging a time for adequate investigation within the next few days. Family doctors who have organized their working programme to allow uninterrupted sessions with their psychiatric patient are convinced the approach is not only more effective, but in the long run, time-saving. Following the initial lengthy interview, the majority of patients with acute neuroses respond favourably to 3–6 individual 20–30 minute sessions at extending intervals over the ensuing 2–3 months.

Prognosis

Although many who suffer acute anxiety state proceed to recovery without medical intervention, clinicians are traditionally as much concerned with support and comfort through an illness as with ultimate prognosis. Psychiatrists believe that insight gained under psychotherapy can protect against recurrence.

Whether treated or not, the most important factor affecting prognosis is the quality of the premorbid personality. Those who have formerly enjoyed good interpersonal relationships through life, particularly within the childhood family, and who have coped adequately with a variety of stresses are likely to effect a satisfactory readjustment. Genetics play little part in the development of the neurosis-prone personality whose weaknesses are the outcome of unfavourable emotional learning. The more neurotic markers in the history, the greater the likelihood of repeated neurotic episodes, and disappointing treatment results. Such markers include: *in childhood:*

prolonged illness, timidity and withdrawal, disturbed relationships especially with parents but also with peers, recollection of childhood as generally unhappy; *in adult life:* distorted marital relationship, unstable work record, nervousness.

Psychiatric trainees are easily tempted to take on a patient declared virtually untreatable by the more experienced. Family doctors are well advised to accept their limitations lest adverse early therapeutic experiences undermine confidence in their ability to treat the treatable.

Relaxation

Many therapeutic variations of behaviour theory have been reported, but are outside the scope of this chapter. There is much, however, to recommend the adoption of induced mental and physical *relaxation,* by means of any of the techniques introduced into the West over recent decades. Initial instruction and training do not of necessity require the active participation of a medical practitioner, for other professionals, e.g. clinical psychologists, have the required skills. The subject is trained in self-induction of the relaxed state with consequent reduction in autonomic nervous activity. There is little doubt now that the most practised and skilled can exert a degree of control over their own blood pressure, pulse rate and metabolic rate which was not until recently believed possible.

Relaxation therapies are of particular value in the chronically anxious and in certain psychosomatic disorders.

Physical methods of treatment

In practice, the value of drug therapy in anxiety states is quite limited. The major tranquillizers such as chlorpromazine, promazine, trifluoperazine, fluphenazine and pimozide are antipsychotics, are not indicated for neuroses, and are in practice seldom so used.

Of all the anti-anxiety agents the most potent in general use have been self-selected alcohol and medically prescribed barbiturates. Rebound depression and possible addiction make *alcohol* an undesirable anti-anxiety agent unless consumption is kept within low limits. Medical advice to desist may or may not be accepted, but the doctor should be wary of advising alcohol to calm the nerves. *Barbiturates* likewise cause rebound depression and dependence/addiction to a degree only recently fully recognized. They induce paradoxical excitement and confusion in a proportion of elderly subjects and can prove fatal taken along with alcohol. In consequence, barbiturate prescribing has declined conspicuously. Psychiatrists have used or advised barbiturates very little, other than for epilepsy, over the twenty years since the hazards of amphetamine/barbiturate mixtures became apparent, and it can now be said with confidence that except for i.v. use in certain specialized intensive treatment programmes, the barbiturates have no real place in the treatment of psychiatric disorders.

Minor tranquillizers have been in vogue for many years for the relief of symptoms of anxiety and depression, so much so that the names of the most commonly prescribed are virtually household words. Insistent demands by patients rather than medical initiative account for contemporary over-prescribing. Repeat prescriptions are provided for years, even without the patient being seen again by the doctor after the initial brief consultation; serious addiction can result.

There are three indications for the use of tranquillizers in neurotic disorders: (1) to tide a patient over an acute situational crisis, in which instance two weeks or less on the drug is sufficient and a month too long, for psychological dependence can develop quite rapidly; (2) as an aid for the chronically anxious individual in whom long-term tranquillizer dependence may be less undesirable than interminable suboptimal efficiency; (3) to dampen anxiety so intense that concentration and coherent thinking are impaired to a degree that renders psychotherapy impossible.

Diazepam is the most widely prescribed of the minor tranquillizers, the drawbacks of which are insufficiently recognized. Foremost are the hazards of dependence and, with long-term use, true addiction (*see* p. 488). Induced impairment of co-ordination and delayed reaction time are undesirable for those in control of potentially dangerous machinery, including road vehicles. The drug not rarely induces release of disinhibited and aggressive behaviour. Diazepam in the first trimester of pregnancy is associated with an increased incidence of babies with hare lip and cleft palate. Of particular relevance to all the hazards is the extremely slow elimination of the drug, traces of which can be detected in the blood a month after the last dose. Pharmacological theory would suggest that alternative benzodiazepines of brief half-life—*oxazepam* and *lorazepam*—are safer alternatives. Effort is now directed to the introduction of tranquillizers which do not impair alertness.

Anxiety is very common, drug treatment is much in demand, and pharmaceutical firms can expect their anti-anxiety agents to recover their daunting research and development costs. Promotional literature initially quotes obscure references and unpublished papers. In most countries doctors and patients have the assurance that approval has been given for use by the appropriate watchdog authority: the USA's F.D.A. and the UK's Committee on Safety of Medicines, yet the disadvantages, contraindications and even dangers of today's new drug may only emerge after several years of cumulative experience channelled through central information agencies. The latest drug is popular because its defects have yet to be revealed.

The underlying cause of the massive over-prescribing of tranquillizers for neurotic disorders lies in the inability or disinclination of otherwise hard-pressed clinicians to resist patients' demands. Judicious use of drugs as and when indicated, along with commonsense practical psychological manage-ment achieves results. Medical resistance to emotional involvement with the patient is as much a bar as the prospect of finding the time.

Medical practitioners as psychotherapists

Of all psychiatric patients, those with anxiety states are the least likely to require admission to a psychiatric bed. They are heavily represented at psychiatric outpatient clinics, yet only a small proportion of the total can ever be, or need to be, treated by psychiatrists. Psychological aspects comprise a half of all illness encountered in general practice. If the clinician is unwilling or unable to undertake the required treatment the patient will turn to non-medical sources for help. It may fairly be asked whether the medical practitioner has any particular role to play when psychological therapies can be administered without a medical training. The non-psychiatric clinician can hardly hope to match the level of psychotherapeutic skill which should develop in therapists who concentrate all their efforts in this one area. His training and experience, however, bring to bear a broad biological approach which is invaluable. In practical terms, he can assess the relevance of somatic symptoms and determine whether they are of physical or psychological origin. Judicious selection can be made from the whole range of physical and psychological methods of treatment. The patient is not just a vehicle for the interplay of psychological forces to be modified by psychological manipulation alone. To the medical practitioner, every patient presents a complex interplay of psychological and physical forces amenable in varying degrees to modification either by psychological influence or by effecting alterations in higher brain function through physical interventions; he is not obliged to enter the fight with one hand tied behind his back.

Medical training at least ensures a questioning attitude to claims for psychotherapy, noticeably absent in many who set forth to save the world from its follies after a brief cram course in psychosocial dogma. Medical and nursing experience inculcate a practical sense of urgency and involvement in preference to sitting around discussing theory.

Eradication of counterproductive tendencies

Basic psychotherapeutic theory presents no great difficulty to the intelligent reader. It is when theory is put into practice that personality and attitudes become paramount. We are aware of certain of our quirks, foibles and prejudices, but are blind to many others, quite apparent to acquaintances and colleagues. We should become aware of some which are prejudicial to the successful practice of psychotherapy. The patient has the therapist to guide him, but who holds up the mirror to the therapist? Glaring tactical and emotional errors can be readily identified by experienced colleagues, hence the value of practical in-service training in psychotherapy. The practitioner working in isolation would be well advised to submit videotaped psycho-therapeutic interviews to a trusted and knowledgeable colleague for comment. Common faults include the adoption of: (1) attitudes of superiority to the patient, perhaps as a particular manifestation of a general attitude unconsciously adopted in defence against insecurity in personal relationships; (2) psychological bullying tactics, forgetting that the techniques were developed to help the less fortunate, not to provide weapons for personal dominance; (3) a moralistic approach, particularly damaging in the presence of conflict between desire and conscience; (4) an over-didactic approach which does not allow the patient gradually to arrive at his own decisions; (5) rushing things, thereby not allowing the patient time to gain confidence to bring forth traumatic emotional material; (6) talking too much, thereby overwhelming the patient's initiative; and (7) allowing the patient to ramble on irrelevant topics, thereby avoiding having to face the truth. When this happens a stated time limit to the course of psychotherapy can be helpful; it forces the patient to get down to the vital issues.

Fortunately common sense, empathy, some knowledge of hidden psychological processes, and avoidance of glaring tactical errors can take the practitioner a long way without formal training. Psychiatrists have no monopoly on psychotherapy. Only a minority have a real flair for it, and not every neurotic patient has the capacity to make progress under psychotherapy.

Claims for the efficacy of psychotherapies are but weakly supported by scientific studies, for neither the procedures nor their aims have ever been clearly defined. Those who claim psychotherapeutic expertise can only continue to apply their methods if convinced of their efficacy. When professional status and self-image are founded on the rock of psychotherapeutic expertise there are resistances to the involvement of would-be neutral observers. In logic it cannot be assumed that causal relationships (in this instance between method and benefit) do not exist unless supported by an accumulation of sound scientific evidence; to do so would be to assume a rather outdated arrogance characteristic of an earlier phase of the scientific cultural explosion. Many, if not most, of the acts and decisions of day-to-day medical practice are founded on good faith and of their nature are not susceptible to scientific study. Few would deny the therapeutic value of good doctor/patient relationships, a concept hard indeed to subject to scientific scrutiny. Psychotherapy is but an extension of this relationship in which the personality and motivation of healer, and patient, are more potent than the particular method favoured. Methods range from full psychoanalysis as devised by Freud and his followers, both orthodox and deviant, through a bewildering network of 'schools' to the basic commonsense psychological interventions which experience shows to be of very considerable value in the management of neurotically anxious and depressed patients.

Agoraphobia

Clinical features

Agoraphobia is a quite common specific syndrome, which despite the presence of conspicuous anxiety demands treatments quite different from those for anxiety state.

Agoraphobia (literally—fear of the market place) occurs especially in young women whose alertness, poise and smart appearance on presentation contrast sharply with the appearance and facial expression of most psychiatric patients. Sufferers tend to be effective, well organized and sociable, with no prior history of psychiatric disorder. Characteristically, the very sudden onset follows some stress which involves a threat to the security of the family group, in particular death and illness.

The presenting complaint is of fear on venturing forth from the security of the home, especially if unaccompanied. Anxiety rapidly escalates to panic in crowded shops, the cinema or church, in trains and buses, indeed anywhere that the subject feels hemmed in by strangers. Questioning invariably reveals that the ultimate fear in such situations is of fainting and hence looking foolish. Only under careful enquiry will the patient reveal the further symptom-complex of unreality which frequently coexists and is often the earliest symptom experienced. Agoraphobic patients are reluctant to reveal their alarming experiences of unreality lest they be thought mad. Complaints of 'dizziness' have to be probed further when, with an articulate subject, it will become clear that what is being described is the feeling of being emotionally alienated from the surrounding world. Either the subject feels strange and unreal in a real world (depersonalization), or the world around seems unreal (derealization). Either way, the content of the verbal description can reach bizarre proportions, raising the suspicion of schizophrenia. However, it is important to observe that the patient invariably qualifies by saying or implying, 'It is as if . . .' In other words, insight is maintained. As an alternative term Phobic Anxiety/Depersonalization (PAD) formally recognizes the frequent coexistence of agoraphobic and unreality states.

Ineffective or harmful treatment for agoraphobia

The agoraphobic patient can become a psychological house prisoner for years. Not unnaturally, the severe restriction on social mobility causes great unhappiness, whence arises the common medical error of effecting a diagnosis of depression. Only rarely and unexpectedly will a patient with PAD respond favourably to the more commonly used antidepressant drugs while those of the tricyclic series may even worsen the condition. Electroconvulsive therapy (ECT) given in good faith for the supposed depressive disorder may temporarily ease the depressive affect but is only too liable to induce an acute exacerbation of the pre-existing unreality. It is totally contraindicated in agoraphobic states *unless* symptoms of *endogenous* depression coexist when it should be used with great caution.

Inappropriate treatment either as for anxiety state or depressive disorder commonly results from failure to recognize the PAD syndrome.

Effective treatment of agoraphobia

Unless there is a prior history of jaundice the monoamine oxidase inhibitor, phenelzine, is the first treatment of choice. Soon after its introduction in the late 1950s the drug unfortunately acquired an exaggerated but widely held reputation as a serious hepatotoxic; the risk is there, but it is small. Furthermore, many practitioners avoid prescribing phenelzine on account of the hazards of interaction with certain items of diet. Severe, and very occasionally, fatal crises of hypertension, or less commonly, hypotension, occurred in the drug's early years before the effects of tyramine-containing foodstuffs became clear. Now the dispensing pharmacist provides the patient with a card warning against (1) tyramine-containing foodstuffs, and (2) catecholamine nasal decongestants and bronchial dilators. The printed card only supplements the doctor's careful instructions, including a precaution to maintain the dietary restrictions for *at least a fortnight* after stopping the slowly metabolized drug. Morphine and pethidine in any intervening acute medical emergency can be fatal and likewise must not be given within 2 weeks of stopping the drug.

Phenelzine is manufactured in 15 mg strength tablets only. Initially, the patient should be advised to take one 15 mg tablet of phenelzine lest rare untoward effects such as severe restless agitation ensue in the following 24 hours. In the absence of any such reaction the dose is raised to 15 mg three times a day, the patient being persuaded to maintain this level *despite initial failure to improve*. The efficacy of phenelzine can be potentiated safely by adding L-tryptophan (supplied as large 0·5 g tablets) at 3 g/day in divided doses. It is essential to see the patient again at about 10–14 days to counter sagging morale and encourage continuance. Only if there is no improvement at all by 5 weeks should the drug be tailed off and stopped in favour of alternative time-consuming treatments under specialist care. Given any level of improvement within the 5 weeks phenelzine is continued at 3–4 tablets/day in divided doses until the maximum response possible is achieved. Thereafter, it is advisable that the patient continue the regime for a further period of 2 months when step-like reductions in daily intake can commence. In the event of a relapse the initially effective dose is resumed, relief being delayed for a week or more. Later the experiment in gradual withdrawal is repeated. Rarely a patient can only be maintained in remission by continuing the drug regime indefinitely. Failure of phenelzine treatment is an indication for referral to a psychiatrist for more complex alternative therapies.

Pharmacogenetics of monoamine oxidase inhibitors (MAOIs)

MAOIs were first introduced into medicine in the treatment of tuberculosis. It was observed that the resultant euphoria was disproportionate to the rate of improvement of the tuberculosis, and the drugs were subsequently shown to have valuable antidepressant properties. Genetically, individuals are either fast or slow acetylators of MAOIs, so it is reasonable to suspect that a proportion of drug failures can be attributed to fast acetylation with consequent ineffective blood concentrations on standard doses. Testing for the MAOI acetylation category of an individual is a relatively simple biochemical procedure, but the practical implications for dose levels are not clear, and such testing is seldom undertaken.

Mind and body—two or one?

A satisfactory response to drug therapy (MAOI) of a pathological mental state (PAD) induced by adverse psychological experience (e.g. bereavement) offers to the reflective clinician an excellent illustration of the two-way interaction between psychological events and states and chemicophysical brain processes, an example made all the more striking when one considers the similarities between psychologically induced depersonalization states and physically induced temporal lobe epilepsy.

Depressive neurosis (syn. reactive depression; exogenous depression)

Depression, like anxiety, is a very common reaction to stress. Which affective response the individual will experience is a function of constitution and, to some extent, of the nature of the stress. Experiences of loss are particularly liable to cause depression.

Differential diagnosis

1. Even quite severe depression cannot be regarded as illness if the provocation has been excessive. For a diagnosis of depressive *neurosis* the reaction must be excessive in relation to the stress which triggered it.

2. Profound affective symptoms of anxiety or depression are not exclusive to the affective disorders, for either can be prominent in psychiatric disorders ranging from schizophrenia to early arteriosclerotic dementia. It is essential to consider and eliminate such alternative psychiatric disorders.

3. Within the affective disorders the differentiation of endogenous from exogenous depression has important treatment implications.

The clinician's assessment of the relative prominence of depression and anxiety usually accords with the patient's reply to the simple question 'Are you more keyed up and tense, or more miserable and down in spirits?' If anxiety is dominant the diagnosis is properly 'anxiety state'. Thus nonpathological depressive reactions, psychiatric syndromes accompanied by depression, endogenous depression, and anxiety state all require consideration in differential diagnosis.

Clinical features

Key features of depressive neurosis are: a tendency for the mood to worsen as the day progresses, difficulty in falling off to sleep at night, blaming others or circumstances for provoking or aggravating the condition, and a mood state which reacts favourably to the day's pleasanter events; familiar company brings relief, with immediate worsening when the patient is alone again. This quality of *reactivity* is hardly seen in endogenous depression.

Unfortunately the term 'reactive depression' also indicates that the onset of the illness is in reaction to adverse experience. To avoid confusion the diagnostic term 'depressive neurosis' is preferable to 'reactive depression'.

Other symptoms common to affective disorders generally are of no help in the differentiation of depressive neurosis: tiredness, anergia, anorexia, weight loss, reduced sex drive, interrupted sleep.

Management

Admission of a neurotically depressed patient to a psychiatric bed is unusual either from general practice or from a psychiatric out-patient clinic. A proportion of parasuicide cases with depressive neurosis, however, do require transfer following intensive care in the medical unit.

Incidence and prevalence statistics show depressive neuroses to be as common as anxiety states, and taken together the two categories of affective neurosis are extremely common. Psychiatric specialists can only treat a small proportion: the burden falls on primary care practitioners.

Drug therapy

Supportive psychotherapy and induction of understanding of relevant cause/ effect sequences are vital whether drugs are used or not. Antidepressant drugs are indicated, dose and duration being as for endogenous depression (*see below*), with expected benefit in some 40–50%. When anxiety is troublesome *either* one of the antidepressants with sedating properties can be selected, e.g. amitriptyline, doxepin or dothiepin, *or* a tranquillizer can be added. Blood levels of drugs in relation to dose vary widely so the use of separate antidepressant and tranquillizing preparations gives a degree of therapeutic flexibility which outweighs the convenience of taking the drugs in combination tablet form.

The drug flupenthixol, introduced into practice as a tranquillizer (i.e. anti-anxiety agent), has interesting antidepressant properties and is now recognized to be especially effective in depressive neurosis. Flupenthixol (0·5 mg tablets) is given in divided doses within a range of 2·0–3·0 mg daily.

Endogenous depression (syn. manic-depressive psychosis— depressed type; depressive psychosis)

Endogenous depression, although one of the group of affective disorders, differs from depressive neurosis in aetiology, course and management. In varying degrees and guises it is a common and very harrowing disorder, often neglected, misdiagnosed or mismanaged, yet it is the most readily treatable of all psychiatric disorders. In its more severe forms, contact with reality gives way to delusional feeling and thinking of psychotic intensity. In the mid-nineteenth century Kraepelin distinguished a group of mental hospital inpatients with certain characteristics; the illnesses occurred as clear-cut attacks between which the subject was unimpaired and able to lead a full normal life in the world outside. The dominant mood when ill was depressive, but in some patients with similar spontaneous onset and resolution the mood was one of pathological elation—the very opposite of depression. In some, elation would characterize one admission and melancholy the next. Kraepelin concluded that depression and mania were different aspects of one and the same disorder, a concept which has stood the test of time as the diagnostic category of manic-depressive psychosis.

Natural history of an episode

Endogenously depressed patients suffer intensely and only rarely lose insight into their own need for treatment. Prior to the 1930s entry to mental hospital was exclusively by certification. Recognition of the absurdity of the procedure for those desperately requesting admission brought changes in the law allowing admission on a voluntary basis. Once in hospital, the overriding clinical management considerations were prevention of suicide, maintenance of nourishment and prevention of exhaustion until spontaneous resolution allowed discharge. Before effective physical treatments were introduced in the 1950s, patients in extremes of abject misery were an everyday sight in mental hospitals, pacing restlessly up and down, wracked with guilt, muttering repeated phrases of hopelessness and despair or, with similar mental content sitting immobile for days and weeks on end. Nowadays with early detection and effective treatment, it is extremely rare to encounter any endogenously depressed patient in such extremity but the picture represents the natural history of a severe attack of manic depressive psychosis, depressed type, which could last from months to several years until terminated by suicide, fatal depressive coma or spontaneous resolution. The change from protective care to effective treatment came with the widespread use of ECT in the late 1940s, followed by the introduction of antidepressant drugs in the late 1950s, until over half of all endogenous depressives referred to psychiatrists were treated without hospital admission. Most episodes are now treatable by non-psychiatric medical practitioners, and the psychiatrist need only be called in for the difficult case.

Aetiology

Whereas depressive *neurosis* is an overreaction to stressful experience, depression *psychosis* usually arises out of the blue for no identifiable external reason. The predisposition is genetically determined as a carefully elicited family history for depression, alcoholism, or suicide will often reveal. Biochemical and clinical research indicate causative reversible cerebral chemical changes, the full pattern of which is yet to unfold. Reduced synaptic levels of neurotransmitter catecholamines or 5-hydroxytryptamine (5-HT, serotonin) characterize episodes of manic-depressive psychosis. Concentrations resume normal levels on spontaneous or induced return to clinical normality. There are alterations in cell concentrations of sodium and potassium which behave likewise, and dopamine seems to be implicated.

Clinical features

Women are twice as vulnerable as men, with an extra loading associated with menstruation, the puerperium and the menarche. Attacks can occur at any age, but whether they occur in childhood in different form is controversial. The speed of onset is characteristic for a given patient in repeated attacks and varies from the very gradual over months, to the very rapid transition from normality to deep despair within 24 hours. For every case of very severe depression of psychotic intensity, there are many cases of lesser intensity, and many more who, though mildly affected, are nevertheless well worth treating. It is estimated that between 1 : 10 and 1 : 20 of the population will have at least one attack in a lifetime.

The presence of both mental and somatic signs and symptoms are indicative of a general impairment of biological functioning. It has never been established how many of the possible listed manifestations have to be present in order to effect the diagnosis. Empathy with the patient's mood is diagnostically critical; one can *feel* the quality and intensity of the depressed mood. Indeed the concordance between psychiatrists in the independent assessment of intensity of depressive mood is extremely high.

Clinically there is slowing of thought, movement and expression. Loss of interest and zest and of the capacity for enjoyment accompany gloom, hopelessness and despair, prominent even in moderately severe episodes, as are feelings of worthlessness, failure and self-blame. Pathological and bizarre guilt feelings and sexual delusions are nowadays mainly confined to the elderly indoctrinated in their earlier years with a capacity for guilt. Thoughts of suicide are inevitable. A specific diurnal rhythm is diagnostic when present: at night the patient falls to sleep without difficulty but wakes early in the small hours of the morning after which sleep is fitful or impossible. Distress is at its most intense in the morning, but at some time between midday and 6 or 7 p.m. the mood lifts and life, if not pleasant, at least becomes tolerable. This characteristic pattern of insomnia and mood change repeats day after day, and the mood does not react favourably to occurrences which would otherwise be pleasurable. In depressive neuroses, in contrast, there is initial insomnia, worsening of mood as the day progresses, reactivity to events, and a tendency to blame other people or circumstances.

Anorexia, weight loss in the untreated, anergia, fatiguability and loss of sexual drive are common in depressions of any type, but bizarre hypochondriacal delusions, classically of rotting bowels, are indicative of severe endogenous depression.

A delusion is a false idea or belief which cannot be corrected by an appeal to reason, and which is inconsistent with the beliefs common within an individual's culture. The expression of delusions indicates a psychotic illness, in which contact with reality is impaired to a degree not seen in neurotic disorders. Even in lesser degrees of illness much of the expressed thought content of the endogenously depressed has delusional quality—the distressed feelings are no longer an understandable response to psychological circumstances.

Mixed exogenous/endogenous depression

The classic differentiation of neurotic and psychotic depression outlined above suggests that depressive illness is simply polarized, but in clinical practice a clear distinction cannot always be effected for patients often present with a mixture of endogenous and exogenous symptoms. This is hardly surprising considering that so many of the population harbour neurotic tendencies which will flare up under stress. An attack of endogenous depression is extremely stressful, for those who have previously endured pain, unhappiness and illness describe it as the worst experience life has to offer. The differentiation is further complicated by the issue of reactive depressive psychosis. Because psychotic endogenous depressive attacks characteristically arise out of the blue with no identifiable precipitating event or circumstance, a false assumption can be made that any excessive depressive reaction to stress is a depressive neurosis. When a clear syndrome of endogenous depression presents, any preceding stress can easily be discounted as the latest and irrelevant manifestation of the truism that 'life is one damned thing after another', for at any moment in a person's life there will have been some recent stress. Gradually it has become accepted that certain severe stresses in the lives of quite stable persons trigger off, not a depressive neurotic reaction, but the chemical changes of psychotic depression. Here again is a striking example of holism; a psychological experience triggers biochemical changes which induce an abnormal psychological state. Bereavement is the most potent precipitant of reactive depressive psychosis. Indeed bereavement is now a far commoner precipitant of mental illness than sexual conflict. The *fin de siècle* sexual repressions of middle-class Europeans have gradually been dispelled, to be replaced by death as the 'great taboo of our time'.

Endogenous depression and physical disease

The presence of somatic symptoms in endogenous depression can set off a fruitless search for physical disease. Conversely, the symptoms may too easily be accepted as depressive in origin and so mask the presence of a physical disease process which is itself the provocation for the psychotic depression. A first attack of endogenous depression in middle age should institute a search for physical illness; the older the patient at the first attack the greater the likelihood of undetected physical pathology. The incidence of malignant and degenerative processes increase with age and a predisposition to psychotic depression which has remained dormant through all life's stresses for over fifty years is unlikely to become manifest in the absence of some unusually potent stress factor. If the stress is psychological or social it will be clearly evident; if not, physical illness is likely. Optimal relief of the symptoms of the physical illness will not be attained without additional treatment of the depressive illness, and the depression will not respond fully unless the physical symptoms are relieved in parallel.

Thus the somatic symptoms of endogenous depression can mimic physical disease, and physical disease can be the precipitant of an attack of endogenous depression. Finally, when the symptoms of some recognized physical disorder seem disproportionate, or treatment fails to bring the degree of relief anticipated, the possibility of a concurrent low-grade depression should not be overlooked.

Management of a first episode

DELAY IN SEEKING HELP

Unless the onset has been abrupt with rapid deterioration, the patient, feeling acutely that his condition is his own fault and evidence of personal inadequacy and failure, may well attempt to fight off the depression for weeks or months before seeking medical help. As depression deepens and initiative becomes impaired the patient is no longer able to seek the necessary help: medical intervention then depends on the initiative of relatives or friends.

THE INTERVIEW

The manner in which the first interview is conducted is critical. The patient must be allowed ample time to give an adequate account of the symptoms for comprehension of prompting questions is slow, thinking is retarded, and responses delayed. The intensity of the mental pain and the desire for help ensure truthfulness and cooperation.

DISPOSAL

The interview terminates with a decision whether to seek early admission, refer to a psychiatric outpatient clinic, or undertake the treatment personally.

Admission. Need for admission does not depend solely on the severity of the illness. Attitudes, and potential for practical supervision and support within the family, are of equal relevance. For patients living alone the threshold of severity warranting admission is lower. Only rarely is compulsory admission justified or desirable.

Outpatient referral. Request for an outpatient appointment should be by telephone with a clear indication of the degree of urgency. An appointment clerk's offer of the next vacancy a fortnight ahead is unacceptable, for the risk of suicide is high over a lengthy waiting period.

If the depression is sufficiently intense to warrant referral or admission three days is the maximum allowable delay. Once under specialist care the risk of suicide becomes negligible.

Management of subsequent attacks

Many people experience only one attack in a lifetime, but recurrence is common enough either immediately after cessation of treatment or months to years later. When medical intervention has proved helpful in the past there will be lesser reluctance to seek medical help and to accept admission again if advised. Following discharge from inpatient or outpatient care the patient must be kept under surveillance until the prospect of post-treatment relapse fades.

It is not always essential to re-refer to specialist services in repeat attacks, for the notes and letters from hospital will have recorded the treatment which previously induced remission. The therapeutic response of a given patient is relatively specific so that the drug and dose which effected recovery in a previous episode is the treatment of first choice for the present episode.

Treatment of the endogenous depressive episode by the non-psychiatrist clinician

INEFFECTIVE DRUG TREATMENT OF ENDOGENOUS DEPRESSION

Nowadays the majority of referred patients diagnosed by the psychiatrist as suffering from endogenous depression have already been under drug treatment from the physician of primary contact. It might be expected that these referred 'treatment failures' would be drug-resistant subjects presenting difficult therapeutic problems, and rightly the province of the specialist. This is rarely so and the great majority have been undertreated, wrongly treated or mismanaged.

The great proportion of patients in endogenous depressive attacks never pass beyond the non-psychiatrist clinician. Doubtless a good number of patients prescribed small doses of antidepresants for unindifferentiated depression respond or resolve, but when any but the mildest endogenous depression presents it is essential to get both diagnosis and treatment right. Reintroduction of the term 'melancholia' might emphasize the difference from other states of depression. Optimal use of the antidepressant drugs at present available has become as important as the search for better drugs.

EFFECTIVE DRUG TREATMENT OF ENDOGENOUS DEPRESSION

The basic principles of drug treatment are:

1. Antidepressant drugs should be prescribed. Even when anxiety levels are high, tranquillizers alone can only bring marginal symptomatic relief confined to the anxiety component.

2. If the patient is conspicuously anxious and agitated either: a tranquillizer may be added to the antidepressant drug, or, alternatively, an

antidepressant drug with sedating properties can be used. If the former tactic is adopted antidepressant/tranquillizer combination tablets are best avoided.

3. It is better to acquire experience of the effects of a few antidepressant drugs than to select at random from the whole range now available.

4. The patient and any accompanying relative need to appreciate that benefit from the antidepressant drug will not be felt until it has been taken regularly for 2–3 weeks, and that in the waiting period the patient will probably feel worse with drug side effects added to the still unrelieved depression.

5. Potentially effective drug dosage must be quickly achieved and maintained *despite side-effects.* G.Ps tend to use low doses to avoid side-effects, while psychiatrists use high doses, even for outpatients, to increase the prospects of success.

6. Expected side-effects should be discussed, with advice to tolerate common harmless ones and report any others, which though less common could be potentially harmful. Intolerable side-effects are an indication for lowering of dose for not infrequently patients with low tolerance eventually respond to maintenance of apparently suboptimal dose levels.

7. Explanations and advice must be given slowly and repeated to allow comprehension by a cerebrally retarded subject distracted by pathological emotion. Verbal recommendations can be backed up by a written note of the drug schedule, the expected side-effects, and the time and place of the next appointment.

8. The patient should be seen at weekly intervals until improvement appears, to allow adjustment of dose levels and to persuade the patient (in whom hope may be almost dead) to persist with the apparently ineffectual treatment. If the patient fails to attend efforts must be made to re-effect contact.

Once improvement has started longer intervals can be allowed between contacts until remission seems secure.

9. Rapid deterioration at any stage calls for speedy psychiatric referral.

10. No tactic ensures failure more effectively than a hurried interview, a prescription without explanation and evasion of the need to follow the patient through.

DURATION OF DRUG THERAPY

The drug of first choice should be stopped if, by *4 weeks* there is no sign of improvement. Given any improvement the drug is continued until maximum benefit is consolidated after which the dose can be reduced by weekly steps to half the initial level. Thereafter it is desirable to persuade the patient to continue the reduced medication for at least a further 2 months in order to reduce the prospect of speedy relapse. When the time comes to stop altogether the drug should not be withdrawn suddenly, but be reduced in steps over the final 2 weeks, so that any deterioration can be swiftly countered by a drug increase to be maintained over a further 2 months, when the withdrawal experiment can be repeated. It is not easy to judge the required duration of drug treatment following recovery. By and large it is better to err on the generous side for both dose and duration.

FAILURE OF DRUG THERAPY

When the drug of first choice has induced no benefit within 28 days, the patient can either be referred, or another antidepressant drug can be exhibited, preferably a drug of quite different chemical structure. Failure of two successive antidepressant drugs over a 2-month period in a milder depression is a clear indication for referral.

ECT

Of endogenous depressive episodes 70–75% can be dispelled by antidepressant drugs within 2–8 weeks. Prior to the introduction of antidepressant drugs, ECT terminated 90% of attacks of endogenous depression. When antidepressant drug therapy has failed to effect recovery and suffering is still intense ECT can be very effective in two-thirds of the drug failure group.

Antidepressant drugs

Introduced in the late 1950s, the first antidepressant drugs were the tricyclic compounds *imipramine* and *amitriptyline*, the latter having sedating properties of particular value in the agitated anxious endogenous depressive. Much effort has since been made by the pharmaceutical industry to devise improved antidepressants. Improvement has many facets: fewer and less distressing side-effects, elimination or reduction of toxic effects, less frequent medication, faster action, maintained recovery. Progress has been made in reducing side-effects, but faster action of a new antidepressant is more often claimed than substantiated. Maintenance in remission of the chronically relapsing or repeating depression is a special issue (*see* p. 468).

In a minority of patients relief of depression appears to be drug specific and the patient may have to face months of trial and disappointment before success is achieved. Once the effective antidepressant therapy for that patient has been identified it becomes the treatment of first choice in any subsequent attack.

Fortunately for most patients in first attacks of endogenous depression the range of potentially effective antidepressant drugs is wide. The choice often hinges more on the type and intensity of expected side-effects, which according to circumstances may be to the patient's benefit, e.g. the drowsiness of mianserin in severe insomnia, or detriment, e.g. the tachycardia of tricyclic antidepressants in cardiac disease.

TRICYCLIC ANTIDEPRESSANTS

Side-effects. The tricyclic antidepressants all have similar anticholinergic side-effects, commonly tachycardia, dry mouth, sweating and focusing difficulty, all of which tend to decrease in intensity over the first few weeks. Amitriptyline can give rise to troublesome daytime drowsiness. Hesitancy of micturition may prove a problem in older men with prostatic enlargement in whom acute retention may develop. Glaucoma is an absolute contraindication.

Dosage. Dosage is similar for *imipramine* and *amitriptyline,* the aim being to achieve and maintain a dose level of 150 mg/day taken in divided doses three times a day. It is best to start the patient at half this dose for the first 3 days lest the sudden experience of side-effects prove alarming. Amitriptyline is available in a once-daily delayed release form, best given at bedtime so that the maximum sedating effect occurs when most needed.

When the time comes to withdraw treatment it should not be done suddenly, but gradually reduced over 2–3 weeks, for the tricyclic antidepressants are vasodilators with rebound vasoconstriction on sudden withdrawal and the possibility of cerebral or cardiac infarct in susceptible subjects. Tricyclic antidepressant drugs are eliminated in 3 or 4 days.

Both imipramine and amitriptyline are safe and effective, the major disadvantages being the intensity of the common side-effects and the effects of the tachycardia on impaired cardiac function.

Of the newer tricyclics *dothiepin* and *doxepin* are alternatives to amitriptyline when depressive illness is characterized by motor agitation and restlessness rather than retardation. Their side-effects are less troublesome and they may act more quickly. The usual achieved dose levels are: Dothiepin 75–150 mg/day in divided doses, to a maximum of 450 mg/day. Tablet strengths 25, 75 mg. Doxepin 150–300 mg/day in divided doses. Tablet strengths 10, 25, 50, 75 mg.

NON-TRICYCLIC ANTIDEPRESSANTS

Mianserin. This is a newer non-tricyclic antidepressant with the particular advantages of minimal anticholinergic side-effects. It is indicated when organic disease affects any of the anticholinergic side-effect target organs and is the drug of choice in the presence of cardiac impairment.

The usual dose range lies between 80 and 200 mg/day in divided doses, three times a day. Tablet strengths 10, 20 and 30 mg.

Phenelzine. The MAOI phenelzine may be effective in a proportion of endogenous depressives when other antidepressants have failed to achieve remission. Although an MAOI may be started some 3 or 4 days after withdrawal of a tricyclic antidepressant, the longer clearance time of MAOIs requires a full 2-week interval after MAOI withdrawal before other antidepressants are started.

There are numerous other antidepressant drugs, but when two of the above have been tried successively over some 2 months without resultant remission it is time to refer to a psychiatrist.

L-Tryptophan. As a treatment of endogenous depression L-tryptophan can prove remarkably successful on occasions and has the merits of absolute safety and freedom from drug incompatabilities. The essential amino acid L-tryptophan is converted to tryptamine, the precursor of 5-HT; and, at much higher levels of intake than any normal diet could provide, may act by restoring synaptic 5-HT to normal levels.

The 0·5 g tablets can be rather difficult to swallow. To achieve therapeutic levels 6–12 tablets (3–6 g) are required daily in divided doses. Improvement is unlikely until the third or fourth week of treatment.

Used simultaneously L-tryptophan can give a boost to the effect of antidepressant drugs, phenelzine in particular.

ADVICE ON E.C.T.

Despite emotional assaults on ECT from antipsychiatric groups, the physician of primary contact would do well to encourage his patient to trust the psychiatrist's judgement on the desirability of a course of ECT. The induced remission rate is higher than with antidepressant drugs. When the latter have failed, ECT comes into its own. Whether given on an outpatient or inpatient basis, it is effective across all ages, is one of the most dramatically successful therapies in medicine, is remarkably safe, and any memory defects it causes are impermanent.

Over-treatment with any antidepressant therapy, including ECT may propel the patient right through normal mood into hypomania or mania.

TREATMENT OF MIXED ENDOGENOUS/EXOGENOUS DEPRESSION

It is necessary, using antidepressant drugs, to achieve and maintain a measure of relief from the psychotic component before attempting psychotherapeutic amelioration of the neurotic maladjustment. Complete eradication of depression is unlikely until both exogenous and endogenous components have responded to appropriate treatments.

Pseudoneurotic preoccupations and worries may well develop *during* an endogenous depressive episode, but, being part of the overall syndrome, they shrink to normal proportions on recovery from the depressive illness.

Sorting out the shifting importance of exogenous and endogenous processes in depressive illness and treating accordingly demands close vigil and keen clinical judgement.

Prophylactic therapy

Treatment of the attack of endogenous depression has become increasingly effective over the past 30 years. Unfortunately, depression is not always limited to one or two episodes in a lifetime. A small proportion of the whole go on to have repeated attacks with spells of complete remission, while a few become bogged into chronic intractable depression of varying degrees of intensity and need specialist help and treatment.

With each attack the family doctor became involved, either in treatment or arranging referral or admission. Now instead he is more often in a partnership with the psychiatrist in the maintenance of prophylactic therapy.

LONG-TERM ANTIDEPRESSANT DRUG THERAPY

Some patients can only be maintained in remission by *continuous medication with the antidepressant drug* which effected recovery, any attempt at drug withdrawal or dose reduction below an established minimum resulting in the re-emergence of depressive symptoms. They are antidepressant drug dependent as a diabetic is insulin dependent, and in no sense addicted. It seems likely that some more or less permanent cerebral biochemical change has taken place, which can only be held in correction by continuous drug therapy.

LONG-TERM LITHIUM THERAPY

Lithium therapy is a major breakthrough, introducing for the first time an effective prophylactic against attacks of manic-depressive psychosis, whether the pathological mood swings be towards mania or depression.

Lithium salts had been advocated for various ills from time to time for over a century before their use became established after 1949 when Cade in Australia reported their efficacy in the treatment of acute mania. Contrary to expectation lithium is not an effective treatment for attacks of manic-depressive (endogenous) depression, but is effective in preventing further attacks whether of depression or mania. Its use in prophylaxis began to spread from the late 1960s and early 1970s, until a decade later between 1 in 1000–2000 of the UK population were variously estimated to be on regular lithium intake. More effective extra mural treatment of depression and lithium-induced prevention of repeat admissions taken together probably account for the significant reduction in the number of depressives under psychiatric inpatient care.

Most general practitioners will by now have patients who, after many years of repeated manic depressive episodes, have been maintained in remission on lithium for over a decade.

Maintained lithium therapy is at its most effective in bipolar manic depressive psychosis, i.e. when both depressive and manic episodes have occurred. Good results are still to be expected however, with a history of unipolar illness, i.e. when all attacks have been either depressive or manic. Complete remission is not always attainable, but lithium therapy is still well worth while if it reduces frequency, severity and duration of attacks and restores antidepressant drug or ECT responsiveness in the treatment of the now milder episodes.

The lightest of the metals, lithium is used extensively in industry, requires no complex pharmaceutical preparation and is in consequence cheap. Laboratory estimation of plasma lithium levels, which must always be available, is a relatively quick and straightforward procedure.

Preparations of lithium. Lithium intake to maintain optimum blood levels usually ranges between 500 and 1250 mg/day. It can be taken either as *lithium carbonate* (250 or 500 mg tablets) in divided doses over the day, or as one of the *delayed release preparations* (300 or 400 mg tablets) which offer the convenience of once-daily dosage. The peaking of daily blood levels with the latter may be undesirable, and the tablet strengths available do not allow the finer dose adjustments possible with lithium carbonate.

Selection of patients for lithium therapy. Lithium therapy is intended for long-term use and as the drug is not entirely without drawbacks and potential dangers the decision to start is not lightly taken.

Many patients had accumulated very long histories of depressive attacks by the time lithium prophylaxis was first introduced, and by now most have been under lithium protection for many years. Decisions now have to be taken on the advisability of lithium protection for patients who have had fewer episodes. Few would consider instituting lithium therapy after two attacks, but beyond that number the decision turns on the frequency, intensity and duration of the attacks, and their effect on the quality of the patient's life.

Once lithium-induced remission has been maintained for a number of years the only way to determine a continuing need for protection is by withdrawal of lithium cover. Relapse is so much the rule in patients with histories of many pre-lithium attacks that the price in suffering has to be weighed against the faint prospect of satisfactory progress without lithium. When prior attacks have been few in number and well spaced in time lithium may be stopped eventually without detriment; some would say it had never been indicated in the first place.

Supervision and tactics. Lithium prophylaxis is best started under specialist supervision in hospital. The patient can be admitted for the purpose when in remission, unless already in hospital recovering under treatment from an attack of manic depressive psychosis. The patient is screened for the contraindications of moderate to severe renal, cardiac or thyroid dysfunction. Once reasonably stable plasma lithium levels have been achieved, with frequent biochemical monitoring, the patient is discharged to psychiatric outpatient care.

The frequency of visits and plasma lithium estimations gradually decreases to once every three months provided plasma levels and clinical state remain satisfactory. Blood samples are despatched to the laboratory a few days in advance so that the report is to hand for the outpatient visit when any required dose adjustment can be advised. Interim plasma lithium estimates are needed following dose changes until the lithium concentration settles at the new level. When dose and plasma levels have remained stable for a year or two many patients pass entirely to general practitioner care.

Optimum plasma levels. It is apparent that for most patients the optimum range of plasma lithium levels is not as high as was formerly considered necessary. The present aim is maintenance at steady levels between 0·5 and 0·8 mmol/l. Toxic symptoms are more likely above 1·2 mmol/l and very likely above 2·0 mmol/l. Some patients show low tolerance and develop toxicity at levels as low as 0·2 or 0·3 mmol/l. It is not necessary to abandon lithium therapy on this account when it is really needed. The appropriate action is to maintain suboptimal plasma levels with small doses for a month or more and raise dose and plasma levels by small steps within the limits of increasing tolerance until therapeutic levels are achieved, a procedure which may take 6 months or a year.

Side-effects and toxic effects. Lithium reduces kidney tubular water resorption so that mild polyuria and polydipsia are invariable and can be ignored. Ataxia is an occasional side-effect. The coarse tremor of toxicity is in itself harmless, but warns of impending vomiting or diarrhoea.

Diarrhoea and vomiting are potentially dangerous toxic effects which the patient must be instructed to report to the doctor immediately, for the resulting dehydration increases the already toxic level of plasma lithium to compound a situation of rapidly escalating gravity. Conversely, dehydration from any cause, including incautious use of diuretics, will quickly raise the concentration of plasma lithium and induce toxic vomiting and diarrhoea to worsen the dehydration. Either way the patient is soon into the vicious spiral of fluid loss and rising plasma lithium levels.

Very rarely, severe toxicity of sudden onset may result from rapidly rising plasma lithium levels in a patient in whom dosage and plasma levels have previously been stable. The most dangerous cause to consider is sudden renal failure.

Management of mild toxicity. When toxic effects are mild the following steps are taken: either stop or lower the lithium intake and send off a blood sample straight away requesting a report by phone. The aim is to continue or restart the lithium at a subtoxic dose level with biochemical monitoring. How this is to be effected depends on the clinical state and reports of daily plasma lithium levels. If in doubt how to proceed the psychiatrist should be called in. On no account should the lithium therapy be abandoned because of the temporary crisis of mild toxic effects.

Management of severe toxicity. In the event of more severe vomiting or diarrhoea, whatever the supposed cause the lithium must be stopped immediately and the patient admitted to a medical ward as a matter of emergency.

As long as a toxic reaction is not associated with any irreversible organ pathology even a severe toxic crisis need not be regarded as an absolute contraindication to resumption of lithium therapy. If it is clear that lithium has been protecting the patient from the misery of repeated episodes of endogenous depression, with the attendant suicide risk, only the most cogent reasons for withdrawing the protection are admissible.

Diuretics. If diuretics have to be used the sodium loss will cause retention of lithium. Hence, lithium dosage must be reduced and lithium plasma levels estimated at frequent intervals.

Thyroid function. Lithium can depress thyroid function, and as the resultant hypothyroidism can prove irreversible thyroid function tests should be carried out at intervals. Just what the intervals should be is uncertain for thyroid function can become irreversibly impaired between routine tests at 6- or 12-month intervals. The most cautious psychiatrists advocate repeat testing at intervals of 2 months.

Mania and hypomania

These are much less common than the depressive manifestations of manic-depressive psychosis. Episodes are either spontaneous in origin or due to over-treatment of endogenous depression. Due to the subjects' almost total lack of insight admission rates and compulsory admission rates are higher than for any other diagnostic group in psychiatry. The manic psychoses respond well to inpatient treatments, usually starting with one of the quicker acting major tranquillizers to effect control while the slower acting lithium builds up its effect over a week or so.

9.4 HYSTERIA AND RELATED DISORDERS

A diagnostic trap

Regrettably common as a diagnostic trap is the assumption that the presence of psychiatric symptoms rules out physical illness. Whereas psychiatrists rarely miss the presence of significant physical illness, the same cannot be said of medical practitioners in general. Never is the 'either physical or psychiatric' fallacy more disastrous than in the presence of hysterical symptoms.

Such classic hysterical conversion symptoms as blindness, paralyses, and areas of anaesthesia are seldom seen now, though hysterical amnesia is occasionally encountered. Very common, however, is the presentation of symptoms in an hysterical manner, a situation which poses the question: are the symptoms all psychologically induced or are some at least caused by physical illness?

Not a disease entity

It is best to look on hysteria not as a disease entity but rather as the manner in which people of appropriate disposition react to stress. Feminists complain that the hysterical personality represents male psychiatrists' concept of women, but attention-seeking self-dramatization is by no means confined to the female sex. Certain professions attract and indeed require people who display the essential characteristics: emotional display, a need to be the centre of attention and to provoke and manipulate the emotional responses of an audience. The constant playing of roles is at variance with development of a true self in depth. To compensate for relative emotional shallowness the histrionic person lives vicariously through the provocation of emotional responses in others. In modest degree such traits are very normal, and contribute only in part to the overall personality. Medically, the contribution of excessive histrionic tendencies creates problems in diagnosis and management. Characteristically, symptoms are described in exaggerated terms—'terrible' pain, 'dreadful' tiredness—and they make little sense in terms of anatomy and physiology. Oddly, the patient may not seem to be deeply concerned, despite the dramatic display of suffering. Attempts at probing for further details of a symptom are countered by half statements, evasions, contradictions or change of topic. The doctor has only to mention a possible symptom for the patient to have it. Throughout, the patient is ever watchful, ever ready to create misunderstandings, to place the doctor on the defensive, to provoke an emotional reaction. At physical examination such simple requests as 'hold your hands straight out in front of you' or 'tell me if this feels sharp' are perversely misunderstood.

It is not easy when someone is apparently playing the fool like this to maintain clinical objectivity, to accept that no-one comes to a doctor solely to waste his time. If the physical symptom mime is *entirely* psychogenic some indentifiable stress will have overwhelmed the subject's psychological tolerance; the experience has been blanked out mentally by conversion into physical symptoms. Physical illness attracts sympathy—it provokes others to emotional responses of concern. The sick person occupies the centre of the stage, the childlike dependence of invalidity satisfies the desires of the immature. The longer diagnosis and management remain a puzzle to the professional, the longer the unhealthy satisfactions continue for the patient.

Management

The principles of psychological treatment and management of the hysteric are easier to declaim than to follow. Such patient must not be allowed to evade real issues and need gradually and step by step to be brought to acceptance of how they have been manipulating their world to accord with childlike fantasies of reality. At every turn, every move. the patient will evade, distort, exaggerate, conceal, distract, and attack, indeed engage in any and every imaginable self-defensive ploy. The successful therapist must display considerable persistence and capacity to absorb punishment.

There is little or no place for drug therapy in the management of uncomplicated psychogenic hysteria.

Malingering

The differentiation of hysteria from malingering is based on the supposition that in the former the subject is unaware of the motives which drive the behaviour, while the malingerer has made a conscious decision to deceive for gain. Not surprisingly, there is a grey area of diagnostic uncertainty, a playground for opposing lawyers and expert witnesses in civil action for damages and compensation claims.

Acute hysterical reaction to stress

The immediate provocative stress can be almost ludicrously obvious to the observer, as when the bridegroom does not turn up for the wedding ceremony and is brought into the casualty department having been found wandering, disorientated for time, place and person, not even knowing who he is.

Given time and kindly management psychogenic hysterical symptoms usually resolve within hours or days without heroic professional intervention. When a person of intelligence and integrity presents with such symptoms great care is necessary, for neurotic reactions are defences against unacceptable experience. When an individual of normally stable personality retreats as far as to develop crude hysterical escape mechanisms the stress, for that person, has been quite intolerable. Thus, ill-considered attempts to turn the patient face to face with the intolerable can result in suicide.

Cases of psychogenic hysteria of sudden onset which do not quickly resolve spontaneously require specialist treatment. Gently uncovering with the patient the life events which underlie the unhealthy pattern of response is a skilled and protracted activity.

Hysterical presentation of physical disease

In the earliest stages of CNS disorder hysterical symptoms can well mask the physical diagnosis. Indeed, neurological signs may only develop months later. It is as though the patient were dimly aware of the implications of the earliest symptoms and escaped into hysterical retreat from the unfaceable. Hysteria is *the* commonest presentation of multiple sclerosis and it may be that the earliest brain pathology of the disease affects those neural circuits involved in the promotion of hysterical behaviour.

Hysterical presentation of mental illness

Hysterical manifestations can supplant the natural anxiety and depression which are common early symptoms of mental disorders ranging from schizophrenia to arteriosclerotic dementia. Of particular diagnostic difficulty is the attack of endogenous depression, the true nature of which is hidden under a froth of hysterical exaggeration, distortion and evasion. A plausible psychogenesis can well blind even the most skilled observer to the true cause of the disorder.

'Hysteria' should never be accepted at its face value, especially when hysterical manifestations present for the first time in a person of stable personality. Even when a psychological precipitant is identified the patient must be subjected to as rigorous an investigation for physical illness or alternative psychiatric diagnosis as the undemanding patient who gives a straightforward history of symptoms and co-operates sensibly during the physical examination.

The patient with persistent hysterical personality traits is as prone to illness as anyone else, and should never be denied serious diagnostic scrutiny because of previous histrionic crises. Such persons have cried 'wolf' too often, to their detriment when serious and treatable illness does occur.

Pathological defences of doctors and nurses

Young nurses are particularly liable to go sick with hysterically determined physical symptoms and their medical knowledge allows a relatively sophisticated mimicry of physical illness syndromes so that a confident diagnosis of psychogenic disorder becomes exceptionally difficult. The sudden transition from the sheltered life of school and home to an environment of suffering and death defeats adaptive mechanisms. In contrast, the medical student's introduction to harsh human realities is more gradual, contacts with patients are of briefer duration and the high intellectual content not only reduces the likelihood of hysterical retreat but protects the student from the full impact of the human distress around him. Medical jokes take the sting out of the unpleasantness. One cannot weep for every dying child and continue to function efficiently, yet medical training can launch a pachyderm with repressed rather than suppressed capacity for empathy on patients whose sufferings are to be his concern for the next forty years. There is a very real temptation for the clinician to retreat from the patient into *excessive* involvement with research, teaching, technical procedures, the library, laboratory investigation, and above all the British clinician's devil of escalating committee involvement. The doctors' retreats include alcoholism and suicide.

The nurse's shock reaction, unless an expression of general personal inadequacy, does not indicate that a nursing career is unsuitable. Better in the long run a compassionate nurse who wilted temporarily under the first impact than a selfishly indifferent one never at risk. Attempts to demonstrate that the hysterical symptoms are a fraudulent deceit serve no useful purpose. The nurse should stay off duty and be given sympathetic and fairly intensive psychological help. The quasi-physical symptoms require investigation along the usual medical lines. Assurance that no serious physical illness is present must lead into a dialogue at common sense level around the shock experience of being thrown in at the deep end at a still tender stage of personal development. Assurances that the reaction is fairly common and well understood, and that the stress lessens with experience are all helpful. In the mutual talking through of unhealthy neurotic reactions a point of breakthrough occurs when the sufferer can be induced to raise a wry smile— a sure indication that a level of objective distancing from the personal dilemma has been achieved, by which stage the neurotic symptoms decline. As soon as the nurse is able, work should be resumed. Nurse training requires a series of limited periods across a range of professional settings and it should prove possible to arrange one of the emotionally less demanding postings on first return from sickness.

Hypochondriasis

Hypochondriasis is similar to hysteria in its mimicry of physical illness, but differs in persistent, fearful belief in the presence of undetected serious physical disease. The fear is quite impervious to medical investigations and reassurance which are, nevertheless, repeatedly sought. The belief system is quasi-delusional. Mental suffering is intense in marked contrast to the emotionally shallow attention-seeking invalid role playing of the hysteric. Repeated physical investigations of the hypochondriac's physical symptoms are therapeutically quite unproductive (unless some 'real' organic illness develops), but it must be admitted that psychiatric treatment has little to offer beyond sympathetic support. In the recent past, relief could be obtained by leucotomy, a treatment now under-used because of supposed popular antagonism, ill-inspired by leaders of the anti-psychiatry subspeciality of the anti-medicine movement.

Münchausen syndrome

Münchausen syndrome is so called for its parallel to accounts of the fantastic liar Freiherr von Münchausen (1720–97). The person displaying the syndrome as now understood seeks admission to hospital for investigation of simulated physical illness, prolongs admission as long as possible, disappears, turns up at another hospital, possibly under a different name, and repeats the pattern as a way of life. If detected, the subject moves on rather than undergo psychiatric investigation.

Deliberately induced disability

The syndrome of deliberately induced disability is commoner than is realized, manifest particularly as skin disorder, bleeding or local infection, all of obscure aetiology. Patients with the syndrome are prepared to go to extraordinary lengths to gain admission and investigation. The self-induced skin lesions are not dangerous, but those who provoke orificial bleeding can become gradually exsanguinated, before admission, down to Hb levels of 2·0–3·0 g/100 ml. Successive pustular stump infections can enforce a series of operations starting with amputation of a terminal phalanx, progressing even to forequarter amputation before the true cause becomes apparent with the development of a whitlow on the remaining hand. Syringe and faecally contaminated needle are used to create deep-seated abscesses and joint infections. Personal experience of work in hospitals leads to considerable expertise in method and concealment. How many serious self-inflicted disabilities go undetected is not known but it is likely that the true aetiology is unsuspected in the majority, while the number of lesser instances must be legion. Deliberate parental induction of disability in children is a recognized variant.

Detection depends primarily on considering the possibility. Invalidation in any degree evokes sympathetic attention and presents opportunities for manipulation and domination to the point of tyranny. Such regression is at its most bizarre in the serious case of deliberately induced disability and self-mutilation. If the patient can be brought face to face with proof of detection the perverse behaviour may stop, allowing an opportunity to tackle the underlying deep-seated distortion of personality development through intensive psychotherapy.

9.5   SCHIZOPHRENIA

The trend to community care

The non-psychiatric clinician will encounter a new case of schizophrenia only rarely but cannot avoid involvement in the care of established schizophrenics living outside the mental hospital. One in every hundred of the population will develop this most serious of mental illnesses. In parts of the USA the incidence would appear to be up to three times higher, but many so diagnosed in the USA would not be considered schizophrenic in Europe. The peak age incidence lies in the later teens and early twenties with survival prospects little short of normal. A generation ago one-half would stay in hospital indefinitely, one-quarter, despite continuing impairment, could get by in the outside world, and one-quarter would remit. Earlier detection with more effective initial therapy and management have improved the situation, so that now only 1 in 10 stays on in hospital under really long-term care. Of those discharged from hospital, the majority still require community nursing, social and medical supervision over extended periods if relapse is to be avoided.

Other medical specialists will from time to time receive established schizophrenics into outpatient or inpatient care for non-psychiatric illness and should understand the principles of management and the need for maintenance drug therapy.

Diagnosis

The diagnosis of schizophrenia is based intellectually on the detection of an unspecified number of the well known signs and symptoms described and listed in textbooks of psychiatry. However, as with so many psychiatric disorders, there is an emotional 'feel' to each category of disturbance, conveyed from the patient to the enquiring observer which is well-nigh diagnostic in itself. The anxious, depressed or manic moods of affective disorders are readily detected through the mechanism of empathy. Most people have at times experienced these moods in lesser degree so have some idea of what it must be like to feel them at pathological intensity. It is truly said that after an hour with a depressed patient one feels life is thoroughly miserable; after like time in a manic's company life is all present joy with a future of limitless possibilities. But after having tried to enter the world of the schizophrenic the feeling is 'either this person is out of his mind or I am'.

The split mind

The reflex arc provides one model for an understanding of the basic processes of mental life at higher level. Sensory input of information from the environment passes into a complex central sorting process by which immediate experience is compared with emotion-laden memories of similar experiences in the past so that sensation is distorted into perception. The motor response appropriate to the perception of the environmental event is the behavioural output, which includes speech, gesture and expression. The term schizophrenia implies splitting of the mind, and it is because the splitting occurs between sensory awareness, central processing and behavioural response that it is well nigh impossible for a mentally fit person to enter the schizophrenic's world. Only in schizophrenia does such splitting occur. In other psychiatric disorders the world is seen, felt and reacted to with inner consistency appropriate to the prevailing mood.

Maintenance drugs in community care

At the end of an initial period of intensive inpatient therapy the decision as to whether a schizophrenic patient is fit for discharge depends on the patient's contact with reality and ability to cope in a practical way with life outside, irrespective of persisting schizophrenic symptoms and signs.

Insulin coma therapy was the standard hospital treatment for the new case of schizophrenia up to twenty years ago, finally abandoned, not because it was considered useless, but rather because newly introduced major tranquillizers achieved similar or better results more simply. Chlorpromazine was the first to be introduced, subsequently followed by alternatives of broadly similar effect—pericyazine, perphenazine, promazine, trifluoperazine, thioridazine and haloperidol. It is now standard practice to use major tranqillizing drugs in the intensive treatment of the new case; ECT has its place when extremes of either excitement or withdrawal fail to respond adequately to drug therapy. One drawback of the major tranquillizers is their tendency to impair initiative when used in sufficiently high doses to relieve positive psychotic manifestations. In this event it is useful to give pimozide, either in addition or as an alternative. Pimozide is prepared in 2, 4 and 10 mg strength tablets, and is taken to a total of up to 10 mg/day in single or divided doses.

The most widely used major tranquillizer in schizophrenia is fluphenazine, as 1, 2·5 or 5 mg tablets, given orally in divided doses to a total of 15 mg daily. It is then relatively simple prior to discharge to substitute one of the delayed release fluphenazine preparations, either the enanthate or the decanoate, both available in ampoules of 25 mg/ml oily injection for intramuscular use. An initial injection of 0·5 ml will reveal any tendency to provoke extrapyramidal side-effects. Thereafter an effective dose regime for the individual will be found within the wide range from 0·5 ml (12·5 mg) every 3 weeks, to 4 ml (100 mg) every 10 days. An alternative drug is flupenthixol, 3 mg tablets, given in divided doses up to 18 mg/day. Thereafter, flupenthixol decanoate (20 mg/ml, and 100 mg/ml) can, after a smaller test dose, be given i.m. every 2–4 weeks in doses between 20 and 100 mg. Regular repeat i.m. injections of a delayed release tranquillizer allow discharge and maintenance in partial remission of any patients who would otherwise relapse quickly on their own, for lack of insight, erratic behaviour and delusional thinking make for poor compliance in regular drug self-administration. Should a relapse occur when the patient is on a delayed release preparation non-compliance in drug administration can be ruled out as a possible causative variable.

Family attitudes can make or break

Few psychiatrists doubt the value of intensive use of major tranquillizers in effecting control in the acute stages of schizophrenia, and of delayed release preparations once the patient leaves hospital. However, not all schizophrenics require drug therapy indefinitely in order to prevent deterioration.

Patients whose initial positive response to intensive drug therapy has been insufficient to allow discharge are commonly maintained as long-term in-patients on supervised oral tranquillizer therapy. Where the hospital offers an optimum environment of stimulating activities and favourable staff attitudes there comes a time when drugs can be withdrawn without detriment. When a patient has been discharged, the need for maintenance drug therapy depends likewise on the quality of the environment. Prospects are good when relatives adopt an easygoing, undemanding, yet affectionate attitude, and it may well be possible for a patient returned to such an emotional environment to dispense with drug therapy altogether without detriment. Relapse and readmission rates are much higher when relatives adopt attitudes either of smothering anxious overprotection or carping rejection. The schizophrenic, with impaired emotional capacity, cannot tolerate intense relationships, and fares best when those around can be held at an emotional distance. Lodgings and jobs providing residential accommodation may prove more favourable than life at home with the family.

The multidisciplinary approach

It must be appreciated that long-term supervision of the discharged schizophrenic requires the co-ordinated involvement of a number of professionals: the hospital-based psychiatrist in the outpatient clinic; the family practitioner watchful for drug side-effects and well placed to assess the emotional quality of the patient's home; the social worker especially involved in arranging suitable work and accommodation and supporting the family; and the community nurse who can take over the routine i.m. injections for schizophrenics within a given area.

It is in the patient's interests that the professionals involved—psychiatrist, G.P., nurse and social worker, maintain contact with each other across the community/hospital boundary whenever possible.

Work and accommodation

The level of work which the established schizophrenic can manage is often unrelated to domestic self-sufficiency. It is not uncommon for one patient to live and sleep at home yet attend a hospital's industrial therapy or occupational therapy department by day, while another can be in quite demanding full employment in the outside world yet have to return to hospital every night and at weekends. Where there is choice, employment and accommodation should be tailored separately to fit each patient's needs at the time. Apart from those in whom the acute attack resolves quickly, only a few patients progress to social independence and full employment, and with the passage of time the prospect of such progression becomes more remote. About one in every two hundred of the population is under supervision as an established schizophrenic living outside hospital.

Better in hospital or out?

The community-supported schizophrenic may require spells of inpatient care and treatment from time to time, and it might be maintained that permanent inpatient status would be preferable. Long-term inpatients, irrespective of diagnosis, are at risk of becoming increasingly institutionalized after some two years in hospital. Apathy and loss of initiative have to be countered by strenuous efforts to maintain a stimulating environment. Yet the schizophrenic kept out of hospital is not always the better for it. Whether hospital or community life is best for a given patient at a given time requires careful unprejudiced assessment.

9.6   THE UNCO-OPERATIVE PATIENT

The more unco-operative the patient the more difficult does therapeutic management become. The barriers arise from various sources.

Causes of impaired co-operation

1. The attitude of the clinician.
2. The attitude and personality of the patient.
3. The influence of relatives and friends.
4. The nature of the illness.

The clinician's attitude

Winning the patient's confidence at the initial interview is critical to all that follows. Forceful, dogmatic, superior or bullying attitudes are absolutely contraindicated. Most psychiatric patients are extremely sensitive to any hint of rejection and respond by withdrawal, counter-hostility or resentment, in any of which states the patient is unable to confide vital information required for diagnosis and management.

A talkative patient, especially at a first interview, is under pressure to pour out the problem as personally experienced, and what emerges is often a most disorderly and disjointed account. Despite the medical desire to construct a tidy history with each item recorded under its appropriate heading, it is as well to allow this initial unburdening to continue relatively unchecked until it is exhausted, for much is to be learned diagnostically from its style and content. Subsequently, the history can be filled out through judicious questioning and promptings. Ideally, three closely related histories are needed: a clinical psychiatric history, a medical history and a formulation of relevant psychopathology. The more inclusive the enquiries, the less the chance of errors in assessment, and the greater the patient's confidence in the clinician's competence. Most therapeutic errors stem from diagnostic error due to failure to complete a comprehensive enquiry.

The attitude and personality of the patient

The patient's initial attitude is usually guarded. Anticipation of adverse reception rouses considerable anxiety. Past experiences of doctors, hospitals and illnesses can help or hinder according to the emotional quality of the memories. Such personality characteristics as volubility, suspicion, aggressiveness or poor intelligence distort the therapeutic relationship. It is the clinician's job to detect such factors and make due allowance.

The influence of relatives and friends

However well meant, the influence of relatives and friends can decide whether the patient presents early or late in the illness, particularly when psychosis is present. The reactions of those in contact can profoundly influence the attitudes of the sick person towards medical treatment. Prejudiced and ignorant advice from these sources undermines professional therapeutic efforts, and so it is essential, if the patient agrees, to involve the relatives initially as informants, and at interviews thereafter to explain to them what is happening and is likely to happen.

The nature of the illness

Patients with endogenous depression are among the most co-operative of all psychiatric patients. Neurotics vary considerably, the most difficult being the hysterics. Co-operation with the clinician is at its poorest in mania, some cases of schizophrenia, hysteria, alcoholism and drug addiction and in the psychopathic and sociopathic whether with superadded psychosis or not. The lack of cooperation of the demented has a more passive quality.

Medical confidence that prescribed drugs are being taken is usually justifiable in endogenous depressives, but the clinician should be guarded with neurotic patients for studies have revealed a surprising degree of failure to comply. Spot laboratory checks of blood or urine can detect whether the drugs are being taken or, depending on rates of elimination, whether they have been recently taken. They are of lesser value when the clinician wants to know if the drugs have been taken regularly in the prescribed doses. Causes of unrevealed rejection of drug recommendations include: failure of the clinician to explain the action and side-effects, failure of the drug to effect benefit, fear of 'drugs' (largely induced by media journalism), pride in self-reliance and, more subtly, repressed hostility in relationship with a father figure or an hysterical need to demonstrate the doctor's incompetence. Given laboratory evidence of non-compliance the clinician should reveal his knowledge to the patient. Attempts with the patient to discover why the drug regime is rejected can lead to modification of therapy if necessary and to better patient compliance.

Compulsion

Legal control of compulsory admission for psychiatric care varies widely between societies, but in all the aim is similar—to protect the subject's civil rights while giving sanction for necessary compulsory detention to protect public and/or patient and allow treatment to be given even against the patient's will if considered necessary for the patient's welfare.

Non-psychiatrists are most likely to become involved as signatories of emergency orders of one sort or another to allow admission and detention for a limited period, after which many patients are sufficiently settled to stay on willingly to complete their treatment. Stringent legal safeguards control longer term detention. If the doctor acts in good faith, exercises due care and judgement, he is unlikely to suffer any legal repercussions.

It is important that no-one should lay a hand on the patient *before* the emergency order is completed and signed. Even to touch a patient without consent, implied or overt, is technically an assault.

Compulsion is required for only a very small proportion (5%) of all psychiatric admissions. Many patients whose behaviour and attitudes would seem to indicate a need for compulsory admission will, when handled with tact and understanding, enter hospital voluntarily. It is the psychiatrist and psychiatric nurses who have the patient 'eating out of their hands' after others have unwittingly worked him up into a 'certifiable' state. Over-persuasion is counterproductive, leading to demands to leave hospital in the first few days which must be granted or countered by the embarrassment of an emergency order made in hospital.

Compulsory admission is almost invariably necessary for the control and treatment of the very treatable manic patient, who, due to total lack of insight, will not comply with persuasions to accept admission and will not take prescribed drugs unless under close hospital supervision.

When insight is lost in dementia the decision whether to admit under compulsion depends on the law's requirements. In countries where a prospective inpatient is required to make a positive verbal or written statement of willingness to be admitted, then compulsion may prove necessary. If the legal requirement is that the patient does not actively object then most dements can be admitted on the grounds that admission is passively accepted. With any patient, if in doubt one should *not* certify. It is particularly rash and undesirable to admit any person under compulsion solely on the basis of expressed religion convictions, even when they are suspected of being delusional; further evidence of mental illness is essential before such action is taken.

Violence

The level of violence within a society is reflected to some extent in the behaviour of the mentally ill, particularly those whose condition tends towards disinhibited behaviour. Admission of unstable disinhibited person-alities has increased as the number of inpatient depressives has fallen. In the late 1950s an 'open doors' policy was introduced, initiating more permissive staff attitudes, enhancement of the hospital environment, and a living style for the patients, both acute and long stay, which approximated more to the freedom of the world outside. It was shown that violence to property and person and suicide actually decreased thereafter within psychiatric hospitals, with no compensatory increase in untoward behaviour by patients now free to pass outwith the hospital to benefit from contact with the real world to which an increasing number would return. How long such policies can be maintained under contemporary trends in social behaviour is uncertain. What *is* certain is that by day and after dark one of the safest places to walk within a city is in the grounds of its psychiatric hospital!

Many psychiatrists have spent a whole working lifetime with psychiatric patients of every type in wards, outpatients, homes and institutions without ever being subjected to any sort of assault. A minority through mismanagement of a delicate situation or ill-luck have been less fortunate. All psychiatrists have had their touch-and-go moments—the immigrant armed with an axe, the paranoid woman with a knife in her handbag. Professional experience of assault would be more common were it not for the sensitivity and understanding extended to the emotionally disturbed, and the confidence which comes with experience.

9.7 SELF-DESTRUCTIVE BEHAVIOURS

Suicide is relatively uncommon, there being 1 case annually per 10 000 of the population in the UK and USA. Certain factors should put the doctor on his guard, as follows.

Predicting suicide

Suicide is highly imitative not only as an act but in the manner in which it is carried out. A particularly bizarre, well publicized suicide can trigger similar acts. Local news of a suicide puts other vulnerable subjects in the area at risk. Suicides tend to occur in small batches. A proportion of those who have previously attempted suicide will eventually commit suicide by design or misfortune. Schizophrenics and unstable psychopathic persons subject to sudden mood changes are at risk for impulsive self-destruction. Endogenous depressives are at considerable risk if an arranged appointment with a psychiatrist is delayed, but once under competent specialist care the risk appears to be minimized. It is not true that those who express suicidal intentions will not commit the act.

Nevertheless, despite identification of the vulnerable, not all such subjects would be willing to accept psychiatric help if so advised. The timing of the act is usually impulsively determined and hence unpredictable. Stress reactions and mood states which would not culminate in suicide will do so when alcohol has released behavioural inhibitions. The clinician should ensure that repeat prescriptions for large quantities of drugs do not put the weapon into the hands of the predisposed.

The involved family

A suicide in the family is the most harrowing of all bereavements to come to terms with. Too frequently, the family's need for psychotherapeutic support is ignored. Guilt feelings, regret and sorrow conflict with marginally admitted counter-hostility direct to the person whose inconsiderate act brought such suffering and shame on them. The agony of ambivalence may never resolve without the opportunity to express the true feelings to a non-condemnatory and trusted person. The family doctor's involvement as psychotherapist cannot start too soon. *Multiple family suicide* is fortunately rare, occurs with some schizophrenics, but is characteristically associated with endogenous depressions in which delusional feelings of hopelessness and gloom for the future make it is a kindness for the family, before initiative is sapped, to kill them all before killing oneself.

A plausible psychopathology can conceal the presence of an episode of genetically determined manic depressive psychosis, depressed type. Inevitable failure to respond to intensive and protracted psychotherapy confirms the patient's despair. A tragic outcome serves to emphasize the importance of refined diagnoses of depressive disorders which distinguishes those likely to benefit from psychological therapies from others for whom only physical therapies can effect a resolution. Repeated or protracted failure of treatment for severe depression increases the risk of suicide very considerably.

Attempted suicide (parasuicide)

The epidemic

The contemporary social epidemic of parasuicide commenced along with the permissive era around 1963, ushering a ten-fold increase in this form of disinhibited imitative behaviour over the ensuing fifteen years. There is some evidence that the peak may now have passed. From single-drug overdose there has been increasing self-poisoning with multiple drugs, often following alcohol intake. The highest incidence and the greatest rate of increase has been in females, especially between 15 and 30 years of age. In rural populations the rate of increase has equalled that in urban areas, but with a much lower initial level the rural incidence in the epidemic has never reached that of urban areas prior to the epidemic.

Each week parasuicide admissions peak on Friday and Saturday nights when, often with drink taken, emotional storms flare up between youngsters and parents, boyfriends and girlfriends, between cohabitees, and between spouses. The suicide attempt is usually interpreted as a cry for help, but emotional blackmail is a prominent feature of many impulsive suicide gestures—'Now look what you've driven me to; you had better be more considerate in future. . .'.

Emergency treatment of parasuicidal overdose

Most attempts at suicide are by deliberate swallowing of one or more therapeutic drugs prescribed for the patient, a member of the family, or bought over the counter. The general practitioner has to size up the situation quickly and try to determine what drugs have been taken and in what amounts. Tragedies have occurred through the GP underestimating the potential seriousness of the poisoning. However trivial the attempt appears to be, it is wise to recontact the patient an hour later.

After calling the ambulance, gastric lavage is undertaken if less than 4 hours have passed since the overdose was taken. Exceptions are drugs which delay gastric emptying in which case lavage is still worthwhile up to 12 hours in poisoning by *tricyclic antidepressants, atropine* and *salicylates.*

Carbon monoxide poisoning from coal gas or vehicle exhaust is less common. If the equipment is available emergency treatment is by 100% oxygen at 2–3 atmospheres maintained to reduce the cerebral hypoxia which can induce irreversible dementia.

The burden falls consecutively on the family, family practitioner, casualty department, ITU, and medical ward. Once the dangerous medical crisis is over, psychiatrist, social worker or psychologist, and GP become involved in what may emerge as a complex tangle of distorted personal relationships and social difficulties. Ideally, the desperate gesture, with involvement of so many trained personnel, might have been prevented had help been sought in time by the patient or the family.

Should a psychiatrist be called in?

It has been customary in the UK to request a psychiatrist's opinion on all hospitalized parasuicides, but it is increasingly the practice that casualty officers and residents assess the patient's psychological state and social circumstances, directing accordingly to psychiatric admission ward or outpatient clinic, to social worker, clinical psychologist, GP, or to no-one. Given postgraduate psychiatric experience the practice is sound; otherwise tragedies could occur.

Personality strength and degree of stress
THE EMOTIONALLY IMMATURE

A fair proportion of all parasuicides occur in *emotionally shallow, immature* subjects. An acute crisis in disturbed closed interpersonal relationships is the usual precipitant of the suicide attempt, which ranges from minimal gesture to life-threatening multiple poisoning. Once recovered in hospital from the physical crisis such a patient is often psychologically calm, alert, smiling, blandly indifferent to the upset occasioned to so many people, unaware of the danger of their recent physical state, and without appreciation of the skilful intervention which returned them to life. Either the provocative tiff has been made up, or the blackmail effect has triumphed. The successful learned behaviour which earned attention and gained personal dominance can become a habit. Many parasuicides of this kind turn down offered treatment, or accept an appointment and fail to turn up. Most, if willing, would benefit from help from social worker or psychologist, for there are no specifically medical aspects of follow-up treatment.

THE EMOTIONALLY MATURE

A proportion of the attempts at suicide in reaction to acute stress occur in persons of *relatively well-integrated personality*. Their threshold of experiential tolerance is higher than in the constitutionally unstable and not unnaturally the provocative stress, whether sudden, long-drawn out or cumulative, is of exceptional severity. Psychological help, intensive and sustained, is not only indicated but liable to yield results.

The endogenous depressive parasuicide

It is extremely important to detect the less obvious cases of endogenous depression and other psychoses for whom discharge home without psychiatric follow-up arrangements delays effective treatment until subsequent deterioration forces attention. The risk of suicide is high. The burden of parasuicides is heavy and hospital staffs can easily come to regard the case load as an imposition. With so many instances of self-induced poisoning for apparently trivial causes the clinician is tempted to bracket them all as 'nuisances'. He does so to the peril of the minority who urgently require special psychiatric treatments. For their sakes there is still a strong case for a psychiatrist's assessment of all parasuicides.

Alcoholism

Alcoholism has been on the increase since 1950, the incidence having gradually declined over the prior century. Its incidence is a function of national rates of alcohol consumption. In the UK the rates for women are now one-third of the male rate and rising. Alcoholism occurs as a chronic addiction state or as the curious 'bout drinking' of several days' duration with periods of normal social drinking in between.

Clinicians should be aware there is a considerably higher than average incidence of alcoholism and drug addiction in doctors, medical students, pharmacists, nurses and hospital workers generally.

The hospital clinician will be involved in the treatment of delirium tremens and other physical complications of alcohol addiction, but the treatment of the addict with a view to inducing subsequent sobriety is best left to the psychiatrist. Inpatient treatment has been traditional, but now outpatient therapy, either individual or group, is having some success. Even one whole day of intensive individual psychotherapy by a multidisciplinary team is claimed to be as effective as prolonged inpatient psychological and social therapy.

Chlormethiazole is used in alcoholism in the treatment of acute withdrawal symptoms. It is a drug of addiction and its use should be confined within a maximum of 7 days. The growing practice of prescribing chlormethiazole over longer periods in general practice management of the alcoholic is not advisable. Chlormethiazole overdose when alcohol has been taken is extremely dangerous.

Persuasion and compulsion

The non-psychiatrist's major contribution is to persuade the alcoholic to accept the reality of the addiction and seek treatment. Over-persuasion is fruitless for success is only possible with a willing patient. The addict who takes the initiative in seeking treatment is self-selected for a possibly successful outcome. Compulsory admission for an alcoholic may be required for concurrent mentally sick behaviour. Very occasionally the certified patient 'sees the light' while still detained and agrees to treatment of the drink problem, but by and large compulsory admission for treatment is futile.

An unreliable historian

Outcome hinges on the *attitude* of the patient. Shallow declarations of good intentions are not sufficient. The capacity of the alcoholic to engage in deception and self-deception is well recognized, but few without experience of alcoholics are prepared for its extent. Nothing that the alcoholic or suspected alcoholic has to say about his drinking can be accepted at its face value. In the self-deceptive stage the alcoholic denies deteriorating marital and family relationships, failing work efficiency and deteriorating financial status. Only relative unbiased informants from within and outwith the family circle can give a reliable account.

The longer the delay in seeking treatment the greater the degree of cumulative irreversible damage to liver and brain. By the time the alcoholic is admitted in hepatic failure or with dementia and Korsakov's syndrome sobriety can only prevent further deterioration; resumption of drinking is fatal.

Suspicions of insobriety even under inpatient treatment are usually well founded. Once discharged from hospital patients' reports are unreliable unless backed up by independent evidence. 'Once an alcoholic always an alcoholic' means that however long sobriety is maintained, even with the help of AA and similar supporting organizations and services, the first drink in an unguarded moment will, with rare exceptions, escalate to resumption of the addiction.

The addiction-prone personality

Alcoholism is slow self-destruction, emotional, intellectual, social and physical. There are doubts as to whether or to what extent alcohol itself is crucial to the addiction. Genetic influences play a part for boy children of alcoholic fathers, adopted as babies, have, as adults, a higher incidence of alcoholism than the natural sons of the adopting parents. Pathological gambling has the characteristics of the non-physical aspects of alcoholism—the periods of abstinence, the first bet escalating to near financial ruin, the indifference to the repercussions on family and social life, the dawning insight and desperate attempts to stop. There is a view that vulnerability to addiction is, in part at least, a genetically determined personality characteristic whether expressed as alcohol, narcotic and other drug addictions or as purely psychological addiction. There is much ignorance about the psychopathology of alcoholism reflected in the diversity of therapeutic practices and theories of causation.

Narcotic addiction

Much of what has been said above about addiction applies with equal or greater force to narcotic addiction, the incidence of which may at any time rise to epidemic proportions, especially among the young. One-third of all narcotic addicts die before they reach their mid-twenties, by which age a further third are still addicted; one-third have overcome the addiction and are leading normal lives.

Manifestations which alert the observant physician include wayward or bizarre behaviour, introspective withdrawal, physical signs of narcotic poisoning and punctured antecubital veins.

Marihuana smoking is as harmful as one cares to believe it is.

Dependence and addiction to therapeutic drugs

A distinction must be made between addiction to therapeutic drugs and drug dependence, which is common. In addiction, usually but not invariably, dose has to be raised to maintain effect and withdrawal ushers in severe psychological and physical symptoms. In drug dependence an effective dose level, once achieved, maintains its effects. Withdrawal leads to return of the symptoms for which the drug was originally prescribed. The young diabetic is not addicted to, but is dependent on, insulin. Likewise, the patient whose anxiety is relieved by a tranquillizer is drug dependent.

IATROGENIC TRANQUILLIZER ADDICTION

With long-term use tranquillizer addiction can develop insidiously, even with average therapeutic doses. Recognition of such cases is on the increase.

It is dangerous to stop the tranquillizer abruptly. Instead it is advisable to seek admission for any such patient who is unable to face the experience unaided yet wishes to become free. The physical and psychological symptoms of withdrawal can be extremely harrowing, and it is claimed by patients with experience of both to be worse than narcotic withdrawal.

9.8 PERSONALITY AND BEHAVIOUR DISORDERS

Sociopathic and psychopathic disorders

Ever since first introduced, the concept of the psychopath has roused controversy. Is psychopathic behaviour indicative of mental illness or is it just plain old-fashioned badness? It is seen at its most vicious in certain cases of murder, rape and grievous bodily harm. Disputation peaks when murder is a capital crime and psychopathy is advanced in defence.

Psychopathy classically presents in three forms: (1) aggressive psychopathy; (2) inadequate psychopathy; (3) creative psychopathy.

Aggressive psychopathy

The condition is characterized by lack of foresight and indifference to the feelings and rights of others. A person with such persistent features of personality is at least a disturbing influence in personal, family, work and social activities, and at worst a public menace. For every psychopath entangled with the law for serious offences there are any number of citizens who display psychopathic behaviour in lesser degrees; they will be represented in any cross-section of patients presenting for medical services.

It can be maintained that the 20% of the population who have 80% of the accidents—the accident prone—are to some extent psychopathic. Certainly they display the quality of impulsive lack of foresight (and on the roads, especially if possessed of psychopathic callousness, such persons constitute a major hazard to themselves and to others). The addition of excess alcohol intake creates what must be the most potent pre-homicidal/self-destructive state in peacetime society.

The terms 'psychopathic' and 'sociopathic' are almost synonymous, the latter stressing more the behaviour as it affects the wider public. Genetic influences play only a minor part; the condition appears to arise from particularly unfavourable childhood experience.

The inadequate psychopath

Persons displaying this form are just unable to cope with life without leaning on other people of more robust temperament. The concept shades over into chronic neuroticism. By no means all persons with persistent neurotic traits are inadequate, for persistent neurotic weaknesses can be compensated by stronger facets of personality. It is when the latter are absent that chronic neuroticism becomes near-total personal inadequacy. Psychopaths of this passive type are easily led, and easily led into trouble.

The creative psychopath

This form is less common and only mentioned here for completeness.

Differential diagnosis of aggressive psychopathy

Temporal lobe epilepsy (TLE)

Impulsively aggressive behaviour can be a manifestation of temporal lobe epilepsy. Amnesia for the episode is common, but the patient who accepts what is reported of the episode will show concern and even take the initiative in seeking medical help, in contrast to the emotional indifference of the psychopath. Other features of TLE will be present, and in many cases a clear onset date for the attacks can be elicited.

Drugs

Certain *drugs* can provoke impulsive and unacceptable behaviour. Alcohol is the obvious one, but narcotics, LSD, mescaline and other hallucinogenics are less common causes. The occasional disinhibition induced by diazepam may have a sociopathic quality. Psychopathy may well underline and be the root cause of some addictions.

To establish a diagnosis of psychopathy the behaviour must be representative of *persistent* traits of personality.

Differential diagnosis of inadequate psychopathy

Mental deficiency

Personal and social inadequacy are features of a proportion of mental defectives and are inversely related to intelligence level. It is advisable to have the IQ measured by a psychologist when inadequacy is associated with apparent mental dullness.

Simple schizophrenia

In this type of schizophrenia positive symptoms are absent. The negative symptoms are the pathological lack of drive and initiative deepening until the patient just sits around vacantly doing nothing. Although onset is gradual in late teens the change in personality contrasts with the fixed personality traits of the psychopath.

Psychopaths as psychiatric patients

As psychiatric patients' psychopaths and sociopaths are on the increase and pose a therapeutic challenge to which we have no real answer. As their behaviour causes distress to others and not to themselves there is little motivation to seek help unless in a crisis of their own making which finally causes personal stress. They commonly seek or are referred to the psychiatrist when proceedings are imminent for criminal behaviour, as psychopathic alcoholics and drug addicts *in extremis,* as parasuicides, or when marriage is about to break up. (Paradoxically, it is the spouse, usually the wife, who, being normal, first begins to crack and seek help.) About half of all acute male psychiatric admissions under the age of 35 enter hospital for such reasons. A reliable history from the general practitioner and other informants reveals the prior existence of a number of unfavourable factors drawn from: emotional and material neglect in childhood, poor work record, unstable personal relationships with parents, peers and spouse if married, court appearances, drunkenness, suicide attempts. Once in hospital they prove unco-operative, upset other patients, break the basic hospital rules, cheek the nurses, come and go as they please and finally leave when they are ready. Their stay yields them no benefit except in rare instances. Nursing staff are prepared to accept all sorts of aberrant behaviour from patients who are identifiably mentally ill, but, not unreasonably, resent the stressful and futile role imposed on them by the psychopathically behaviour-disordered. A psychiatric ward unit can contain only a very limited number of patients with sociopathic behaviour. In larger numbers they virtually take over. Inpatient 'treatment' of psychopathic patients as applied to date has little to offer. The occasional success makes all the effort a little more worthwhile.

When from the content of a court report or through psychotherapy the subject with psychopathic tendencies learns how earlier experience dictates subsequent attitudes and behaviour the knowledge is seized as a welcome determinist excuse for similar behaviour in the future. Efforts to change would involve painful self-scrutiny; it is much less stressful to continue to displace unresolved hostility on to others.

It will be appreciated that psychopathic traits are at one extreme of a continuum with the over-inhibited, conflict-ridden neurotic at the other. Traditional psychotherapy aims to weaken the hold of repressed superego function in the latter. Psychopathic tendencies require a strengthening of superego function. How the aim of increased self-discipline is to be achieved still baffles psychiatrists, prison and probation officers, social workers, priests, friends, relatives and academic theorists.

Psychopaths are particularly liable to develop psychoses of sudden onset. The episodes are often short-lived with spontaneous resolution. When of longer duration inpatient treatment is indicated. As with patients long categorized as 'neurotic' or 'hysterical' the psychopathic patient stands in danger of relatives' and doctors' blindness to intercurrent physical or psychiatric illness; assessment is difficult in face of the chronic state. 'Oh, it's just him again with his usual carry-ons.'

Psychopaths as medical patients

In medical patients in the wider sense the presence of psychopathic traits undermines treatment in proportion to the intensity of the personality disorder. As historians the psychopathic are untruthful and misleading, but their presentation of complaints lacks the manipulative coyness of the role-playing hysteric. The psychopath does have charm in plenty and can impress the gullible, for a time at least.

Even under the close supervision of inpatient care psychopathic traits make for unreliability and careless lack of co-operation. Out of hospital they are poor attenders, though their explanations and excuses are plausible enough on the first few occasions. Drug compliance is not to be assumed, advice is ignored. They default from care as suddenly as they originally sought it.

The doctor can only cope as best he can, while realizing the limitations imposed by the patient's personality. In the longer term there is hope for the psychopath. The condition would appear to be a delayed emotional maturation in a physically and intellectually matured young adult. Usually by the mid-thirties emotional development catches up and the 'patient', if he really is a 'patient' at all, settles down. Psychopathic behaviour is not common beyond the age of thirty five.

The unstable teenager
Compared with the bafflement and gloom engendered by the prospect of attempting treatment of the psychopath there is room for therapeutic optimism with the unstable teenager.

Some come to psychiatric care following an attempt at suicide or a remand report on a young offender. Many are referred by the family doctor, and more would be referred were the effects of treatment more widely appreciated.

A typical story is of a wayward youngster at loggerheads with parents, insistently demanding a high degree of personal freedom of action which cannot be handled. Beneath the hostility and defiance hides a deeply unhappy human being, tossed hither and thither by conflicting emotions, all at sea in the transition from childhood to the adult world. Once the barriers are down the insecure teenager is only too anxious to confide fears and doubts to a sympathetic, non-condemnatory neutral.

Others have opted out between school and the challenges of establishing the self in the workaday world beyond. They sit around parasitically at home, contributing neither to their keep nor to the work of the home until in desperation the parents seek medical help. The loss of initiative and inexplicable idleness raise a suspicion of schizophrenia and a period of inpatient observation may be required before the diagnostic issue can be resolved.

Treatment
Fairly intensive psychotherapy pays off whether given by family doctor, clinical psychologist, social worker or psychiatrist. The therapist is amply rewarded by the pleasure and satisfaction of useful involvement in the processes whereby the young patient works through the fears and conflicts and passes with growing confidence towards adulthood.

When rebellion, withdrawal, conflicts or family frictions are less tractable, admission to psychiatric hospital is advisable. The anticipated duration of stay is considerably longer than the average 7 weeks for the general run of acute psychiatric illnesses, and some indication of the anticipated longer stay should be given. Once in hospital, the patient is not only given individual and group psychotherapy but is exposed to a structured programme designed to encourage more healthy and realistic management of personal and social relationships within the working, recreational, social and living environment of the hospital. Parental visits and spells at home give indications of the rate of progress. The process cannot be hurried and little can be expected within a matter of weeks. The average duration of stay for results with this group is more of the order of 6 months. The effort is well spent.

9.9 PSYCHIATRIC DISORDERS OF WOMEN

The heaviest burden of mental illness falls on women. In every category of psychiatric disorder with the exceptions of alcoholism and aggressively psychopathic behaviour the incidence is higher in women than in men.

The psychiatric disturbances associated with female reproductive function are those occurring with menstruation, the menopause, pregnancy and the puerperium.

Premenstrual tension (PMT)

This is extremely common in the week to ten days prior to menstruation and distressing enough to drive many sufferers to seek medical help.

Symptoms

The symptoms include: bloated feelings due to water retention, lower abdominal pain; tension, anxiety or depression; irritability, lethargy and somatic symptoms. Existing psychosomatic and psychiatric symptoms become exaggerated. Blood pressure is elevated, weight increases, rings and shoes become tight.

Cause

The condition is caused by insufficient progesterone production by the adrenals and ovaries with consequent water retention and potassium depletion.

Treatment

Diuretics, even with added potassium, though capable of relieving somatic symptoms have little effect on the psychological component, which is due to Na/K imbalance. When symptoms are relatively mild restriction of fluids and extra dietary salt may bring relief, otherwise it is necessary to correct the Na/K imbalance caused by the deficiency of progesterone.

Progesterone is ineffective orally so must be given during the 7–10 days before menstruation, either as rectal or vaginal suppositories 200–400 mg daily, or by deep intramuscular injection of an oily suspension daily or every second day, in doses of 50–100 mg. Although usually effective the modes of administration are somewhat unpleasant and in time a change can be made to implantation of progesterone which will maintain its effect for 3–9 months before repetition; any irregular menstrual bleeding induced can be regarded as harmless.

Synthetic progestogens are taken by mouth. The effects vary from one individual to another because the progestogen can be converted to any of a range of steroids, so that it acts as: an oestrogen, causing nausea and worsening of the PMT; as an anabolic hormone, causing weight gain; as a testosterone, causing the developing of male characteristics, or it can act favourably as an aldosterone antagonist preventing water retention. The best progestogen preparation with the least adverse effects in a given patient may only be found after a period of trial and error.

Oral contraceptives, in combined oestrogen/progesterone, or progesterone only, preparations can be beneficial.

The menopause

Women are particularly liable to develop mental illness during the menopause, a time of somatic and emotional distress of sudden or gradual onset which can last any time up to 5 years.

Psychological symptoms of moderate irritability, fatigue, anxiety or mild depression are so common and expected that few women feel a need to turn to medical services for relief. At greater symptom intensity antidepressants or tranquillizers are indicated in conjunction with psychological support.

Psychological effects

The menopause is a time not only of hormonal imbalance but of psychological crisis, one of those anxious transition periods that occur at key times throughout life when former attitudes and expectations are no longer appropriate and a fresh orientation is still to be worked out. For many women the menopause is an experience of loss of much that has given life meaning. Loss of reproductive functioning and feared loss of sexual attractiveness often come as children grow away from the home. The childless woman is going to remain childless for ever.

There are compensations and freedoms to the postmenopausal life which the woman in transition may only see dimly if at all as she baulks at the question, 'What am I going to do with the rest of my life?' She can be helped to see and work her way through.

Postmenopausal tension state

A common disorder which has received little attention in the psychiatric literature is the postmenopausal state characterized by extreme and protracted tension and anxiety which predominates over lesser feelings of depression. Whether the state is essentially endogenous or exogenous is not clear but it is extremely difficult to treat. Antidepressant drugs, tranquillizers, relaxation therapy, psychotherapy—all may promote minor degrees of temporary relief. In these cases oestrogen therapy may prove particularly beneficial when given over repeated short periods of limited total duration at the lowest effective dose, e.g. ethinyloestradiol 0·05 mg–0·1 mg t.d.s. for 3 weeks out of 4 over 2 or 3 months, reduced to twice a day, then once a day over a total of 6–9 months. Alternatively, stilboestrol 0·125–0·5 mg b.d. can be used in a similar manner.

Endogenous depression in the menopause

The incidence of endogenous depression is twice as high in females as in males at any age, but in females the incidence has a definite peak at the menopause. The essential clinical manifestations and treatment of endogenous depression, or other psychosis, at the menopause have no special features, except that the added presence of psychological symptoms of the menopause confuse the diagnosis and extend the treatment requirements.

Pregnancy

Pregnancy has long been considered *the* time in a woman's life when she is exceptionally free of psychiatric illness. While this is true for the major psychoses the same cannot be said for the neuroses.

Neurotic illness in pregnancy

The prospect of childbirth presents an exceptional challenge to the capacity for adaptation, the success of which depends on emotional maturity and stability as influenced by attitudes to childbearing and to the pregnancy, stability of the relationship with the father within or outwith marriage, his attitude and behaviour, attitudes of parents, and practical socioeconomic problems like housing and domestic finances.

Adverse psychological reaction can be expressed as anxiety, depression, emotional lability and mood swings, fearful anticipation of labour and of fetal abnormality, any of which at greater intensity creates an overt neurosis.

1. Women neurotically disturbed before pregnancy continue their neurosis into pregnancy and the puerperium.

2. One pregnant woman in ten develops a neurotic reaction in the first trimester which usually resolves spontaneously after the third month, only to re-emerge in the puerperium.

3. A further one in twenty becomes neurotically disturbed in the second or third trimester. These latter, being sufficiently robust psychologically to weather the psychological effects of pregnancy itself, only become neurotic in response to some unrelated major stress such as serious family illness or a death.

Psychiatric drugs in pregnancy—effects on the fetus and newborn child

In the first trimester barbiturates and *diazepam* increase the incidence of cleft palate and harelip.

In the second and third trimesters phenothiazines used long term in high dose can cause retinal damage in the fetus. *Lithium* crosses the placenta and can cause goitre in the fetus.

Sedatives, tranquillizers and *hypnotics* all cross the placental barrier and if present at the time of delivery may provoke delay in the initiation of respiration in the newly born. *Barbiturates* depress respiration, and are a cause of unresponsiveness after birth. *Diazepam* and *chlordiazepoxide* rapidly cross the placenta, depress activity of the newborn and can cause hypothermia and hypotonia.

It is advisable to use tranquillizers, sedatives and hypnotics with extreme caution or not at all in early and late pregnancy.

Lithium—post-delivery

Lithium plasma levels can rise considerably following delivery, necessitating a lowering of dose from that which previously maintained steady levels.

Therapeutic abortion

Legal requirements and restrictions vary widely from one country to another, and the decision of the individual doctor is influenced as much by personal, philosophical, moral, religious and social convictions as by objective assessment of the clinical issues involved.

Pregnant women in search of abortion are extremely insistent and react to firm resistance with hostility. In practice their primary medical advisers know the likely opinions of different psychiatrists and refer accordingly.

The incidence of psychiatric illness after therapeutic abortion is very much less than after pregnancy (one-tenth).

The puerperium

There is a considerable increase in psychiatric admissions in the first 2 weeks of the puerperium and a great increase in psychiatric referrals.

Mild reactions

Mild disturbances of mood are very common in the days following parturition and include the well-known 'fourth day blues' attributable to the combined effects of hormonal changes and realization of the restrictions imposed by responsibility for a helpless baby.

Neuroses

At 3–6 months postpartum one woman in six is suffering from depressive neurosis. Most of this group were not neurotically disturbed in later pregnancy, but many suffered from depressive neuroses in the first trimester.

In summary there are two patterns of neurotic reaction associated with childbearing:

1. Neurotic developments in the first trimester which resolve but carry a fairly high chance of re-emergence as protracted depressive neuroses in the puerperium.

2. Neurotic reactions of the later stages of pregnancy which usually follow some major stress not associated with the pregnancy.

Treatment of depressive neurosis in the puerperium requires an appropriate balance of psychotherapy, environmental manipulation and use of antidepressant drugs.

Psychoses

Endogenous depression is the most common of the puerperal psychoses. Schizophrenia and mania are of lesser incidence, and only rarely is delirium now seen. Most psychiatrists maintain that there are no special qualities to any of the psychoses occurring in the puerperium while others emphasize a mild delirious quality in the early stages. As the issue has no treatment implications it need not be pursued here. Puerperal psychoses can be regarded as examples of well-recognized psychotic syndromes which happen to occur with increased incidence in the puerperium.

It is not clear why a particular pregnancy is followed by a puerperal psychosis. Maternal psychosis may follow only one, not necessarily the first, birth within a large family of children, and it is unusual to find any outstanding physical or psychological stress in that pregnancy, labour or puerperium. Moreover, puerperal psychosis is not particularly associated with illegitimate birth, stillbirth or twin birth. Past psychiatric history and premorbid personality are very similar in women with puerperal and non-puerperal psychoses. Endogenous processes would appear to play a greater role than psychological and environmental factors in the genesis of puerperal psychoses.

The mother/child bond

Only a small proportion of mothers with postpartum psychiatric disorder are admitted to a psychiatric bed. When circumstances allow and the receiving hospital makes provision it is advantageous to have the baby admitted with her. Nursing staff attend to the baby's needs when the mother is acutely ill, but she maintains contact. Increasingly as her state improves she becomes involved under supervision in the care of the infant. In this way she gradually takes over with increasing confidence and the vital period of early bonding between mother and child is not disrupted.

9.10 PSYCHOGERIATRICS

The increasing population aged over 65, with its high incidence of mental illness creates a major medical and social commitment which justifies the adoption of psychogeriatrics as a clinical subspecialty by one psychiatrist in ten. The mental illnesses of the elderly in addition to dementia include endogenous depression, neuroses, paranoid psychoses and delirium.

Prevention

Factors associated with old age psychiatric illness, whether provocative or aggravating, include deafness, blindness, loneliness, poverty and physical ill health.

Deafness

Deafness in most instances can be helped by provision of a hearing aid. Many old people are curiously reluctant to use an aid, choosing perversely to remain cut off from human contact. Deafness, often a source of amusement to others, is psychologically more disabling than sympathy-attracting impairment of sight, for deafness isolates from human communication while defective eyesight only impairs perception of the physical world. Many old people complain that the hearing aid supplied is useless or distressing through distortion of sound. Although the ageing nervous system has impaired adaptive capacity, it will adapt if exposed to mildly disturbing sensation for long enough. Just as no one is expected to overcome the initial discomfort of dentures if they are only inserted at meal times, so wearing the hearing aid only for special occasions will not allow adaptive filtering of the initial unpleasant quality of sound. The elderly deaf subject should be persuaded to wear the aid and keep it switched on from getting up until going to bed, reassurance being given that with persistence the maximum benefit possible will be obtained.

Defective vision

Defective vision requires investigation and appropriate treatment, for though not as isolating as deafness it can tip the balance towards mental illness when other provocative factors are present. Not uncommonly, the elderly person with spectacles fails to realize that gradually worsening vision is not just another of age's burdens to be borne, but is an indication for repeat sight testing and supply of different lenses. In default, the subject should be chivvied into taking the necessary action. Cataract, glaucoma, and other ocular pathologies are less likely to be overlooked. Glaucoma is a contraindication to the use of tricyclic antidepressants with their anti-cholinergic side-effects.

Poverty

It is easier to say that poverty is associated with mental illness in old age than to do anything positive about it. In countries with adequate welfare provision no one should be in serious poverty but many elderly people are not in receipt of what is due to them either because, having been brought up to believe strongly in economic self-reliance, their pride will not allow them to take advantage of 'charity', or because the bureaucratic ramifications of welfare provision, difficult enough to disentangle at any age, are quite beyond the grasp of the ageing brain.

Where social agencies have overlooked the problems of a particular old person, the doctor, once called on to deal with a medical crisis, can alert them. In some NHS general practices in the UK it is the custom to visit every elderly person on the doctor's list at intervals of 1 or 2 months. Such regular visiting, as opposed to responding to a request to be seen, is invaluable in detecting early physical, psychiatric and health-threatening social problems, and initiating steps to limit or correct impending trouble before crisis intervention is needed. As an alternative, a health visitor calls regularly every few months and alerts the doctor or appropriate social agency. Health visitors in the UK are especially sensitive to developing mental illness.

Whatever the merits in some societies of personal payment by the patient for medical services rendered, such a service is inadequate for the preventive needs of the geriatric population.

Loneliness

Loneliness in old age is a major precipitant of mental illness. In many contemporary Western societies family cohesion has weakened. Younger relatives are highly mobile in the search for better jobs, and the elderly are re-housed in the isolation of remote housing developments. Soaring transport costs keep them virtually housebound. Hard-pressed social agencies can only effect contact in a crisis. Ideally, all elderly persons living alone would benefit from surveillance, with persuasion and provision of transport, to attend available social diversions in the neighbourhood.

The factor common to special sense impairment, poverty and loneliness is social isolation to which, as a further provocative cause of mental illness, must be added physical ill health.

Physical illness

In the elderly physical illness increasingly takes the form of malignant disease or organ degeneration which at best can only be slowed down by medical intervention. Degenerative disease creates chronic physical impairment, immobility, and decreased ability to carry out essential household tasks and shopping. Hospitalization comes early when social disability presses hard, but at least highlights provocative social problems which can be given full consideration in the subsequent rehabilitation programme.

In vulnerable elderly subjects physical illness can be the final stress which precipitates psychiatric illness.

The ageing personality

The person who remains bright, alert, interested in other peoples' lives and unselfish into real old age is exceptional.

As people age short-term memory declines while older memories persist. The memory distortion, allied to failing vigour, with decreasing pleasure and interest in present events, accounts for the manner in which old people increasingly live in and prattle about the past. Thinking slows down, comprehension becomes impaired, and initiative declines. Coping with day-to-day practical tasks becomes more difficult. Personality alters; unfortunately the less desirable features of previous personality tend to come to the fore and the old person, somewhat less lovable and less loved, can all too easily become demanding, difficult and querulous.

The psychiatric illnesses of old age
The chronic organic psychoses (the dementias)
SENILE DEMENTIA

Most old people never regress beyond the stage outlined above, but with every decade of increasing age after the mid-60s an increasing proportion decline further with ever increasing perceptual, emotional and intellectual impairment proceeding hand in hand with deteriorating behaviour and personal habits. Senile dementia has begun and will inevitably run its progressive course to gross defects of recent memory and intellect, disorientation in time and place and misidentification of people, shamelessly dirty eating and toilet habits, slovenly dress, self-neglect and emotional fatuity.

The non-specialist doctor, if not already aware of the deterioration, will be approached by relatives or social agencies. The need for hospitalization does not depend only on the stage of progression of the dementia. Account must be taken of social support available, the tolerance level of the family, the presence of children in the home, whether the housewife is also employed—in general, the ability and willingness of the family to carry on, balanced against the burden the family can be expected to bear. Sooner or later, hospitalization can no longer be avoided, the onset of shameless incontinence often forcing the family beyond the limit of toleration.

Difficulties involved with the admission include: guilt on the part of key relatives (daughters especially) which must be talked out, availability of a hospital bed, and the question of compulsory admission. Shortfall in provision of an adequate number of hospital beds for long-term care of the elderly dements resident in a hospital's service area places quite unacceptable burdens on families. Every possible assistance should be mobilized while awaiting a vacancy. Not only are the numbers of elderly dements increasing, but their life expectancy as inpatients is also increasing; in consequence the wait for a death vacancy is lengthening. Hospital psychogeriatric day care goes some way to easing the relatives' burden until advancing deterioration makes admission imperative. The doctor saddled with such a problem may, by maintaining pressure on the hospital, gain earlier admission for his dementing patient. Meanwhile the admission of some other patient in urgent need is put back. Strategically, the solution is contingent on the problem being given the medicopolitical priority it deserves. In essence, senile dementia is a common slow mode of death in which the brain is the organ which degenerates ahead of others. Very fortunately, personal suffering is not a feature of senile dementia, for bland and fatuous emotional flattening accompanies the other manifestations throughout. No known treatment will critically influence the inevitable and gradual process of deterioration. The comfort of the patient and acceptance by the relatives depend on high standards of nursing care.

THE PRESENILE DEMENTIAS

The presenile dementias, Alzheimer's and Pick's diseases, with onset in the 50s, are relatively uncommon. Management is as for senile dementia.

ARTERIOSCLEROTIC DEMENTIA

This is the other major category of old age dementia. Cerebral arteriosclerosis can occur without generalized arteriosclerosis. In contrast to the gradual progression of senile dementia the deterioration proceeds by steps, a succession of cerebral infarcts, each with short-lived acute confusion and subsequent local neurological defect, the nature of which depends on the site of damage. The effects of repeated infarcts cumulate and dementia commences. The patient is initially aware of the mental deterioration and reacts with feelings of anxiety or depression which can be sufficiently distressing to require appropriate therapy with tranquillizing or anti-depressant drugs. As dementia deepens, emotional flattening brings a kindly indifference. Care is otherwise as for senile dementia. Ultimately, unless a fatal infarct intervenes, hospitalization becomes imperative.

Claims made for the value of vasodilators in arteriosclerotic dementia are unsupported by sound scientific evidence. There are possible harmful effects to be considered, especially postural hypotension, causing critical oxygen starvation of an already damaged brain.

TREATABLE DEMENTIAS

It is too easy to assume that any dementia in an elderly subject is irremediable, for there are dementias which are treatable, as caused by benign and some malignant cerebral tumours, hypothyroidism, vitamin B_{12} deficiency and neurosyphilis (GPI)—a relatively uncommon cause of dementia, which accounted for 10% of all male psychiatric admissions only a generation ago. Cardiac insufficiency, anaemias, and other non-cerebral conditions causing diminished oxygen transport will aggravate established dementia, or precipitate the vulnerable subject into dementia. Geriatric dementing patients must be screened for treatable states as early as possible, for the dementing process implies cumulative irreversible brain damage.

Delirium

Delirium is the clinical syndrome of the *acute* organic reaction. The physical causes are legion. The acute infections are now much less common than formerly. Drugs implicated include L-dopa, opiates, anaesthetic agents, tricyclic antidepressants (overdose) and withdrawal of alcohol and barbiturates.

Clinically, delirium occurs in any degree from mild confusion with restless anxiety to the classic syndrome of: (1) acute confusion with disorientation for time and place and misidentification of persons, (2) visual hallucinations, and (3) an affective state varying between fear and panic, with appropriate motor excitement.

The state lasts from 2 to 10 days.

The presence of mild delirium complicates management and treatment of the causative physical disorder. When the physical disorder is of a serious nature exhaustion from concurrent delirium can well tip the scales towards a fatal outcome.

Delirium can occur at any age but the elderly are particularly vulnerable. Thus the occurrence and intensity of a delirium is a function of age and the suddenness and severity of the physical provocation.

TREATMENT OF DELIRIUM

Therapeutic attack is directed to the delirium *and* to its physical cause. *Severe delirium* in the elderly is life-threatening and demands swift and effective treatment.

In the elderly it is advisable to start any drug treatment with a small dose, to test effectiveness and side-effects, and then proceed as indicated to the higher dose levels. Pharmacokinetics in the elderly are such that adequate cell drug concentrations are achieved with lower than average drug doses.

Chlorpromazine or promazine should be given orally or intramuscularly in a relatively small dose of 25–30 mg. If there are no adverse effects and there is no improvement the drug should be repeated in a dose of 50–100 mg. As an alternative intramuscular trifluoperazine can be used in 1 mg doses repeated to a total of 5 mg/day. When life is threatened and speed of response is vital promazine can be given intravenously in doses of 50 mg, repeated to a total of 300 mg daily.

Benzodiazepines can be given in relatively large dose—chlordiazepoxide 25–50 mg or diazepam 20–40 mg.

Psychological factors in treatment are important in the milder case, or when drugs are once effecting control of a more severe delirium.

PREVENTION AND TREATMENT OF THE PSYCHOGENIC ELEMENT IN DELIRIUM

Delirium can be provoked by psychological circumstances such as the stress of continuous shellfire or aerial bombardment, or experimentally under conditions of prolonged sensory deprivation in an isolation chamber. In lesser degree isolation and fear-provoking experience can, particularly in the elderly, induce mild purely psychogenic delirium.

The principles of prevention and treatment of the psychogenic element of a delirious state are important for nurses. On admission the nurse introduces herself by name, shows where the toilets are, and explains something of the ward routine and personnel, slowly, clearly and simply. Befriended, helped and orientated the patient's natural agitation and worry about coming into hospital are considerably allayed. Orientating information has to be repeated tactfully at intervals to ensure grasp of whereabouts, day and time, and who is who. Such humane and commonsense tactics greatly reduce the prospect of delirium and contain its intensity once established.

Nursing ignorance, neglect and mismanagement are common aggravating factors of any psychiatric disorder evident in a general hospital ward patient, culminating in panic calls for psychiatric intervention in a crisis which need never have arisen and which subsides if the nurses can appreciate and apply the specialist's recommendations for psychological management. In default, such patients calm very quickly without any medication after transfer to the care of psychiatric nurses.

Neurosis

Neurosis in old age is rare as a new development, but age brings little prospect of improvement for the chronically neurotic. Indeed, with failing cerebral functions, the subject's ability to contain the neurosis diminishes and its manifestations create an unusually demanding, endlessly complaining old person, very trying to those attempting to give support and help.

Endogenous depression in the elderly

A really severe attack of endogenous depression can mimic a dementia. Due to self-absorption in suffering events do not register so there is a defect of recent memory and even a degree of disorientation arising from the patient's emotional indifference to the environment. The more prominent the depressive syndrome and the younger the patient, the less does the clinician consider the diagnosis of organic dementia. Once into the age group in which organic dementia becomes increasingly common, the pseudo-dementia accompanying endogenous depression, especially when depressive symptomatology is not conspicuous, can easily lead to a mistaken diagnosis of dementia, with consequent failure to treat a very treatable condition. When endogenous depression occurs in the actual presence of organic dementia, it must be treated in its own right to relieve the patient's distress. Endogenous depression is common in the elderly and, especially when it is a first attack, a search must be mounted for the covert physical disease which is so often the precipitant.

TREATMENT

Elderly subjects with endogenous depression are no less treatable than younger subjects. Interestingly, given physical screening, ECT is remarkably safe even with patients in their 80s. Because of the high incidence of physical disorders in the elderly discretion is required in the choice of antidepressant drug. Antidepressants with conspicuous anticholinergic effects should be avoided. The drug of choice is mianserin—a newer antidepressant with minimal anticholinergic effects. There is natural concern about dose levels in elderly subjects, but given adequate supervision, the rule holds that higher, but still tolerable, dose levels are likeliest to effect a remission. Excessive caution leads to failure and prolongation of the psychotic episode (*see* p. 463).

When depression is severe and the patient lives alone, admission to a psychiatric bed is advisable. Only rarely is there any sustained resistance from a depressive patient advised to enter hospital voluntarily for care and treatment.

In episodes of lesser severity, and when the patient is living with sensible relatives, treatment without admission is quite practicable. The key relative has to become more involved than usual. It is the practice to outline the treatment programme to patient and relative together, and give the latter responsibility for drug administration as detailed in a schedule especially written for the patient. Contact must be maintained at regular intervals of not more than a week until a positive response allows less frequent consultations until remission is achieved.

Failure of the drug of first choice over a 4-week period is an indication for referral to a psychiatrist.

Paranoid psychoses

Paranoid psychoses are less common, but if treatment is approached in the right way, gratifying results can be achieved.

Paranoid mood, though not infrequent as a feature of dementias, depressions and neuroses in old age, also stands out as a syndrome in its own right. The person is seized by a primary delusion of persecution on which is built an elaborate but plausible structure of plots, interference and harassment carried on secretly by persons known (neighbours) or unknown. The police may have been approached to have the persecution stopped.

The entire delusional system is encapsulated, i.e. it does not 'spill over' and affect other aspects of the patient's functioning. It is quite possible to spend long periods in the person's company without receiving any hint of abnormality, until by chance one touches on some relevant topic and the psychosis bursts through. The persecutory delusions appear to be very firmly held, so it is odd that the person will incongruously accept the status of 'patient' and allow referral to a psychiatric clinic. It may take some time before the patient is ready to reveal the delusions to a doctor, and once revealed they should never be challenged head on. An attitude of sympathetic concern, short of connivance, gains the patient's confidence. The emotional intensity which drives the delusions can be reduced by major tranquillizers. It is quite useless to prescribe the drugs with an explanation that they are for the delusions, for this implies disbelief in the reality of the reported happenings. It can be put to the patient rather that the persecutions must be unnerving, and that some tablets might have a settling effect. Trifluoperazine, initially in doses of 10 mg daily, raised as required by 5 mg/day at weekly intervals until a response is obtained, is a widely used neuroleptic (i.e. major tranquillizer) which lowers the emotional tension and allows the force of the delusions to subside.

These patients characteristically attend regularly for assessment and dose regulation. In time the initially effective dose level is cautiously reduced to an effective maintenance level which may have to be taken indefinitely.

9.11 LIAISON PSYCHIATRY AND PSYCHOSOMATIC MEDICINE

Liaison psychiatry is a new term introduced to cover psychiatric consultations requested for patients under the care of other hospital specialists. Medical requests to assess parasuicide cases apart, the greatest number of such requests originate from two specialities: *obstetrics and gynaecology*— on account of the psychologically and hormonally induced emotional disorders associated with menstruation and child bearing, and for opinions on the advisability of abortion and sterilization. *Geriatric medicine*— especially for help in choosing appropriate care for the considerable proportion of elderly patients who have both physical and psychiatric disorders.

SURGERY

The incidence of postoperative psychiatric disorder as recorded is remarkably low, yet a casual visit to a surgical ward will reveal that up to 10% of the patients display overt psychiatric disturbance: depression, paranoid attitudes, delirium, and pre- and postoperative anxiety and depression of pathological degree. The arc of surgical vision seems at times almost to exclude perception of pathological manifestations which cannot be cut with the knife.

The request: Notes should be prepared on the salient history and observations prompting the request. An exhaustive all-embracing account is not required or expected. Brief notes should be presented under a number of headings:

Degree of urgency: Whether clinical urgency, or urgency to clear a bed.

The immediate clinical situation
1. Behaviour and expressed feelings.
2. Medical condition and current treatment with *details of drugs.*

The background
1. Relevant family or childhood history.
2. Personality and past psychiatric disorder.
3. Particular recent events or situations which might have contributed.
4. Social factors of possible importance at home and at work. Too often the psychiatrist arrives on the ward having received a message at second hand to find medically orientated notes only, nurses who have just come on duty and give an inadequate hearsay account of nursing observations, while the resident doctor may be either off duty or urgently occupied elsewhere. Helpful notes left for the psychiatrist's perusal do allow a start to be made. Their preparation before a consultation is common medical practice and courtesy.

Psychosomatic medicine

If the term psychosomatic is assumed to mean that psychological events and states influence bodily physicochemical processes then there is no state of ill health that is not psychosomatic. Not infrequently, in scientific studies of psychiatric inpatients, orthopaedic accident cases have been chosen as the comparative inpatient psychologically normal control group. The practice became suspect with growing appreciation of the personality characteristics of the accident prone. It may be difficult for the mechanistically orientated clinician to appreciate the potency of psychological influence on somatic function, but, for example, rapid death of the Australian aborigine following formal ostracizing by the elders is now well documented. It is hardly surprising then that the personality characteristics and state of mind of the patient, mediated through physicochemical processes, profoundly affect the body's reactions to insult.

In common medical usage the term 'psychosomatic disorders' covers a range of illnesses, basically physical but overtly responsive to psychological influences; migraine, epilepsy, asthma, peptic ulcer, benign hypertension, ulcerative colitis.

The principle weapon of therapeutic attack varies from patient to patient and from time to time. When psychological aggravation in prominent treatment is directed towards reduction of tension and anxiety. The methods employed are largely as for anxiety state—tranquillizing drugs, psychotherapy and techniques for self-induction of relaxation. Biofeedback is a line of treatment for experts.

It is far from easy to be sure how far any psychological therapy is effective, for physical therapies are usually in use simultaneously and many psychosomatic conditions wax and wane spontaneously. Not infrequently induced insight into unrecognized conflicts and sources of anxiety improve psychological wellbeing without affecting the psychosomatic disorder either way.

A particular difficulty arises when the psychiatrist can uncover no evidence of psychological malaise as a plausible explanation of a referred patient's symptoms, and likewise the physician's investigations reveal no physical cause. The patient is left in the air, puzzled, angry even, and worried that there might be an obscure and as yet undetected physical cause. Discharge is followed by re-referral and *faute de mieux* the patient usually finds a haven with the psychiatrist.

SLEEP AND INSOMNIA

Hypnotic dependence—prevention and management

Complaints of insomnia are extremely common, increase with age, and are by no means confined to subjects with psychiatric illness. Preoccupation with insomnia and its relief is a modern fad reminiscent of Victorian 'bowel-fixation'. Sleep laboratory studies reveal that reports of sleeplessness are greatly exaggerated when compared with the objective evidence of night-long EEG recordings. The subject who literally does not 'sleep a wink all night' does not repeat the experience the next night, and reported failure to sleep for nights on end is shown to be quite false.

It is all too easy to start a patient on drug treatment for insomnia. Habituation develops rapidly and it is easier to re-prescribe than to withstand insistent demands. In this way hypnotics are prescribed for years on end. Six hundred million hypnotic tablets or capsules are dispensed annually in the UK, while in the USA with four times the population the figure is ten times as great at six thousand million. It is widely recognized that far too many people are unnecessarily on regular hypnotics for too long.

There are occasions when hypnotics really are helpful, but they should only be supplied for a very limited period, as short as one or two nights and not more than four to tide over the acute insomnia associated with the shock of bereavement or other acute traumatic experience, or cover changes of night and day shift work, jet-lag, and upsetting change of environment. Apprehension, noise and unfamiliarity are more than sufficient to induce insomnia on the night of admission to hospital. Too often the hypnotic, once started, is continued throughout the patient's stay, recorded in the discharge letter and re-prescribed indefinitely by the general practitioner.

Certainly it is unpleasant for a patient to suffer the severe insomnia which follows for one or two nights after enforced withdrawal or voluntary relinquishment of hypnotics after weeks or months of use. The worst is soon over, however, and a normal sleep pattern is quickly re-established without recourse to hypnotics again.

Fortunately, the massive prescribing of addictive barbiturates for day and night sedation has been reduced to a trickle. What the profession has achieved with a drug of addiction can be repeated with drugs of dependence.

Insomnia in psychiatric illness

Neuroses

In anxiety and depressive neuroses the patient characteristically has difficulty falling off to sleep after retiring to bed. A small dose of a quick acting, rapidly eliminated tranquillizer blankets cerebral over-arousal and sleep follows. Useful drugs are lorazepam (1 mg tablets) 1–2 mg nocte, or oxazepam (10 mg tablets) 10 or 20 mg nocte, or flurazepam 15 mg nocte, all of which have a shorter half-life than nitrazepam. Flurazepam, like nitrazepam, may leave a hangover effect the following morning.

In the elderly there is still a place for chloral in the form of the relatively weak chloral hydrate variant, dichloral phenazone.

Psychoses

Extremes of insomnia characterize acute mania and delirium tremens, conditions which require immediate inpatient care.

ENDOGENOUS DEPRESSION

While the prescribing of a hypnotic may be a psychologically justifiable gesture in endogenous depression little is to be expected of it. Terminal insomnia (early waking) is a component of the depressive syndrome and will resolve after two or three weeks when antidepressant treatment begins to relieve the depression. Thereafter hypnotics are not required.

FOR FURTHER READING

*Brown D. and Pedder J. (1979) *Introduction to Psychotherapy*. London, Tavistock.

Bruch H. (1974) *Learning Psychotherapy*. Cambridge (Mass.), Harvard University Press.

*Cohen J. and Clark J. H. (1979) *Medicine, Mind and Man*. Reading, Freeman.

Dalton K. (1969) *The Menstrual Cycle*. London, Pelican.

Freeman A. M., Sack R. L. and Berger P. A. (eds.) (1979) *Psychiatry for the Primary Care Physician*. Baltimore, Williams & Wilkins.

Garfield S. L. (1980) *Psychotherapy. An Eclectic Approach*. New York, Wiley.

*Goldberg D. and Huxley P. (1980) *Mental Illness in the Community. The Pathway to Psychiatric Care*. London, Tavistock.

*Hart B. (1943) *The Psychology of Insanity*. London, Cambridge University Press.
A little classic, 1st edition 1912. The title belies the content: mental mechanisms.

Lader M. H. (1975) *The Psycho-physiology of Mental Illness*. London, Routledge & Kegan Paul.

Menninger K. (1975) *Whatever Became of Sin?* London, Hodder & Stoughton (1973 Hawthorn Books Inc.).

*_Mental Disorders: Glossary and guide to their classification in accordance with the Ninth Revision of the International Classification of Diseases_ (1978), Geneva, WHO (Reprinted 1980 with minor corrections).
Gives brief descriptions of the syndromes.
Pitt B. (1974) _Psychogeriatrics._ London, Churchill Livingstone.
*Rafaelson O. and Hollister L. E. (1979) _Psychotherapeutic Drugs._ Copenhagen, Munksgaard International.
Sadler M. (ed.) (1978) _Mental Illness in Pregnancy and the Puerperium._ Oxford, Oxford University Press.
*Silverstone T. and Turner P. (1982) _Drug Treatment in Psychiatry,_ 3rd ed. London, Routledge & Kegan Paul.
van Praag H. M. (ed.) (1979) _Management of Schizophrenia._ Assen (Netherlands), Van Gorcum.
Watts C. A. H. (1966) _Depressive Disorders in the Community._ Bristol, Wright.
The first study of depression in general practice.

*Indicates essential reading.

Index